VARCAROLIS'
Manual of Psychiatric Nursing Care
An Interprofessional Approach

WITHDRAWN

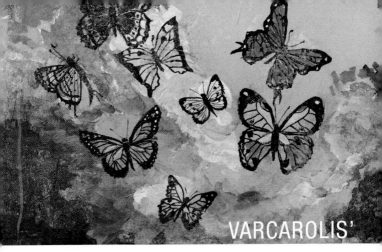

VARCAROLIS'

Manual of Psychiatric Nursing Care

An Interprofessional Approach

7TH EDITION

Margaret Jordan Halter, PhD, APRN
Former Clinical Nurse Specialist, Cleveland Clinic Akron General, Akron, Ohio
Former Faculty, Malone College, Canton, Ohio
University of Akron, Akron, Ohio
The Ohio State University, Columbus, Ohio
Former Associate Dean, Ashland University, Mansfield, Ohio

Christina A. Fratena, MSN, APRN, CNS-BC, PMHCNS-BC
Clinical Nurse Specialist, SpringHaven Counseling Center, Dundee, Ohio
Faculty, Malone University, Canton, Ohio
Former Faculty, University of Akron, Akron, Ohio
Former Clinical Nurse Specialist, Aultman Hospital, Canton, Ohio

ELSEVIER

4367

KH

Elsevier
3251 Riverport Lane
St. Louis, Missouri 63043

Varcarolis' Manual of Psychiatric Nursing Care: **ISBN:** 978-0-323-79305-6
An Interprofessional Approach, Seventh Edition

Notices

Practitioners and researchers must always rely on their own experience and knowledge in evaluating and using any information, methods, compounds or experiments described herein. Because of rapid advances in the medical sciences, in particular, independent verification of diagnoses and drug dosages should be made. To the fullest extent of the law, no responsibility is assumed by Elsevier, authors, editors or contributors for any injury and/or damage to persons or property as a matter of products liability, negligence or otherwise, or from any use or operation of any methods, products, instructions, or ideas contained in the material herein.

Previous editions copyrighted 2019, 2015, 2011, 2006, 2004, and 2000.
Library of Congress Control Number: 2021941697

Content Strategist: Yvonne Alexopoulos
Content Development Specialist: Lisa Newton
Publishing Services Manager: Deepthi Unni
Project Manager: Radjan Lourde Selvanadin
Design Direction: Brian Salisbury

Printed in India

Last digit is the print number:
9   8   7   6   5   4   3   2   1

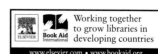

Working together
to grow libraries in
developing countries

www.elsevier.com • www.bookaid.org

8/22/22

This book is dedicated to:

People who are living with and recovering from mental illness.

Nursing students and registered nurses who support recovery from mental illness.

Reviewers

J'Andra Antisdel, MSN, RN-BC
Visiting Clinical Assistant Professor
Indiana University South Bend
South Bend, Indiana

Josephine M. Britanico, MSN, RN, PNP
Assistant Professor of Nursing
Borough of Manhattan Community College/City University of New York
New York City, New York

Debra Forbes, MSN, RN
Associate Professor of Nursing
Kirkwood Community College
Cedar Rapids, Iowa

Chris Paxos, PharmD, BCPP, BCPS, BCGP
Director of Pharmacotherapy
Professor of Pharmacy Practice
Northeast Ohio Medical University, College of Pharmacy
Rootstown, Ohio
Associate Professor of Psychiatry
Northeast Ohio Medical University, College of Medicine
Rootstown, Ohio

Preface

As with previous editions, the seventh edition of the *Varcarolis' Manual of Psychiatric Nursing Care* supports students and practitioners in planning realistic, evidence-based, and individualized nursing care for their patients. This thoroughly updated edition of the *Manual* provides readers with a foundation for clinical work in contemporary psychiatric settings. The chapters are logically and intuitively arranged in four parts:

- Part I provides a snapshot of basic psychiatric nursing concepts and tools. These chapters focus on the nursing process, therapeutic relationships, and therapeutic communication.
- Part II explores specific diagnostic groups, an overview of major disorders within these groups, and guidelines for developing and providing psychiatric nursing care.
- Part III discusses psychiatric crises such as suicide and family violence and outlines the nursing process as it pertains to these crises.
- Part IV is devoted to treatment modalities for psychiatric disorders that are provided by advanced practice professionals such as psychiatric nurse practitioners and psychiatrists. This section begins with essential pharmacotherapy regarding specific classifications of drugs such as antipsychotics and antidepressants. These chapters are followed by common brain stimulation therapies, such as electroconvulsive therapy and vagus nerve stimulation. Finally, a summary of psychological therapies such as cognitive–behavioral therapy is described.

The organization of the clinical chapters mirrors the *Diagnostic and Statistical Manual of Mental Disorders*, 5th edition *(DSM-5)*. Although classical references have been retained, citations are thoroughly updated.

In this edition, we use the International Council of Nurses' nursing diagnosis classification system. This system uses logical, understandable, and interprofessional terminology to describe responses to psychiatric disorders.

Acknowledgments

Thanks to my Elsevier family for coordinating and completing another successful project! Kudos to Yvonne Alexopoulos, senior content strategist, for providing strong feedback and supporting my ideas for this seventh edition. Yvonne is a brilliant person with thought-provoking comments along with a humorous take on thorny issues. As always, cheers go out to Lisa Newton, our content development manager. Lisa responds to emails within an hour, sends positive greetings, and adds a personal touch to nearly all of our communications. A big thanks to Clay Broeker, senior project manager, for pulling all the details together, ensuring consistency, and producing a reader-friendly edition for students and clinical nurses.

In this seventh edition of the *Manual*, we adopted standardized nursing diagnoses from the *International Classification for Nursing Practice (ICNP)*. The *ICNP* was developed and published by the International Council of Nurses (2019), part of the World Health Organization's publications. The ICNP provides an agreed-upon set of terms that are logical, useful, and consistent with other health care disciplines. This system also supports the reuse of clinical data for research, management decisions, quality evaluation, and policy development.

Much of the *Manual* was developed in 2020. This was a year that will be long remembered as the start of the Coronavirus pandemic, which brought countless losses. 2020 also brought with it the loss of this textbook's original editor, Elizabeth (Betsy) Varcarolis. Betsy was a pioneer in the development of a leading undergraduate psychiatric nursing textbook, *Foundations of Psychiatric-Mental Health Nursing*, and later added this *Manual*. Betsy and I went on to introduce the condensed *Essentials of Psychiatric Mental Health Nursing*.

Countless psychiatric nursing students have benefited from Betsy's conversational style of writing about complex topics. Her beliefs about psychiatric nursing have influenced the specialty, state board of nursing examinations, and national certifications and prepared countless students for the provision of strong, interpersonal-based patient care.

I am fortunate to have been Betsy's apprentice and I will miss her as a constant in the world. Cheers to her and a life-well lived.

Peggy Halter

About the cover artwork

"Butterfly Abstract" is by Bradley D. Rankin of Cuyahoga Falls, Ohio. Bradley created this painting for the 2020 annual Art of Recovery event in Akron, Ohio. This event highlights artwork of clients from a local community mental health center. Bradley sends the following message to nurses: "Mental illness recovery is possible with help from family, friends, and professionals. Never give up on a patient."

CHAPTER 1

The Nursing Process

The nursing process is a problem-solving process. It is the basic framework for nursing practice with patients who are experiencing psychiatric disorders or conditions. The National Council of State Boards of Nursing (NCSBN, 2018a, p. 5) defines the nursing process as "a scientific, clinical reasoning approach to client care that includes assessment, analysis, planning, implementation and evaluation." The nursing process is fundamental to patient care and is a basis of this textbook.

A recent trend that may eventually impact the use of the nursing process is the building and expanding of the nursing process through a model of clinical judgment (NCSBN, 2021). Clinical judgment is the outcome of critical thinking and decision making. It is a process that uses nursing knowledge to assess situations, identify a prioritized patient concern, and devise evidence-based solutions to deliver safe client care. This evidence-based model is officially called the NCSBN Clinical Judgment Measurement Model.

Safety and quality care for patients are also prime directives for nurses and nursing education. The national initiative that is centered on patient safety and quality of care is known as *Quality and Safety Education for Nurses (QSEN)*. QSEN competencies are integrated throughout this manual, and specific examples are highlighted along with each standard of practice. Box 1.1 provides a summary of the competencies.

The basis of psychiatric–mental health nursing is the therapeutic relationship. It is within this relationship that

1

Box 1.1 **Quality and Safety Education for Nurses (QSEN) Competencies**

Patient-centered care: Recognize the patient or designee as the source of control and full partner in providing compassionate and coordinated care based on respect for the patient's preferences, values, and needs.

Teamwork and collaboration: Function effectively within nursing and interprofessional teams, fostering open communication, mutual respect, and shared decision making to achieve quality patient care.

Evidence-based practice: Integrate best current evidence with clinical expertise and patient/family preferences and values for delivery of optimal health care.

Quality improvement: Use data to monitor the outcomes of care processes and use improvement methods to design and test changes to continuously improve the quality and safety of health care systems.

Safety: Minimizes risk of harm to patients and providers through both system effectiveness and individual performance.

Informatics: Use information and technology to communicate, manage knowledge, mitigate error, and support decision making.

QSEN Institute. (n.d.). *QSEN competencies.* http://qsen.org/competencies/pre-licensure-ksas

---

care is provided to address healthcare problems, both actual and potential. These problems occur in the context of or as the result of psychiatric disorders, also known as *mental illness* or *mental disorders.*

The *Diagnostic and Statistical Manual of Mental Disorders (DSM)* is the official publication of the American Psychiatric Association (APA) for categorizing psychiatric disorders in the United States. The *DSM* provides clinicians, researchers, insurance companies, pharmaceutical firms, and policy makers with standard criteria for the classification of psychiatric disorders. Clinicians use this publication as a guide for planning care and evaluating patients' treatments.

First published in 1952, the current manual is the fifth edition of the *DSM,* which is known as the *DSM-5* (APA, 2013). This *Manual of Psychiatric Nursing Care* uses the *DSM-5* for organizing the order of clinical chapters and for describing psychiatric disorders.

TERMS USED TO DESCRIBE RECIPIENTS OF CARE IN THIS MANUAL

You may notice that textbooks and instructors use different terms to refer to the recipients of nursing care. These terms are matters of organizational choice, professional beliefs, and even personal preference. Client is one common recipient-of-care term that tends to be used in community-based or private practice settings. A consumer of mental health care is another term frequently used in community-based or private practice settings. One of the most common terms used by health care professionals is patient. The noun patient usually refers to an individual who needs a higher level of care and is being treated for in an acute care setting. While not all students who read this manual will have clinical experiences based in acute care settings, for simplicity and consistency, the term patient will be used in this manual to refer to the recipient of nursing care.

ASSESSMENT

The psychiatric–mental health registered nurse provides a unique and comprehensive assessment of the patient's health status that guides the plan of care. Assessment is both an essential initial activity and one that is ongoing throughout the period of care. The focus and type of information that is gathered are based on the patient's specific condition and by anticipating future needs.

QUALITY AND SAFETY STANDARDS (QSEN) RELATED TO ASSESSMENT

- Patient-centered care: Elicit preferences, values, and expressed needs as part of the clinical interview.
- Informatics: Identify essential information that must be available in a common database to support patient care.

Individuals with psychiatric disorders are encountered by nurses working in psychiatric units. However, symptoms such as depression, suicidal thoughts, anger, disorientation, delusions, and hallucinations are experienced by patients in all settings. These settings include medical-surgical, obstetrical, and intensive care units; outpatient care; extended-care facilities; emergency departments; and community centers. Psychiatric symptoms are not always the result of psychiatric disorders, and they may stem from chemical imbalances, substance use, and other disease processes.

The assessment phase of the nursing process has several primary goals. They are to:

- Establish rapport.
- Determine the chief complaint (i.e., the perception of the problem in the patient's own words).
- Review physical status and obtain baseline vital signs.
- Identify the impact of symptoms on the patient's life (e.g., self-esteem, loss of intimacy, role functioning, change in family dynamics, lifestyle change, and employment issues).
- Identify risk factors that may affect safety (e.g., confusion, suicidal ideation, or homicidal thoughts).
- Gather information related to previous illnesses, treatment, and hospitalizations.
- Identify psychosocial (i.e., psychological and social) aspects of the patient's life (e.g., family relationships, social patterns, interests and abilities, stress factors, substance use, social supports).

It may be helpful if the patient's support system (e.g., family members, friends, and relatives) participates during the data collection if possible and desirable to provide additional information. If law enforcement was involved in the admission, it is important for the nurse to determine the circumstances involved in police intervention.

Past medical and psychiatric history can also supply valuable information. This is particularly important if the patient is experiencing psychosis, is withdrawn and mute, or is too agitated to provide an accurate history. Charts from previous hospitalizations or electronic medical records are extremely helpful. Laboratory reports also provide important information.

While not always practical from a time perspective or for brief encounters, a complete mental status examination may be conducted during the assessment phase of the nursing process. A patient-centered assessment is included in Appendix A. This assessment not only provides structure for a complete mental status examination, it also reinforces terms and important concepts.

Most healthcare facilities provide patient assessments in either paper or electronic format. While these tools are integral for gathering essential data, they can feel impersonal as question after question is asked. With practice, nurses may become proficient with a less formal approach to assessment by clarifying, focusing, and exploring information with the patient. This method allows patients to use their own words to express themselves and enables the nurse to observe a wide range of nonverbal behaviors. A unique style of interviewing congruent with the nurse's personality develops as comfort and experience increase. Box 1.2 presents areas that are typically evaluated during the assessment phase.

Issues for Which Referral May Be Indicated

Patients may be referred to other disciplines within the healthcare team, such as social services or occupational therapy, and might need further investigation when planning long-term care. This is especially important in the case of serious mental illness and if any of the following problems are present:

- Inadequacy of primary support (e.g., due to death, illness, divorce, sexual or physical abuse, neglect of a child, discord with siblings, birth of a sibling)
- Problems related to the social environment (e.g., death or loss of friends, inadequate social support, living alone, difficulty with acculturation, discrimination, life-cycle transition such as retirement)
- Educational problems (e.g., illiteracy, academic concerns, conflict with teachers or classmates, inadequate school environment)
- Occupational problems (e.g., unemployment, job insecurity, stressful work schedule, difficult work conditions, job dissatisfaction, job change, conflict with boss or coworkers)
- Economic problems (e.g., poverty, inadequate finances, insufficient welfare support)
- Barriers to healthcare access (e.g., inadequate services, transportation to facilities unavailable, inadequate health insurance)
- Interaction with the legal system or crime (e.g., arrest, incarceration, litigation, victim of crime)

Box 1.2 **Common Assessment Areas**

Previous psychiatric treatment
Educational background
Occupational background
  Employed? Where? How long?
  Special skills
Social patterns
  Describe family.
  Describe friends.
  With whom does the patient live?
  To whom does the patient go in times of crisis?
  Describe a typical day.
Sexual patterns
  Sexually active? Practices safe sex? Practices birth
    control?
  Sexual orientation
  Sexual difficulties
Interests and abilities
  What does the patient do for leisure?
  What sport, hobby, or leisure activity is the patient
    good at?
Medications
  What medications does the patient take? How often?
    How much?
  What herbal or over-the-counter drugs does the patient
    take? How often? How much?
  What psychiatric medications does the patient take or
    use? How often? How much?
  How many drinks of alcohol does the patient take?
    How often? How much? Last use?
  What recreational drugs does the patient take or use?
    How often? How much? Last use?
  Does the patient identify the use of drugs as a problem?
Coping abilities
  What does the patient do when upset?
  To whom can the patient talk?
  What usually helps to relieve stress?
  What did the patient try this time?

Cultural and Social Assessment

Healthcare providers in the United States work with an increasingly culturally diverse population. Providing effective care necessitates an awareness of and appreciation for an individual's cultural background. All healthcare professionals, especially mental health professionals, need to continually expand their knowledge and understanding of the complexity of the cultural and social factors that influence health and illness. It is especially important to broaden one's understanding of how health and illness are influenced by cultural and social factors.

Spiritual and Religious Assessment

The importance of spirituality and religious beliefs is an often-overlooked element of patient care. Spirituality and religious beliefs have the potential to exert an influence on how people understand meaning and purpose in their lives and how they use critical judgment to solve problems. Box 1.3 offers suggestions for gathering information to better adapt a plan of care to an individual patient's needs.

After the Assessment

After the initial assessment, it is useful to summarize and review the data with the patient. This summary provides patients with assurance that they have been heard. It also allows the patient the opportunity to clarify potential misinformation.

Tell the patient what will happen next. For example, if the initial assessment takes place in the hospital, tell the patient about meetings that will occur with other clinicians. After conducting the initial assessment, the nurse informs the patient when and how often they will meet. If the nurse thinks a referral is necessary (e.g., a psychiatrist or advanced practice nurse, social worker, or medical personnel), this is also discussed with the patient.

Non–English-Speaking Patients

Nearly 22% of the US population does not speak English at home (US Census Bureau, 2019). If a nurse does not speak the patient's language, data gathering may be inaccurate and incomplete, not to mention impossible. The Americans with Disabilities Act of 1990 established federal standards to ensure that communication does not interfere with equal access to healthcare for everyone. All healthcare organizations must provide language interpreters, interpreters trained in sign language, telecommunication devices for the deaf (TDDs), closed-caption decoders

---

Box 1.3 **Brief Cultural, Social, and Spiritual and Religious Assessment**

Cultural Assessment
Language
  What is your primary spoken language?
  How would you rate your ability to speak and understand English?
  Would you like an interpreter?
Communication style
  Observe nonverbal communication (e.g., gestures, posture, eye movement)
  What are your feelings about touch?
  Observe how much eye contact the patient is comfortable with.
  How much or little do people make eye contact in your culture?
Family group
  Describe the members of your family.
  Who makes the decisions in your family?
  Which family members can you confide in?
Health and illness beliefs
  When you become ill, what is the first thing you do to take care of the illness?
  How is this illness viewed by your culture?
  Are there special practices within your culture that address your healthcare problem?
  Are there any restrictions on diet or medical interventions within your cultural beliefs?
  What are the attitudes of mental illness in your culture?
  Who do you go to when you are medically ill?
  Are there special practices within your culture that address psychiatric conditions?

Social Supports
  Are there people outside the family, such as friends and neighbors, that you are close to and feel comfortable confiding in?
  Is there a place where you can go for support (e.g., church, school, work, club)?

Spirituality and Religion
  What importance does spirituality or religion have in your life?
  Do your spiritual or religious beliefs relate to your healthcare? How?
  Does your faith help in stressful situations? How?
  Would you like to have a spiritual advisor or religious leader visit?
  Who or what supplies you with strength and hope?

for televisions, and amplifiers on phones. Translators are made available to provide written information in the patient's own language.

Family members, friends, or neighbors are often used to communicate in emergency medical situations. However, using nonprofessional interpreters may have significant drawbacks. For example, a family interpreter might want to protect the patient and filter out information given to the patient. Conversely, the family member might want to filter out information to the healthcare provider. Using a professional interpreter reduces the risk of wrong procedures, medications errors, and other adverse events.

The following guidelines are recommended when working with an interpreter:

- Address the patient directly rather than speaking to the interpreter.
- Maintain eye contact with the patient to ensure patient involvement and strengthen personal connection.
- Avoid interrupting the patient and interpreter.
- Ask the interpreter to give you verbatim translations.
- Avoid using technical medical terms the interpreter or the patient might not understand.
- Avoid talking or commenting to the interpreter at length. The patient might feel left out and distrustful.
- Ask for permission to discuss intimate or emotionally charged topics first, and prepare the interpreter for the content of the interview.
- Arrange for the interpreter and the patient to meet each other ahead of time, if possible, to establish some rapport.
- Aim for consistency by using the same interpreter for subsequent interactions.

When an interpreter is not immediately available, aids such as picture charts or flash cards can help the nurse and patient communicate important basic information about the patient's immediate needs (e.g., degree of pain or need for toileting). Due to cultural norms or because they want to be helpful, some patients with limited English might seem agreeable and nod "yes" even though they do not understand. Asking questions that require more than a "yes" or "no" answer can provide a better idea of the patient's level of understanding.

ANALYSIS

Based on a comprehensive assessment, psychiatric–mental health registered nurses analyze the data to determine patient problems and potential problems. The term *patient* can be replaced with the words *family, group,* or *community.*

QUALITY AND SAFETY STANDARDS (QSEN) RELATED TO ANALYSIS

Patient-centered care: Integrate understanding of multiple dimensions of patient-centered care, including the patient's needs, preferences, and values, within their cultural parameters.

Nursing Diagnoses

Nursing diagnoses identify unmet needs that are within the nurse's domain to treat. In this textbook, we use the diagnoses provided by *International Classification for Nursing Practice (ICNP)* developed by the International Council of Nurses (2019). This classification system is a part of the World Health Organization (WHO) family of classifications. It provides an agreed upon set of terms that are logical, useful, and consistent with other healthcare disciplines.

A well-chosen and well-stated nursing diagnosis is the basis for selecting therapeutic goals and interventions. A nursing diagnosis is usually composed of the problem, probable cause, and supporting evidence.

An example of a nursing diagnosis is *risk for self-mutilation.* In the case of this diagnosis, the nurse identified several characteristics during the assessment that put the patient at risk for this behavior.

Related Factors (Probable Cause)

The probable cause is linked to the nursing diagnosis with the term *related to.* This term identifies factors that contribute to or are related to the development or maintenance of a patient problem. The probable cause tells us what needs to be addressed to bring about change and identifies what needs to be targeted through nursing interventions. In the case of potential for self-mutilation, the addition of a second part of the patient problem results in:

Risk for self-mutilation related to anxiety

This statement indicates that the nurse and healthcare team will initiate interventions that reduce the patient's anxiety. Anxiety can also be improved by increasing the patient's ability to express tensions verbally rather than act them out physically.

Consider the difference in a plan of care for someone with the same nursing diagnosis, but with a different probable cause. For example, *risk for self-mutilation related to command hallucinations* indicates that the patient is experiencing auditory hallucinations that tell the patient to engage in self-harm. In this case the self-mutilation (e.g., cutting) may relieve the anxiety brought on by the voices. Interventions will again be aimed at decreasing the patient's anxiety by finding a calmer environment or offering an as-needed medication. Teaching distraction techniques such as reading out loud, talking with others, engaging in an activity, and singing lightly may also be useful.

Defining Characteristics (Supporting Evidence)

Two basic types of data provide support for nursing diagnoses—signs and symptoms. Signs are objective or observable information (e.g., a rash, slumped posture, hyperactivity), and symptoms are subjective reports of the patient (e.g., "I'm tired" or "I feel nervous"). Both types of data are the defining characteristics that are linked to the diagnosis and probable cause by the words *as evidenced by.* Supporting data that validate the diagnosis of *risk for self-mutilation related to anxiety* include:
- *Fresh cuts on forearms*
- *Scars on forearms*
- *"I cut myself to calm down."*

Types of Nursing Diagnoses
Problem-Focused Statements
For problem-focused statements, the nurse makes a judgment about a human response to a health condition or life process. An example of a problem-focused statement is:
Anxiety related to losing employment and financial burdens.

Risk Statements
Potential problem statements indicate a vulnerability that carries a high probability of developing negative responses. Nursing diagnoses in this category include preventable occurrences such as falls, self-injury, pressure

ulcers, and infection. This type of nursing diagnosis always begins with the phrase "risk for" followed by supporting evidence. Because the problem has not yet occurred, there is no probable cause (i.e., related to).

An example of a potential problem statement is:

Risk for injury as evidenced by extreme agitation, hyperactivity, less than 2 hours rest at night, poor skin turgor, and abrasions on hands and arms.

Health Promotion Diagnosis

A health promotion diagnosis supports the transition of an individual, family, or community from a specific level of wellness to a higher level of wellness. As with risk statements, health promotion diagnoses do not require a related factor. Instead, the defining characteristics provide evidence of the desire to improve a current state of health. Readiness for effective coping as evidenced by stating "Alcohol is ruining my life" and "I am ready to find other ways to cope with anxiety."

OUTCOMES

Outcomes are patient-centered (e.g., "the patient will") and written in positive terms. As a basis for evaluation, overall outcomes are formulated to reverse the problem stated in the nursing diagnosis. In the case of a patient with impaired coping, an overall outcome would be for the patient to demonstrate improved coping.

QUALITY AND SAFETY STANDARDS (QSEN) RELATED TO OUTCOMES

- Patient-centered care: Integrate understanding of multiple dimensions of patient-centered care.
- Patient-centered care: Engage patients or designated surrogates (e.g., family members) in active partnerships that promote health, safety, well-being, and self-management.
- Quality improvement: Seek information about outcomes of care for populations served in the care setting.

Outcome criteria are ideal outcomes that reflect the maximum level of health that the patient can realistically achieve through nursing interventions. In this clinical companion, overall desired outcome criteria are provided.

Short-term and long-term goals are steps toward the overall outcome(s). These goals are stated in behavioral and measurable terms and might have time factors such as "in 1 week," "by discharge," or "within 2 days." The goals are evaluated and revised as the patient progresses or does not progress. The amount of time needed to attain some of these goals will vary.

A patient with bipolar disorder in a manic phase may be extremely agitated. In this case, the nursing diagnosis may be:

Risk for injury as evidenced by hyperactivity, less than 2 hours rest at night, and poor skin turgor.

The overall outcome for this diagnosis is a reversal of the problem, that is, the patient will be free from injury.

Possible long-term goals and associated short-term goals might include the following:

1. The patient will return to pre-mania level of activity.
   a. The patient will spend 10 minutes in a quiet, non-stimulating area with a nurse each hour during the day (by time/date).
   b. The patient will engage in short 1:1 exchanges with the nurse while walking (by time/date).
2. The patient will sleep 6 to 8 hours per night within 1 week.
   a. The patient will sleep 3 to 4 hours per night with the aid of medication (by time/date).
   b. The patient will identify the connection between sleep loss and mania (by date).
3. The patient will maintain a sufficient daily fluid intake by (date).
   a. The patient will drink a total of 9 cups (women) or 12 cups (men) of liquids (e.g., water, juice, milk, or milkshakes) a day (by date).
   b. The patient's skin turgor will be within normal limits within 24 hours, as evidenced by raised area disappearing in less than 4 seconds when skin over the sternum is pinched and released.

PLANNING

QUALITY AND SAFETY STANDARDS (QSEN) RELATED TO PLANNING

- Patient-centered care: Respect patient preferences for degree of active engagement in the care process toward helping the patient meet needs and goals.
- Evidence-based practice: Base the individualized care plan on evidence-based planning.
- Informatics: Document and plan patient care in an electronic health record.

Once you have completed an assessment and formulated nursing diagnoses, the problems are prioritized. Maslow's Hierarchy of Needs (Fig. 1.1) provides a useful framework for doing so. Physiological needs and safety always come first because they have the potential for the most serious harm. Then the higher-order needs are addressed, including love and belonging and self-esteem. For each problem statement, desired outcomes are developed and interventions for achieving the outcomes are selected.

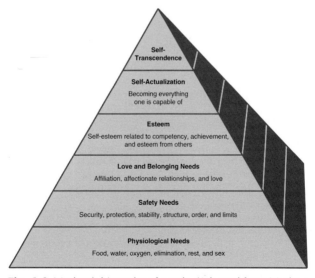

Fig. 1.1 Maslow's hierarchy of needs. (Adapted from Maslow, A. H. [1972]. *The farther reaches of human nature*. Viking.)

The nurse considers the following specific principles when planning interventions:

- *Safe:* Interventions promote safety for the patient, as well as for other patients, staff, and family.
- *Compatible and appropriate:* Interventions are compatible with other therapies and with the patient's personal goals and cultural values, as well as with institutional rules.
- *Realistic and individualized:* Interventions are (1) within the patient's capabilities, given the patient's age, physical strength, condition, and willingness to change; (2) based on the availability of support staff; (3) reflective of the actual available community resources; and (4) within the student's or nurse's capabilities.
- *Evidence-based:* Interventions are based on scientific evidence and principles when available.

Evidence-based interventions and treatments are the gold standard in healthcare. Evidence-based practice for nurses is a combination of clinical skill and the use of clinically relevant research in the delivery of effective patient-centered care. Using the best available research, incorporating patient preferences, and making sound clinical judgment and skills provide an optimal patient-centered nurse–patient relationship.

IMPLEMENTATION

QUALITY AND SAFETY STANDARDS (QSEN) RELATED TO IMPLEMENTATION

- Patient-centered care:
  - Provide patient-centered care with sensitivity and respect for the diversity of human experience.
  - Recognize the boundaries of therapeutic relationships.
  - Participate in building consensus or resolving conflict in the context of patient care.
- Safety: During the interventions minimize the risk of harm to patients and providers through both system effectiveness and individual performance.
- Teamwork and collaboration:
  - Initiate requests for help when appropriate to the situation.
  - Integrate the contributions of others who play a role in helping the patient or family achieve health goals to ensure quality patient care.

Implementation includes the actions that nurses take to carry out the nursing measures identified in the care plan to achieve the expected outcome criteria. When carrying out nursing interventions, additional information is gathered, and further refinements of the care plan may be made.

The psychiatric–mental health registered nurse implements the plan with evidence-based interventions whenever possible, using community resources, and collaborating with the interprofessional team. According to the American Nurses Association, American Psychiatric Nurses Association, and the International Society of Psychiatric-Mental Health Nurses (2014), basic-level interventions include the following:

1. Coordination of care
2. Health teaching and health promotion
3. Pharmacological, biological, and integrative therapies
4. Milieu therapy
5. Therapeutic relationship and counseling

In addition to these five interventions, psychiatric–mental health advanced practice registered nurses are qualified to provide three higher-level interventions:

6. Consultation
7. Prescriptive authority and treatment
8. Psychotherapy

EVALUATION

QUALITY AND SAFETY STANDARDS (QSEN) RELATED TO IMPLEMENTATION

Quality improvement: Seek information about outcomes for populations served in the care setting.

Evaluation is an ongoing process that includes evaluating the effectiveness of plans and strategies and documenting the results. Desired outcome evaluation occurs in the context of the entire plan of care and represents a comprehensive approach to determining the success of the plan.

In addition to addressing the success of desired outcomes, nursing students may evaluate long-term and short-term goals. These goals can have three possible outcomes: The goal is met, not met, or partially met. Consider a previous example of a nursing diagnosis:

Risk for injury as evidenced by hyperactivity, less than 2 hours rest at night, poor skin turgor, and abrasions on hands and arms.

Evaluation of the short-term goals might be documented as follows:

1. The patient will spend 10 minutes in a quiet, nonstimulating area with a nurse each hour during the day.

   Goal partially met: After 2 days, patient continues restless and purposeless pacing and is only able to stay quiet with nurse for 4 to 6 minutes per hour.

2. The patient will sleep 3 to 4 hours at night with the aid of medication (by time/date).

   Goal met: Within 3 nights, the patient was able to sleep 4.5 hours with the aid of a short-term benzodiazepine.

3. The patient will drink 8 oz of fluid (e.g., juice, milk, milkshake) every hour.

   Goal met: Patient takes frequent sips of fluid provided in cups with lids equaling 8 oz an hour during the hours of 9 a.m. to 4 p.m., with reminders from nursing staff.

4. The patient's skin turgor will be within normal limits within 24 hours, as evidenced by raised area disappearing in less than 4 seconds when skin over the sternum is gathered and released.

   Goal not met: At 8:00 a.m., patient's skin turgor still poor. Raised area from gathered skin over sternum disappeared 4 seconds after release. Evaluate need for increasing daytime fluids from 9 a.m. to 9 p.m.

IN THE CHAPTERS THAT FOLLOW

This clinical reference guide is intended to help nurses and nursing students develop a patient-centered plan of care. The chapters in Parts II and III of this manual present specific *DSM-5* psychiatric disorders and psychiatric crises that might require nursing interventions. For each disorder or phenomenon, the most common plans of care are presented. Suggested outcomes are offered for each nursing diagnosis, and specific nursing assessments and actions are provided with supporting rationales. Students and nurses may select those interventions that are appropriate for their patients and modify where necessary to meet the patients' unique needs.

The remaining chapters provide information to support nursing care through an overview of medical treatment modalities. Part IV is devoted to pharmacotherapy such as antidepressants and antianxiety agents. Part V focuses on nonpharmacological approaches such as psychotherapy (i.e., talk therapy) and brain stimulation therapies.

CHAPTER 2

Therapeutic Relationships

Psychiatric–mental health nursing is based on principles of *science*. Knowledge of anatomy, physiology, and chemistry is the basis for providing safe and effective biological treatments. Knowledge of pharmacotherapy—a medication's mechanism of action, indications for use, and adverse effects based on evidence-based studies and trials—is vital to nursing practice. However, it is the caring relationship and the development of the interpersonal skills needed to enhance and maintain such a relationship that make up the *art* of psychiatric nursing. This art comes to life through the therapeutic relationship where caring and healing can occur.

NURSE–PATIENT RELATIONSHIP

The nurse–patient relationship is the basis of all psychiatric–mental health nursing treatment approaches, regardless of the specific goals. We all have distinct gifts—unique personality traits and talents—that we can learn to use creatively to form positive bonds with others. The use of these gifts to promote healing in others is referred to as the *therapeutic use of self*. A positive therapeutic alliance, which is collaborative and respectful, is one of the best predictors of positive outcomes in therapy (Gordon & Beresin, 2016).

Talk Therapy

Basic-level psychiatric–mental health nurses use counseling techniques in the context of the therapeutic relationship. Counseling is a supportive face-to-face process that helps individuals to problem solve, resolve personal conflicts, and feel supported. Education and learning are also included under the counseling umbrella.

A formalized approach to talk therapy that is based on theoretical models is called *psychotherapy*. Health care providers with advanced training, such as psychiatric–mental health advanced practice registered nurses, psychiatrists, social workers, counselors, and psychologists, are licensed to practice psychotherapy. Evidence suggests that psychotherapy within a therapeutic partnership actually changes brain chemistry in much the same way as medication. Thus the best treatment for most psychiatric disorders is a combination of medication and psychotherapy.

Goals and Functions

A therapeutic nurse–patient relationship has specific goals and functions, including the following:
- Facilitating communication of thoughts and feelings
- Assisting with problem solving to help facilitate activities of daily living
- Exploring self-defeating behaviors and testing alternative behaviors
- Promoting self-care and independence
- Providing education about medications and symptom management
- Promoting recovery

PERSONAL VERSUS THERAPEUTIC RELATIONSHIPS

Throughout life, we meet people in a variety of settings and share a variety of experiences. With some individuals, we develop long-term relationships. With others, the relationship lasts only a short time. Naturally, the kinds of relationships we develop vary from person to person and from situation to situation.

Personal Relationships

A personal or social relationship is an association that is initiated for the purpose of friendship, socialization, enjoyment, or accomplishment of a task. Mutual needs are met during social interaction. People may give advice and sometimes help meet basic needs such as lending money. During social interactions, roles may shift. For example, one day you may be the listener, and one day you may be listened to. Within a personal relationship, there is little emphasis on the evaluation of the interaction, although we sometimes reflect on what we have said or done. In the following example, notice the casual friend-like tone of the nurse:

Patient: "Oh, I just hate to be alone. It's getting me down, and sometimes it hurts so much."

Nurse: "I know how you feel. I don't like being alone either. Getting on TikTok or Instagram might help you feel less alone, it does me." (In this nontherapeutic response, the nurse is minimizing the patient's feelings and giving advice prematurely.)

Therapeutic Relationships

In a therapeutic relationship, the nurse uses communication skills, understanding of human behaviors, and personal strengths to enhance the patient's growth. Patients more easily engage in the relationship when the clinicians address their concerns, respect patients as partners in decision making, and use straightforward language. The focus of the relationship is on the patient's ideas, experiences, and feelings. Together, the nurse and the patient identify areas that need exploration and periodically evaluate the degree of the patient's progress.

Although the nurse may take on a variety of roles (e.g., teacher, counselor, socializing agent, liaison), the relationship is consistently focused on the patient's problem and needs. The nurse's needs are met outside the relationship.

Nursing students have the opportunity to develop therapeutic nurse–patient relationships with the support of both clinical faculty and nursing staff. This clinical supervision is a mentoring relationship characterized by feedback and evaluation. Typically, students experience a gradual increase in autonomy and responsibility.

Like staff nurses, nursing students may struggle with the boundaries between personal and therapeutic relationships, because there is a fine line between the two. In fact, students often feel more comfortable being a friend because it is a more familiar role, especially with patients close to their own age. When this occurs, students need to make it clear (to themselves and the patient) that the relationship is a therapeutic one.

A therapeutic relationship does *not* mean that the nurse is not friendly. Talking about everyday topics (e.g., television, weather, and children's photos) is not forbidden.

In fact, a small amount of self-disclosure on the nurse's part may strengthen the therapeutic relationship by helping establish rapport. For example, your patient is your age and asks you about nursing school. Briefly sharing your views on nursing school will increase the trust in the relationship. Can you imagine saying, "We won't be talking about me"? On the other hand, multiple questions about such topics as your dating life should result in redirection and clarification of roles.

In a therapeutic relationship, the patient's problems and concerns are explored. Consider the response of the nurse in this situation compared with the previous example of the nurse suggesting social media as a response to loneliness:

Patient: "Oh, I just hate to be alone. It's getting me down, and sometimes it hurts so much."

Nurse: "Loneliness can be painful. What is going on now that you are feeling so alone?"

Professional Boundaries and Roles

Professional boundaries exist to protect patients. Boundaries are the expected and accepted social, physical, and psychological boundaries that separate nurses from patients. This separation is essential considering the power differential between the nurse and the patient. This differential also exists between the nursing student and patient, even if you do not feel powerful. For example, you have read the patient's chart, you are there to help, you will soon be a registered nurse, and you are not a patient. These qualities put nursing students in a position of some authority, particularly from the patient's perspective.

Blurring of Boundaries

Boundaries are always at risk for becoming blurred. One way to judge whether boundaries are being blurred is by gauging the level of involvement. Nurses who are under-involved with patients may be at the least disinterested and neglectful, and at the worst be guilty of patient abandonment (National Council of State Boards of Nursing, 2018b). Over-involvement may result in actions that could result in loss of the registered nurse license such as boundary violations (e.g., disclosing personal patient information) and professional sexual misconduct (e.g., propositioning a patient). A more common type of blurred boundaries is boundary crossings.

Boundary Crossings

Boundary crossings are the least serious form of over-involvement. They tend to give the impression of "something's not quite right," but they do not actually violate ethical standards. In fact, some boundary crossing may actually support the work being done by the patient.

Two common circumstances in which boundaries are crossed are (1) when the relationship slips into a personal context and (2) when the nurse's needs such as the need for attention, affection, and emotional support are met at the expense of the patient's needs.

A personal context for a nurse–patient relationship is evident in the following exchange:

Patient: "Well I decided not to go to that dumb group. 'Hi, I'm so-and-so, and I'm an alcoholic.' Who cares?" (The patient sits slumped in a chair, chewing gum and nonchalantly looking around.)

Nurse (in an impassioned tone): "You seem to always sabotage your chances at getting better. You need AA to get in control of your life. Last week you were going to go, and now you've disappointed everyone."

In this case, the patient reminds the nurse of her mother, who was an alcoholic. The nurse sorts her feelings out and realizes the feelings of disappointment and failure belonged with her mother and not the patient. The nurse starts out the next session with the following approach:

Nurse: "I was thinking about yesterday, and I realize the decision to go to AA or find other help is solely up to you. Let's talk about what happened to change your mind about going to the meeting."

When Values and Beliefs Do Not Match

It is important for nurses to understand that our personal values and beliefs are not right for everyone. It is helpful to realize that our values and beliefs (1) reflect our own culture or subculture, (2) are derived from a range of choices, and (3) are those we have chosen for ourselves from a variety of influences and role models. Our values and beliefs guide us in making decisions and taking actions that we hope will make our lives meaningful, rewarding, and fulfilled.

Working with other people whose values and beliefs are different can be a challenge. Topics that cause controversy in society in general—including political ideology, religion, gender roles, abortion, war, drugs, alcohol, and sex—also can cause conflict between nurses and patients. What happens when the nurse's values and beliefs are different from those of a patient? Consider the following examples of possible conflicts:

- The patient is planning to have an abortion, which is in opposition to the nurse's belief that life begins at conception.
- The nurse values cleanliness, whereas the patient believes that showering more than once a week wastes water and harms the environment.
- The nurse believes in feminism and values women's rights. The nurse resents the female patient who defers to her husband's judgment.

Self-awareness supports patient-centered care and requires that we understand what we value and those beliefs that guide our behavior. Being self-aware helps us to accept the uniqueness and differences of others.

PEPLAU'S NURSE–PATIENT RELATIONSHIP

Hildegard Peplau introduced the concept of the nurse–patient relationship in 1952 in her groundbreaking book *Interpersonal Relations in Nursing*. This model of the nurse–patient relationship has become well accepted as an important tool for all nursing practice. A professional nurse–patient relationship consists of a nurse who has skills and expertise and a patient who wants to feel better again, understand the illness and its treatment alternatives, alleviate suffering, find solutions to problems, improve quality of life.

Peplau (1999) described the nurse–patient relationship as evolving through three distinct and overlapping phases. An additional preorientation phase, during which the nurse prepares for the orientation phase, is also included:

1. Preorientation phase
2. Orientation phase
3. Working phase
4. Termination phase

Most likely, you will not have time to experience all the phases of the nurse–patient relationship in your often brief psychiatric–mental health nursing rotation. However, it is important to be aware of these phases to recognize, practice, and use them later. In some psychiatric environments, it may even be possible to move through all the phases in one clinical day interaction, though to a less thorough degree.

Preorientation Phase

The preorientation phase begins with preparing for your assignment. The patient chart is a rich source of information, including mental and physical evaluation, progress notes, and patient orders. You will probably be required to research your patient's condition, learn about prescribed medications, and understand laboratory results.

Staff may be available to share more anecdotal information or provide tips on how to best interact with your patient. Be aware that in some psychiatric settings, such as a state psychiatric hospital, the staff and/or your instructor may recommend talking with the patient before reading the chart to reduce any bias that may occur.

Another task before meeting the patient is recognizing your own thoughts and feelings. Nursing students usually have many concerns and experience anxiety, especially on their first clinical day. These universal concerns include being afraid of those with psychiatric problems, of saying the wrong thing, and of not knowing what to do in response to certain patient behaviors. Table 2.1 identifies patient behaviors and gives examples of possible reactions and suggested responses.

Experienced faculty and staff monitor the unit atmosphere and have a sense for behaviors that indicate escalating tension. They are trained in crisis interventions, and formal security is often available on-site to give the staff support. Your instructor will set the ground rules for safety during the first clinical day. These rules may include not going into a patient's room alone, staying where others are around in an open area, and reporting signs (i.e., what you observe) and symptoms (i.e., what a patient says) of escalating anxiety.

Orientation Phase

The orientation phase is the first time the nurse and the patient meet. Specific tasks of the orientation phase follow.

Table 2.1 **Patient Behaviors, Possible Reactions, and Useful Responses**

Possible Reactions	Useful Responses
If the patient threatens suicide	
The nurse may feel overwhelmed and be frightened.	The nurse assesses whether the patient has a plan and the lethality of the plan. The nurse tells the patient that this is serious, that the nurse does not want harm to come to the patient, and that this information needs to be shared with other staff.
The nurse may wonder if this threat is manipulation.	The nurse and patient can then discuss the thoughts, feelings, and circumstances that led up to suicidal thoughts.
If the patient asks the nurse to keep a secret	
The nurse may feel conflicted due to a desire for the patient to feel safe and accepted.	The nurse cannot make this promise. The information may be important to the health or safety of the patient or others: "I cannot make that promise. It might be important for me to share it with other staff."
If the patient asks the nurse personal questions	
The nurse may think that it is rude not to answer.	The nurse may or may not answer the patient's query. The nurse may choose to answer a simple question with a brief response and then refocus on the patient. For example, "Yes, I have been enjoying nursing school. Let's talk about what is happening with your housing situation."
The nurse may feel put on the spot and want to leave the situation.	
The nurse may recognize that the patient is trying to deflect the focus of the discussion.	
If the patient makes sexual advances	
The nurse feels uncomfortable but may feel disappointed in having to "damage" the therapeutic relationship.	The nurse sets clear limits and boundaries: "I'm not comfortable with [name the behavior]. This is a professional relationship. We will focus on your problems and concerns."
	The nurse might leave to give the patient time to reflect and gain control, saying: say: "I am going to leave for a bit. I'll be back at [time] to check on how you're doing."

Continued

Table 2.1 **Patient Behaviors, Possible Reactions, and Useful Responses—cont'd**

Possible Reactions	Useful Responses
If the patient cries	
The nurse may feel uncomfortable, experience increased anxiety, or feel somehow responsible for making the person cry.	The nurse should stay with the patient and let the patient know that it is alright to cry. "You are upset about your brother's death." "What are you thinking right now?"
If the patient does not want to talk	
A nurse who is new to this situation may feel rejected, incompetent, or disappointed in the clinical experience.	The nurse might spend short, frequent periods (e.g., 5 minutes) with the patient throughout the day: "Our 5 minutes is up. I'll be back at 10 a.m. and stay with you 5 more minutes." This gives the patient the opportunity to understand that the nurse is reliable and returns on time consistently. It also gives the patient time to feel less threatened.
If the patient gives the nurse a present	
The nurse may feel uncomfortable when offered a gift.	Organizations often have guidelines on this. General advice: If the gift is expensive or money, the only response is to graciously refuse. If it is inexpensive, it is often appropriate to graciously accept, particularly toward the end of the treatment period. However, in some settings, the acceptance of any gift may be discouraged.
If a patient interrupts a conversation with another patient	
The nurse may feel a conflict and does not want to seem rude. Sometimes the nurse tries to engage both patients in conversation.	By maintaining a focus on the original patient, the nurse demonstrates that the session is important: "I am with Mr. Duff for the next 20 minutes. At 10 a.m. we can talk."

Introductions

The first task of the orientation phase is introductions. The patient needs to know about the nurse (i.e., who the nurse is and the nurse's background) and the purpose of the meetings. For example, a student might supply the following information:

Student: "Hello, Ms. Chang; I am Bob Jacobs. I'm a registered nursing student from Fairlawn University. I am in my psychiatric rotation and will be coming here for the next six Thursdays. I would like to spend time with you until you are discharged. I'm here as a support person for you as you work on your treatment goals."

Knowing what the patient would like to be called is also essential—names and titles are meaningful to most people. In the previous example, the student began by using a formal title of Ms. Chang. After checking the patient's identification band and reading it out loud, "Dorothy Chang," the student should ask, "What would you like to be called?"

Establishing Rapport

A major emphasis during the first few encounters with the patient is on providing an atmosphere in which trust and understanding, or rapport, can grow. As in any relationship, you can nurture rapport by demonstrating genuineness, empathy, and unconditional positive regard. Being consistent, helping in problem solving, and providing support are also essential aspects of establishing and maintaining rapport.

Specifying a Contract

A contract emphasizes the patient's participation and responsibility because it shows that the nurse does something *with* the patient rather than *for* the patient. The contract, either stated, written, or both, contains the place, time, date, and duration of the meetings. Termination of the relationship is also discussed.

Explaining Confidentiality

The patient has a right to know (1) who else will be given the information shared with the nurse and (2) that the information may be shared with specific people such as a clinical supervisor, the healthcare provider, the staff, or other students in conference. The patient also needs to know that the information will not be shared with relatives, friends, or others outside the treatment team, except in extreme situations. Extreme situations include child or elder abuse and threats of self-harm or harm to others.

Working Phase

A strong working relationship allows the patient to safely experience increased levels of anxiety and recognize dysfunctional responses. New and more adaptive coping behaviors can be practiced within the context of the working phase.

A major focus of the working phase is on recognizing ineffective ways of coping and replacing them with healthier methods of coping. Sometimes the patient's coping methods were developed to survive in a chaotic and dysfunctional family environment. Although coping methods may have worked for the patient at an earlier age, they may now interfere with the patient's healthy functioning and interpersonal relationships.

Another important aspect of this working relationship is patient education. To facilitate this education, become familiar with biological factors (e.g., genetic, biochemical) and psychological factors (e.g., cognitive distortions, learned helplessness) that may be the basis of a patient's psychiatric disorders. Understanding medications, laboratory work and results, and other treatments is also essential. This knowledge prepares you to help your patients to learn, which in turn prepares them to take the lead role in their own care.

Termination Phase

The termination phase is the final phase of the nurse–patient relationship. Termination may occur when the patient is discharged, when the student's clinical rotation ends, or another time based on the student's learning needs and the patient's wishes to continue meeting. The tasks of termination include the following:

- Summarizing the goals and objectives achieved
- Discussing ways for the patient to incorporate new coping strategies into daily life
- Identifying future goals and plans

- Evaluating the patient's understanding of the psychiatric condition, treatment (e.g., medication and psychotherapy), and follow-up care

If a nurse senses that the patient is reluctant to be discharged, it is important to address this reluctance. A general question—such as "How do you feel about being discharged?"—may provide the opening necessary for the patient to describe feelings.

Part of the termination process is to discuss the patient's plans for the future. If the termination is the result of a discharge, part of these plans has usually been discussed by the psychiatrist or advanced practice provider, including follow-up care and referrals. Registered nurses generally reinforce those plans and emphasize understanding of medications and recognizing when symptoms are increasing. Self-help groups can also be encouraged.

FACTORS THAT PROMOTE A PATIENT'S GROWTH

Personal characteristics of the nurse that promote change and growth in patients are (1) genuineness, (2) empathy, and (3) positive regard. These are some of the intangibles that are at the heart of the art of nursing and patient-centered care.

Genuineness

Genuineness refers to the nurse's ability to be open, honest, and authentic in interactions with patients. Being genuine is a key ingredient in building trust. When a person is genuine, others get the sense that what is displayed on the outside of the person is congruent with who the person is on the inside. Nurses convey genuineness by listening to and communicating clearly with patients. Being genuine in a therapeutic relationship implies the ability to use therapeutic communication tools in an appropriately spontaneous manner rather than rigidly or in a parrot-like fashion.

Empathy

Empathy occurs when the helping person attempts to understand the world from the patient's perspective. This understanding is in contrast to sympathy, which involves feeling pity or sorrow for others. Although these are considered nurturing human traits, they may not be particularly useful in a therapeutic relationship.

The following examples clarify the distinction between empathy and sympathy. A friend tells you that her mother was just diagnosed with inoperable cancer. Your friend then begins to cry and pounds the table with her fist.

Sympathetic response: "I feel so bad for you *(tearing up)*. I know how close you are to your mom. She is such an amazing person. Oh, I am so sorry." (You hug your friend.)

Empathetic response: "This must be devastating for you *(silence)*. It must seem so unfair. What thoughts and feelings are you having?" (You stay with your friend and listen.)

Empathy is not a technique but rather an attitude that conveys respect, acceptance, and validation of the patient's strengths. Empathy may be one of the most important qualities that a psychiatric–mental health nurse can possess.

Positive Regard

Positive regard implies respect. It is the ability to view another person as being worthy of caring about and as someone who has strengths and achievement potential. Positive regard is usually communicated indirectly by attitudes and actions rather than directly by words.

Attitudes

One way to convey positive regard, or respect, is having a positive attitude about working with the patient. The nurse takes the patient and the relationship seriously. The experience is viewed not as "a job," or "part of a course," but as an opportunity to work with patients to help them develop personal resources and actualize more of their potential in living.

Actions

Some actions that manifest positive regard are attending, suspending value judgments, and helping patients develop resources.

Attending. Attending behavior is the foundation of a therapeutic relationship. To succeed, nurses must pay attention to their patients in culturally and individually appropriate ways. Attending is a special kind of listening that refers to an intensity of presence or being with the patient. At times, simply being with another person during a painful time can make a difference.

Suspending Value Judgments. As previously discussed, everyone has values and beliefs. Using our personal value system to judge patients' thoughts, feelings, or behaviors is not helpful or productive. For example, if a patient is using drugs or is involved in risky sexual behavior, the nurse recognizes that these behaviors are unhealthy. Rather than labeling these activities as good or bad, the nurse helps the patient explore the thoughts and feelings that influence this behavior. Judgment on the part of the nurse will most likely interfere with further exploration.

The first steps in eliminating judgmental thinking and behaviors are to (1) recognize their presence, (2) identify how or where you learned these responses, and (3) construct alternative ways to view the patient's thinking and behavior. Denying judgmental thinking will only compound the problem.

Helping Patients Develop Resources. It is important that patients remain as independent as possible to develop new resources for problem solving, gaining personal support, and planning for the future. The nurse does not do the work the patient is responsible for doing unless it is absolutely necessary and then only as a step toward promoting independence. Consistently encouraging patients to use their own resources helps minimize their feelings of helplessness and dependency. It also validates their ability to bring about change and practice self-advocacy.

CHAPTER 3

Therapeutic Communication

Humans have an innate need to relate to others. Our advanced ability to communicate with others gives substance and meaning to our lives. All our actions, words, and facial expressions convey meaning to others. We cannot *not* communicate. Even silence is charged with meaning and may convey acceptance, anger, or thoughtfulness. Strong communication is the foundation for happy and productive relationships. On the other hand, ineffective communication may result in anxiety and negative feelings, and even dangerous mistakes.

In the provision of nursing care, communication takes on a new emphasis. Goal-directed, and scientifically based communication is referred to as *therapeutic communication*.

The ability to form patient-centered therapeutic relationships is fundamental to effective nursing care. Therapeutic communication is central to the formation of patient-centered therapeutic relationships. *Patient-centered* refers to the patient as a full partner in care whose values, preferences, and needs are respected (Quality and Safety Education for Nurses, 2012). Determining levels of pain in a postoperative patient; listening as parents express feelings of fear concerning their child's diagnosis; and understanding, without words, the needs of an intubated patient in the intensive care unit are essential skills in providing quality nursing care.

Ideally, therapeutic communication is a professional ability you learned and practiced early in your nursing education. In psychiatric–mental health nursing, communication skills take on a different and new emphasis. Psychiatric disorders cause physical symptoms (e.g., fatigue, loss of appetite, insomnia) and emotional symptoms (e.g., sadness, anger, hopelessness, euphoria) that affect a patient's ability to relate to others.

It is often during the psychiatric clinical rotation that students appreciate the usefulness of therapeutic communication. They begin to rely on techniques that may have once seemed artificial. For example, restating sounds so simplistic, the student may hesitate to use this technique:

Patient: "At the moment they told me my daughter would never be able to walk like her twin sister, I felt like I couldn't go on."

Student: *(restates the patient's words after a short silence)* "You felt like you couldn't go on."

That technique, and the empathy it conveys, is supportive in such a situation. Developing therapeutic communication skills takes time, and with continued practice, you will find your own style and rhythm. Eventually, these techniques will become a part of the way you instinctively communicate with others in the clinical setting.

Saying the Wrong Thing

Nursing students are often concerned that they may say the wrong thing, especially when learning to apply therapeutic techniques. Will you say the "wrong thing"? Yes, you probably will. That is how we all learn to find more useful and effective ways of helping individuals reach their goals.

Will saying the wrong thing be harmful to the patient? Consider that symptoms of psychiatric disorders—irritability, agitation, negativity, little communication, or being hypertalkative—often frustrate and alienate friends and family. It is likely that the interactions the patient had been having were not always pleasant. Patients tend to appreciate a well-meaning person who conveys genuine acceptance, respect, and concern for their situation. Even if you make mistakes in communication there is little chance that the comments will do actual harm.

VERBAL AND NONVERBAL COMMUNICATION

Verbal Communication

Verbal communication consists of all the words a person speaks. We live in a society of symbols, and our main social symbols are words. Words are the symbols for emotions and mental images. Talking is our link to one another and the primary instrument of instruction. Talking is a need, an art, and one of the most personal aspects of our private lives.

Nonverbal Communication

Have you heard, "It's not what you say but how you say it"? While this expression is not 100% true, it is the nonverbal behaviors that may be sending much of the real message through. Other common examples of nonverbal communication are physical appearance, body posture, eye contact, hand gestures, sighs, fidgeting, and yawning. Table 3.1 identifies examples of nonverbal behaviors.

Vocal quality, or paralinguistics, is an aspect of nonverbal communication. It encompasses voice volume, pitch, rate, and fluency. Speaking in soft and gentle tones is likely to encourage a person to share thoughts and feelings. Speaking in a rapid, high-pitched tone may convey anxiety and create it in the patient. Emphasis on certain words also conveys meaning. Consider, for example, how drastically tonal quality and inflection can affect communication in a simple sentence like "I will see you tonight."

1. "*I* will see you tonight." (I will be the one who sees you tonight.)
2. "I *will* see you tonight." (No matter what happens, or whether you like it or not, I will see you tonight.)
3. "I will see *you* tonight." (Even though others are present, it is you I want to see.)
4. "I will see you *tonight*." (It is definite, tonight is the night we will meet.)

Interaction of Verbal and Nonverbal Communication

Spoken words represent our public selves. They can be straightforward or used to distort, conceal, or disguise true feelings. Nonverbal behaviors include a wide range of human activities, from body movements to facial expressions to physical responses to messages received from others. How a person listens, uses silence, and uses the sense of touch may also convey important information about the private self that is not available from conversation alone.

Messages are not always simple. They can appear to be one thing when in fact they are another. Often, people have greater conscious awareness of their verbal messages

Table 3.1 **Nonverbal Behaviors**

Behavior	Nonverbal Cues	Example
Body behaviors	Posture, body movements, gestures, gait	The patient is slumped in a chair, face in hands, and occasionally taps the right foot.
Facial expressions	Frowns, smiles, grimaces, raised eyebrows, pursed lips, licking of lips, tongue movements	The patient scowls when speaking to the nurse, but when alone, smiles and giggles.
Eye expression and gaze behavior	Lowering brows, intimidating gaze	The patient's eyes harden with suspicion.
Voice-related behaviors	Tone, pitch, level, intensity, inflection, stuttering, pauses, silences, fluency	The patient talks in a loud voice with pressured speech.
Observable autonomic physiological responses	Increase in respirations, diaphoresis, pupil dilation, blushing, paleness	When discharge is mentioned, the patient becomes pale, diaphoretic, and respirations increase.
Personal appearance	Grooming, dress, hygiene	The patient is dressed in a wrinkled shirt, stained pants, and dirty socks, and is unshaven.
Physical characteristics	Height, weight, build, complexion, age	The patient is overweight with poor posture.

than their nonverbal behaviors. The verbal message is sometimes referred to as the *content* of the message (what is said), and the nonverbal behavior is called the *process* of the message (nonverbal cues a person gives to substantiate or contradict the verbal message).

When the content is congruent with the process, the communication is more clearly understood and is considered healthy. For example, if a student says, "It's important that I get good grades in this class," that is *content*. If the student has bought the books, takes thorough notes, and has a study buddy and/or tutor, that is *process*. In this case, the content and process are congruent and straightforward, and there is a healthy message. If, however, the verbal message is not reinforced or is in fact contradicted by the nonverbal behavior, the message is confusing. If a student says, "It's important that I get good grades in this class" and does not have the books, skips classes, and does not study, the content and process do not match. The student's verbal and nonverbal behaviors are incongruent.

COMMUNICATION SKILLS FOR NURSES

Therapeutic Communication Techniques

Once you have established a therapeutic relationship, you and your patient can identify specific needs and problems. You can then begin to work with the patient on increasing problem-solving skills, learning new coping behaviors, and experiencing more appropriate and satisfying ways of relating to others. Strong communication skills will facilitate your work. These skills are called *therapeutic communication techniques* and include words and actions that help to achieve health-related goals. Some useful techniques for nurses when communicating with their patients are (1) silence, (2) active listening, (3) clarifying techniques, and (4) questions.

Using Silence

Students and practicing nurses alike may find that when the flow of words stops, they become uncomfortable. They may rush to fill the void with questions or idle conversation. These responses may cut off important thoughts and feelings the patient might be taking time to think about before speaking.

Although there is no specific rule concerning how much silence is too much, silence is worthwhile only as long as it is serving some function and not anxiety provoking to the patient. Knowing when to speak largely depends on the nurse's perception about what is being conveyed through the silence.

Silence may provide meaningful moments of reflection for both participants. It is an opportunity to contemplate thoughtfully what has been said and felt, weigh alternatives, formulate new ideas, and gain a new perspective. When the nurse waits to speak, this allows the patient to break the silence, resulting in the patient sharing thoughts and feelings that may otherwise have been withheld.

Some psychiatric disorders, such as major depressive disorder and schizophrenia, and medications may cause a slowing of thought processes. Patience and gentle prompting can help patients gather their thoughts. For example, "You were saying that you are worried about the side effects of the new antidepressant."

Active Listening

People want more than just a physical presence in human communication. In active listening, nurses fully concentrate, respond, and remember what the patient is saying verbally and nonverbally. By giving the patient undivided attention, the nurse communicates that the patient is not alone. This kind of intervention enhances self-esteem and encourages the patient to direct energy toward finding ways to deal with problems. Serving as a sounding board, the nurse listens as the patient tests thoughts by voicing them outloud.

Clarifying Techniques

Understanding depends on clear communication, which is aided by verifying the nurse's interpretation of the patient's messages. The nurse can request feedback on the accuracy of the message received from verbal and nonverbal cues.

Paraphrasing. Paraphrasing occurs when you restate the basic content of a patient's message in different, usually fewer, words. Using simple, precise, and culturally relevant terms, the nurse may confirm an interpretation of the patient's message. Phrases such as "I'm not sure I understand" or "You seem to be saying…" help the nurse to interpret the message in what may be a bewildering mass of details. It also helps the patient to feel heard and may provide greater focus. The patient may confirm or deny the perceptions nonverbally by nodding or looking bewildered or by direct responses: "Yes, that is what I was trying to say" or "No, I meant…"

Restating. Restating is a clarifying strategy that helps the nurse to understand what the patient is saying. It also lets patients know that they are being heard. Restating differs from paraphrasing in that it involves repeating the same key words the patient has just spoken. If a patient remarks, "My life is empty… it has no meaning," additional information may be gained by restating, "Your life has no meaning?"

Although this is a valuable technique, it should be used sparingly. Patients may interpret frequent and indiscriminate use of restating as inattention or disinterest. Overuse makes restating sound mechanical. To avoid overuse of restating, the nurse can combine restatements with direct questions that encourage descriptions: "What sort of goals do you have for your evening?" "How is your family responding to your illness?"

Reflecting. Reflection assists patients to understand their own thoughts and feelings better. Reflecting may take the form of a question or a simple statement that conveys the nurse's observations of the patient. The nurse might briefly provide an interpretation of the patient's verbal and nonverbal behavior. For example, to reflect a patient's feelings about life, a good beginning might be, "You sound as if you have had many disappointments."

When you reflect, you make the patient aware of inner feelings and encourage the patient to own them. For example, you may say to a patient, "You look sad." Perceiving your concern may allow the patient to spontaneously share feelings. The use of a question in response to the patient's question is another reflective technique. For example:
Patient: "Do think I really need to be hospitalized?"
Nurse: "What do you think, Kelly?"
Patient: "I don't know. That's why I'm asking you."
Nurse: "I'll be willing to share my impression with you. However, you've probably thought about hospitalization and have some feelings about it. I wonder what they are."

Exploring. Exploring is a technique that enables the nurse to examine important ideas, experiences, or relationships more fully. For example, if a patient tells you he does not get along well with his wife, you will want to further explore this area. Possible openers include the following:
"Tell me more about your relationship with your wife."
"Give me an example of how you and your wife don't get along."
Table 3.2 summarizes therapeutic communication techniques.

Table 3.2 **Therapeutic Communication Techniques**

Therapeutic Technique	Description and Example
Silence	Gives the person time to collect thoughts or think through a point. *Encouraging a person to talk by waiting for the answers.*
Accepting	Indicates that the person has been understood. An accepting statement does not necessarily indicate agreement but is nonjudgmental. *"Yes." "Uh-huh." "I follow what you say."*
Giving recognition	Indicates awareness of change and personal efforts. Does not imply good or bad, right or wrong. *"Good morning, Mr. James." "I see you've eaten your whole lunch."*
Offering self	Offers presence, interest, and a desire to understand. Is not offered to get the person to talk or behave in a specific way. *"I would like to spend time with you." "I'll stay here and sit with you awhile."*
Offering general leads	Allows the other person to take direction in the discussion. Indicates that the nurse is interested in what comes next. *"Go on." "And then?" "Tell me about it."*
Giving broad openings	Clarifies that the lead is to be taken by the patient. However, the nurse discourages pleasantries and small talk. *"Where would you like to begin?" "What are you thinking about?"*
Placing the events in time or sequence	Puts events and actions in better perspective. Notes cause-and-effect relationships and identifies patterns of interpersonal difficulties. *"What happened before?" "When did this happen?"*

Making observations	Calls attention to the person's behavior (e.g., trembling, nail biting, restless mannerisms). Encourages the patient to notice the behavior and describe thoughts and feelings for mutual understanding. *"You appear tense." "I notice you're biting your lips." "You appear nervous whenever John enters the room."*
Encouraging description of perception	Increases the nurse's understanding of the patient's perceptions. Talking about feelings and difficulties can lessen the need to act them out inappropriately. *"What are the voices saying?" "What is happening now?" "Tell me when you feel anxious."*
Encouraging comparison	Brings out recurring themes in experiences or interpersonal relationships. Helps the person clarify similarities and differences. *"Has this ever happened before?" "Is this how you felt...?" "Was it something like...?"*
Restating	Repeats the main idea expressed. Gives the patient an idea of what has been communicated. If the message has been misunderstood, the patient can clarify it. *Patient: "I can't sleep. I stay awake all night." Nurse: "You stay awake all night?"*
Reflecting	Directs questions, feelings, and ideas back to the patient. Encourages the patient to accept personal ideas and feelings. Acknowledges patients' right to make decisions and encourages patients to think of themselves capable people. *Patient: "What should I do about my husband's affair?" Nurse: "What do you think you should do?"* or *Patient: "My brother spends all of my money and then has the nerve to ask for more." Nurse: "You feel angry when this happens?"*

Continued

Table 3.2 Therapeutic Communication Techniques—cont'd

Therapeutic Technique	Description and Example
Focusing	Concentrates attention on a single point; useful when the patient jumps from topic to topic. This technique is not helpful if a person is experiencing a severe or panic level of anxiety. *"You've mentioned many things. Let's go back to your thinking of 'ending it all'."*
Exploring	Examines certain ideas, experiences, or relationships more fully. If the patient chooses not to elaborate by answering "no," the nurse does not probe or pry. In such a case, the nurse respects the patient's wishes. *"Would you describe it more fully?" "Could you talk about how it was that you learned your mom was dying of cancer?"*
Giving information	Makes facts the person needs available. Supplies knowledge from which decisions can be made or conclusions drawn. Provides teaching. *"This medication is for..." "The test will determine..."*
Seeking clarification	Helps patients clarify their own thoughts and maximize mutual understanding between nurse and patient. *"I am not sure I follow you." "Give an example of a time you thought everyone hated you."*
Presenting reality	Indicates what is real. The nurse does not argue or try to convince the patient, just describes personal perceptions or facts in the situation. *"That was Dr. Todd, not a man from the Mafia." "That was the sound of a car backfiring."*

Voicing doubt	Expressing uncertainty regarding the reality of the patient's perceptions or conclusions, especially in hallucinations and delusions. Use with caution and only after rapport has been well established. *"Isn't that unusual?" "Really?" "That's hard to believe."*
Verbalizing the implied	Puts into concrete terms what the patient implies, making the patient's communication more explicit. **Patient:** *"I can't talk to you or anyone else. It's a waste of time."* **Nurse:** *"Do you feel that no one understands?"*
Summarizing	Brings together important points of discussion to enhance understanding. *"Have I got this straight?" "You said that…" "During the past hour, you and I have discussed…"*
Translating words into feelings	Responds to the feeling expressed, not just the content. **Patient:** *"I am dead inside."* **Nurse:** *"Are you saying that you feel lifeless? That life seems meaningless?"*
Formulating of a plan of action	Allows the patient to identify alternative actions for interpersonal situations the patient finds disturbing (e.g., when anger or anxiety is provoked). *"What could you do to let anger out harmlessly?" "What are some other ways you can approach your boss?"*

Adapted from Hays, J. S., & Larson, K. (1963). *Interacting with patients.* Macmillan. Copyright 1963 by Macmillan Publishing Company.

Questions

Open-Ended Questions. Open-ended questions encourage patients to share information about experiences, perceptions, or responses to a situation. The following are examples:

- "What are some of the stresses you are under right now?"
- "How would you describe your relationship with your wife?"

Because open-ended questions are not intrusive and do not put the patient on the defensive, they help the clinician elicit information. This technique is especially useful with new patients or when a patient is guarded or resistant to answering questions. Open-ended questions are particularly useful when establishing rapport.

Closed-Ended Questions. Nurses are usually urged to ask open-ended questions to elicit more than a "yes" or "no" response. However, closed-ended questions, when used sparingly, can give you specific and needed information. Closed-ended questions are most useful during an initial assessment or intake interview or to assess the patient's status, "Are the medications helping you?" "Are you hearing voices now?" "Did you seek therapy after your first suicide attempt?"

Nontherapeutic Communication

People often use nontherapeutic or ineffective communication. However, for nurses, using nontherapeutic communication can be particularly problematic because it impairs the nurse–patient interaction and negatively impacts the therapeutic relationship. Table 3.3 summarizes types of nontherapeutic communication and suggests more helpful responses.

Excessive Questioning

Excessive questioning—asking multiple questions (particularly closed-ended) consecutively or rapidly—casts the nurse in the role of interrogator who demands information without respect for the patient's willingness or readiness to respond. This approach conveys a lack of respect for and sensitivity to the patient's needs.

Excessive questioning controls the range and nature of the responses, can easily result in a therapeutic stall, or

Table 3.3 **Nontherapeutic Communication**

Nontherapeutic	Description and Example	More Helpful Response
Giving advice	Assumes the nurse knows best and the patient cannot think independently. Inhibits problem solving and fosters dependency. *"Get out of this situation immediately."*	Encouraging problem solving: *"What were some of the actions you thought you might take?"* *"What are some of the ways you have thought of to meet your goals?"*
Minimizing feelings	The nurse seems unable to understand or empathize with the patient. Feelings or experiences are belittled, which can cause the patient to feel small or insignificant. *"Everyone gets down in the dumps."*	Empathizing and exploring: *"You must be feeling very upset. Are you thinking of hurting yourself?"*
Falsely reassuring	Attempting to provide comfort not based on fact or reality. Causes a person to feel unheard. May cause the patient to stop sharing feelings. *"I wouldn't worry about that." "Everything will be all right."*	Clarifying the patient's message: *"What specifically are you worried about?"* *"What are you concerned might happen?"*
Making value judgments	Can make the patient feel guilty, angry, misunderstood, not supported, or anxious to leave. *"You smoke and your wife has lung cancer?"*	Making observations: *"I notice you are still smoking."*
Asking "why" questions	Critically demands an explanation; often makes the patient feel defensive. *"Why did you stop taking your medication?"*	Giving a broad opening: *"Tell me some of the reasons that led up to quitting your medications."*

Continued

Table 3.3 **Nontherapeutic Communication —cont'd**

Nontherapeutic	Description and Example	More Helpful Response
Excessive questioning	Results in the patient not knowing which question to answer and possibly being confused about what is being asked. *"How's your appetite? Are you losing weight? Are you eating enough?"*	Clarifying: *"Tell me about your eating habits since you've been depressed."*
Giving approval, agreeing	Implies the patient is doing the *right* thing—and that not doing it is wrong. May lead the patient to focus on pleasing the nurse or clinician. *"I'm proud of you for applying for that job." "I agree with your decision."*	Making observations: *"I noticed that you applied for that job."* Asking open-ended questions: *"What led to that decision?"*
Disapproving, disagreeing	Can make a person defensive. *"You really should have shown up for the medication group."*	Exploring: *"How did you decide not to come to your medication group?"* *"How did you arrive at that conclusion?"*
Changing the subject	Invalidates the patient's feelings and needs. Leaves the patient feeling isolated and increases feelings of hopelessness. ***Patient:*** *"I'd like to die."* ***Nurse:*** *"Did you go to Alcoholics Anonymous like we discussed?"*	Validating and exploring: *"This sounds serious. Have you thought of harming yourself?"*

Adapted from Hays, J. S., & Larson, K. (1963). *Interacting with patients.* Macmillan. Copyright 1963 by Macmillan Publishing Company.

may completely shut down an interview. It is a controlling tactic and may reflect the interviewer's lack of security in allowing patients to tell their own stories. It is better to ask more open-ended questions and then follow the patient's lead. For example:

Excessive questioning: "Why did you leave your wife? Did you feel angry with her? What did she do to you? Are you going back to her?"

More therapeutic approach: "Tell me about the situation between you and your wife."

Giving Approval or Disapproval

We often give our friends and family approval when they do something well, but giving praise and approval becomes much more complex in a nurse–patient relationship. Saying, "That is an amazing mask you made in art therapy" is supportive and may, in fact, promote a dialogue about the emotional meaning of the mask. Contrast that comment with, "It makes me happy to see you sitting with Chelsea at lunch." When the patient is doing a behavior to please another person, it is not coming from the individual's own conviction. Thus the new response really is not a change in behavior as much as an act to win approval and acceptance from another.

Disapproval is the opposite side of the same coin. "I was disappointed that you showed up late for group therapy" or "You should quit smoking" are counterproductive for any therapeutic relationship. Statements such as these will cause negative feelings such as shame or resentment and undermine the patient's recovery process.

Giving Advice

We ask for and give advice all the time. In a way, nurses give advice when they teach (e.g., "Take your medication with food."). The nontherapeutic form is when the advice becomes more personal in nature. "If I were you, I would leave your husband" or even "You should find a new job" interferes with the patient's ability to make personal decisions. When a nurse offers patients solutions, the patients eventually begin to think the nurse does not view them as capable of making effective decisions.

Asking "Why" Questions

"Why" demands an explanation and implies wrongdoing. Think of the last time someone asked you why: "Why didn't you go to the funeral?" or "Why did you pick that outfit?" Such questions imply criticism. We may ask our friends or family these questions, and in the context of a solid relationship, the why may be understood more as "What happened?" With people we do not know— especially those who may be anxious or overwhelmed—a why question from a person in authority (e.g., nurse, physician, or teacher) can be experienced as intrusive and judgmental, which serves only to make the person defensive.

ENVIRONMENTAL VARIABLES

Setting

Effective communication can take place almost anywhere. However, the quality of the interaction—whether in a clinic, a clinical unit, an office, or the patient's home—depends on the degree to which the nurse and patient feel safe. Establishing a setting that enhances feelings of security is important to the therapeutic relationship. A healthcare setting, a conference room, or a quiet part of the unit that has relative privacy but is within view of others is ideal.

When care is provided in a home setting, patients may feel safer and more comfortable than in the clinical setting. An additional benefit of a home visit is being able to assess the patient in the context of everyday life.

Telehealth was becoming popular for healthcare delivery, particularly psychiatric services, prior to 2020. The advent of the COVID-19 pandemic dramatically increased the use of and comfort with telepsychiatry, which is likely to remain a popular delivery method.

Nursing care such as counseling, screening, health education, and coordinating services can easily be accomplished electronically. Benefits include increasing access to care and eliminating the stigma associated with visiting psychiatric facilities. A primary disadvantage of telehealth is the elimination of the personal face-to-face presence. Other more easily addressed barriers are limited broadband services in rural areas, lack of equipment in low-income homes, licensing restrictions, and reimbursement policies.

Seating

In all settings, arrange chairs so that conversation can take place in normal tones of voice and so that eye contact can be comfortably maintained or avoided. A nonthreatening physical environment for both nurse and patient includes the following:

- Be at the same height by both sitting or both standing.
- Avoid a face-to-face arrangement when possible; a 90- to 120-degree angle may be less intense, and the patient and nurse can look away from each other without discomfort.
- Provide safety and psychological comfort in terms of exiting the room. The patient is not seated between the nurse and the door, and the nurse is not seated in such a way that the patient feels trapped in the room.
- If possible, avoid having a desk between the nurse and the patient. A desk tends to be a physical and a psychological barrier and also represents a power delineation.

Walking while talking may be an alternative to sitting. Some psychiatric disorders result in hyperactivity and agitation, making sitting extremely uncomfortable. Furthermore, activity reduces depressive symptoms and is usually a healthier option for both the patient and the nurse.

Spacing

The use of personal space is a significant variable when communicating with another person. Generally speaking, distance is based on the following in the United States:

- **Intimate distance** (1.5 feet or less) is reserved for those we trust most and with whom we feel most safe.
- **Personal distance** (1.5–4 feet) is for personal communications such as those with friends or colleagues.
- **Social distance** (4–12 feet) applies to strangers or acquaintances, often in public places or formal social gatherings.
- **Public distance** (12 feet or more) relates to public space (e.g., public speaking).

It is important to note that in individuals with some psychiatric conditions, space should be altered. For example, if a person with schizophrenia is experiencing paranoia, personal and social distance should be increased. Likewise, during an episode of mania and agitation, space should also be increased.

IMPROVING COMMUNICATION SKILLS

Clinical Debriefing

An increasingly popular method of providing clinical supervision is through debriefing. According to the National League for Nursing (2015), debriefing is such an excellent learning method that it should be incorporated into all clinical experiences. Debriefing refers to a critical conversation and reflection regarding an experience that results in growth and learning. Debriefing supports essential learning along a continuum of "knowing what" to "knowing how" and "knowing why."

Process Recordings

A good way to increase communication and interviewing skills is to review your clinical interactions exactly as they occur. Process recordings are written records of a segment of the nurse–patient session that reflect as closely as possible the verbal and nonverbal behaviors of both patient and nurse. Process recordings have some disadvantages because they rely on memory and are subject to distortions. However, you may find them to be useful in identifying communication patterns.

Communication Skills Evaluation

After you have had some introductory clinical experience, you may find the facilitative skills checklist in Table 3.4 is useful for evaluating your progress in developing interviewing skills. Note that some of the items might not be relevant for some of your patients (e.g., numbers 11–13 may not be possible when a patient is experiencing psychosis [disordered thought, delusions, and/or hallucinations]). Self-evaluation of clinical skills is a way to focus on therapeutic improvement. Role-playing can help prepare you for clinical experience and practice effective and professional communication skills.

Table 3.4 **Communication Self-Assessment Checklist**

Instructions: Periodically during your clinical experience, use this checklist to identify areas needed for growth and progress made. Think of your clinical patient experiences. Indicate the extent of your agreement with each of the following statements by marking the scale:

SA = strongly agree, A = agree, NS = not sure, D = disagree, SD = strongly disagree

1. I maintain appropriate eye contact.	SA	A	NS	D	SD
2. Most of my verbal comments follow the lead of the other person.	SA	A	NS	D	SD
3. I encourage others to talk about feelings.	SA	A	NS	D	SD
4. I ask open-ended questions.	SA	A	NS	D	SD
5. I restate and clarify the person's ideas.	SA	A	NS	D	SD
6. I paraphrase the person's nonverbal behaviors.	SA	A	NS	D	SD
7. I summarize in a few words the basic ideas of a long statement made by the person.	SA	A	NS	D	SD
8. I make statements that reflect the person's feelings.	SA	A	NS	D	SD
9. I share my feelings relevant to the discussion when appropriate to do so.	SA	A	NS	D	SD
10. I give feedback.	SA	A	NS	D	SD
11. At least 75% or more of my responses help enhance and facilitate communication.	SA	A	NS	D	SD
12. I assist the person in listing some available alternatives.	SA	A	NS	D	SD
13. I assist the person in identifying some specific and observable goals.	SA	A	NS	D	SD
14. I assist the person in specifying at least one next step that might be taken toward the goal.	SA	A	NS	D	SD

From Myrick, D., & Erney, T. (1984). *Caring and sharing.* Educational Media Corporation.

CHAPTER 4

Neurodevelopmental Disorders

During any given year, 16.5% of children and adolescents living in the United States experience at least one psychiatric disorder (Whitney & Peterson, 2019). About half (49.6%) of these children and adolescents receive treatment for the disorder. Unfortunately, when left untreated, psychiatric conditions may result in devastating consequences for academic, social, and psychological functioning. Furthermore, problems first apparent in childhood and adolescence often continue into adulthood.

The American Psychiatric Association ([APA], 2013) defines neurodevelopmental disorders as a group of conditions with an onset in the early developmental period, often before the child begins school. These disorders result in impairments in personal, social, and academic functioning. The associated deficits range from specific learning limitations to global impairment. The major categories included in the neurodevelopmental disorders chapter in the *Diagnostic and Statistical Manual of Mental Disorders* (APA, 2013) are:

- Intellectual disabilities
- Communication disorders
- Autism spectrum disorder (ASD)
- Attention-deficit/hyperactivity disorder (ADHD)
- Specific learning disorder
- Motor disorders

In addition to these mental health problems, adolescents and children are impacted by most of the same psychiatric conditions as adults, including anxiety disorders, depressive disorders, psychotic disorders, and eating disorders. Nursing students caring for children and adolescents may refer to other chapters in this manual for general care plans related to other psychiatric disorders.

We begin with an overview of assessment techniques and therapeutic methods that are useful when working with children and adolescents. This overview is followed by associated nursing care for two specific neurodevelopmental disorders, ADHD and ASD.

INITIAL ASSESSMENT

In the initial assessment, the nurse asks the child or adolescent about life at home with parents and siblings and life at school with teachers and peers. Children and adolescents are encouraged to describe current concerns. The nurse then asks questions to gain an understanding of their developmental history. Play activities, such as games, drawing, puppets, and free play, are used for younger children who have difficulty responding to a more direct approach. An important part of the first interaction is observing interactions between the child, caregiver, and siblings when possible.

Families are involved in therapy whenever possible. They are given support in parenting skills to help them provide nurturing and to set consistent limits. Family counseling is often a key component of treatment. Parents can learn to use behavioral techniques, monitor medication, collaborate with the school to encourage academic success, and make a home environment that promotes the achievement of normal developmental tasks. In extreme cases where parents are abusive, use substances, or are extremely dysfunctional, the child may require out-of-home placement.

GENERAL INTERVENTIONS WITH CHILDREN

Ideally, treatment of childhood and adolescent disorders uses a multimodal approach of coordinated care. Close work with schools, remediation services, and mental health professionals who provide behavior modification are all a part of the care.

General interventions include the following:
- Rewarding positive behaviors (e.g., using a point system) to reduce maladaptive behaviors
- Play therapy
- Bibliotherapy
- Expressive arts therapy
- Journaling
- Music therapy
- Managing disruptive behaviors with time out or time in a quiet room

Selected Childhood Disorders

Two disorders commonly seen in children and adolescents are discussed in this chapter. ADHD will be presented first along with associated nursing care. This discussion is followed by an overview of ASD and associated nursing care.

ATTENTION-DEFICIT/ HYPERACTIVITY DISORDER

Individuals with ADHD exhibit inattention, impulsiveness, and hyperactivity. It is important to note that some people are inattentive but not hyperactive or impulsive. In the absence of hyperactivity, the diagnosis becomes inattentive-type ADHD, with symptoms such as disorganization, lack of focus, and forgetfulness.

To diagnose an individual with ADHD, symptoms must be present in at least two settings (e.g., at home and school) and occur before the age of 12. The disorder is often initially detected when the child has difficulty adjusting to elementary school. Attention problems and hyperactivity contribute to low frustration tolerance, temper outbursts, labile moods, poor school performance, peer rejection, and low self-esteem.

Peer relationships are strained because of difficulty taking turns, poor social boundaries, intrusive behaviors, and interrupting others. Individuals with inattentive type of ADHD may exhibit high degrees of distractibility and disorganization. They may be unable to complete challenging or tedious tasks, become easily bored, frequently lose things, or require frequent reminders to complete tasks. Children with ADHD are also more likely than their peers to experience enuresis (bed-wetting) along with a similar trend for encopresis (fecal soiling).

Epidemiology

According to a national parent survey, the estimated number of children who have been diagnosed with ADHD is slightly more than 6 million, or about 9.5% (Danielson et al., 2018). Boys are more likely to receive this diagnosis as compared to girls—nearly 13% and nearly 6%, respectively. The estimated prevalence of ADHD in adults is 4.4%, with more men (5.4%) than women affected (3.2%) (Kessler et al., 2006). The median age of onset is 7 years, although some people may go undiagnosed until functional impairments become noticeable in adulthood.

Risk Factors

ADHD tends to run in families. The concordance rate for identical twins is between 51% and 58% (Ebert et al., 2016). Although certain genes are correlated with the disorder, there have been no absolute connections. Very low birth weight triples the risk of ADHD. Maternal smoking and alcohol use, child abuse, neglect, neurotoxin exposure (e.g., lead), and infections (e.g., encephalitis) also increase the risk of ADHD.

ASSESSMENT GUIDELINES
ATTENTION-DEFICIT/HYPERACTIVITY DISORDER

1. Gather data from parents, caregivers, teachers, or other adults involved with the child. Ask about level of physical activity, attention span, talkativeness, frustration tolerance, impulse control, and the ability to follow directions and complete tasks.
2. Assess social skills, friendship history, problem-solving skills, and school performance. Gather this information from the family or caregiver.
3. Assess for comorbidities such as anxiety and depressive symptoms.
4. Assess for indicators of learning disorders, ASD, or intellectual disabilities.
5. Ask about eating and sleeping patterns and monitor these regularly, particularly if the child is being treated with stimulants.

Nursing Diagnoses

The International Classification for Nursing Practice (ICNP; International Council of Nurses [ICN], 2019) provides useful nursing diagnoses for individuals with ADHD. Because children and adolescents with ADHD may display impulsive behaviors, *impaired impulse control* is a primary focus. Conflict with authority figures, refusal to comply with requests, and inappropriate ways of getting needs met are addressed with *impaired coping. Impaired socialization* addresses difficulty making or keeping friends. Interpersonal and academic problems lead to *chronic low self-esteem.* Because parent's or caregiver's participation in therapeutic programs is essential, *impaired family process* applies.

INTERVENTION GUIDELINES

Help the child or adolescent reach full potential by fostering developmental competencies and coping skills:
1. Protect from harm and provide for physical and emotional needs.
2. Provide immediate feedback for unacceptable behaviors.
3. Increase the use of interpersonal skills to maintain satisfying relationships with adults and peers.
4. Provide immediate positive feedback for acceptable behaviors.
5. Increase the child's or adolescent's ability to control impulses.
6. Use role-play to practice responding in acceptable ways when feeling frustrated.
7. Foster the development of a realistic self-identity and self-esteem based on achievements and the formation of realistic goals.
8. Provide support, education, and guidance for parents or caregivers.

Nursing Care for Attention-Deficit/Hyperactivity Disorder
Impaired Impulse Control
Related to
- Neurological dysfunction
- Distractibility

- Lack of self-restraint
- Difficulty in delaying gratification

Desired Outcome The patient will demonstrate improved impulse control.

Assessment/Interventions and *Rationales*

1. Implement techniques for managing disruptive behaviors (Table 4.1). *These techniques are effective in connecting with the child, diffusing potential outbursts, keeping the child safe, and teaching appropriate behaviors.*

2. Set clear, consistent limits in a calm, nonjudgmental manner. Remind the patient of the consequences of acting out. *Patients gain a sense of security with clear limits and calm adults who follow through on a consistent basis.*

3. Avoid power struggles and repeated negotiations about rules and limits. *When limits are realistic and enforceable, manipulation can be minimized.*

4. Use strategic removal if the patient cannot respond to limits (e.g., time out in a quiet room). *Removal allows the patient to express feelings and discuss problems without losing face in front of peers.*

5. Process incidents with the patient to make it a learning experience. *Reality testing, problem solving, and testing new behaviors are necessary to foster cognitive growth.*

6. Use a behavior modification program that rewards the patient for seeking help with handling feelings and controlling impulses to act out. *Consistently reinforcing positive responses results in improved social behavior and increased self-esteem.*

7. Redirect expressions of disruptive feelings into nondestructive, age-appropriate behaviors. Channel excess energy into physical activities. *Learning how to modulate the expression of feelings and use anger constructively are essential for self-control.*

8. Teach mindfulness techniques to increase the patient's ability to remain in the here-and-now rather than jumping from activity to activity. *Mindfulness techniques support the management of impulse control.*

9. Encourage feelings of concern for others and remorse for the results of impulsive actions. *The development of empathy promotes thinking before acting.*

10. Provide prescribed medication and encourage the patient to be involved in monitoring symptoms, side effects, and improvement. *Patients who are actively involved in their care feel empowered and are more likely to adhere to a medication regimen.*

Table 4.1 **Techniques for Managing Disruptive Behaviors in Children**

Technique	Description
Planned ignoring	When behaviors are determined by staff to be attention seeking and not dangerous, they may be ignored.
Use of signals or gestures	Use a word, gesture, or eye contact to remind the child or adolescent to use self-control.
Behavioral contract	A verbal or written agreement between the patient and nurse or other parties (e.g., family, treatment team, teacher) about behaviors, expectations, and needs.
Additional affection	Involves giving a child planned emotional support for a specific problem or engaging in an enjoyable activity.
Use of humor	Use well-timed appropriate kidding as a diversion to help the child or adolescent save face and relieve feelings of guilt or fear.
Collaborative and proactive solutions	Identifies and defines problematic behaviors and specific triggers, and develops a collaborative method for creating mutually agreeable solutions to the specific situation or trigger.
Counseling	Verbal interactions, role-playing, and modeling to teach, coach, or maintain adaptive behavior and provide positive reinforcement.
Clarification as intervention	Help the child or adolescent understand the situation and motivation for the behavior.
Restructuring	Changing the activity in a way that decreases the stimulation or the frustration (e.g., shorten a story or change to a physical activity).
Modeling	Learning behaviors or skills by observation and imitation that can be used in a wide variety of situations.
Role-playing	Acting out a specified script or role to enhance the child's understanding of that role and to learn and practice new behaviors, skills, and specific situations.
Limit setting	Giving direction, stating an expectation, or telling a child what to do or where to go.

Continued

Table 4.1 **Techniques for Managing Disruptive Behaviors in Children**—cont'd

Technique	Description
Redirection	Used after an undesirable or inappropriate behavior to engage or re-engage an individual in an appropriate activity.
Simple restitution	After a behavioral disruption, the child is required or expected to correct the adverse environmental or relational effects of misbehavior (e.g., apologizing to the people harmed, fixing the chairs that are upturned).
Time out in a quiet room	A quiet environment away from other people allows the child or adolescent time to regroup and manage feelings and behavior.
Seclusion and restraint	During extreme circumstances, after less restrictive responses have failed, the child may need protection from impulses to act out or hurt self or others.

Impaired Coping
Related to
- Neurological dysfunction
- Low level of self-confidence
- Fear of failure/humiliation
- Disturbance in ability to release tension
- Highly reactive and difficult to comfort temperament
- Disturbed relationship with parent or caregiver (e.g., lack of trust, abuse, neglect, conflicts, inadequate role models, disorganized family system)
- Deficient support system

Desired Outcome The patient will demonstrate improved coping.

Assessment/Interventions and *Rationales*
1. Use one-to-one or an appropriate level of observation to monitor rising levels of frustration and determine emotional/situational triggers. *External controls are needed for emotional support and to prevent tantrums and rage reactions.*
2. Intervene early to calm the patient, problem solve, and defuse a potential outburst. *Learning can take place before the patient loses control. New solutions and compromises can be proposed.*

3. Avoid power struggles and no-win situations. *Therapeutic goals are lost in power struggles.*
4. Use behavioral techniques to reward tolerating frustration, delaying gratification, and responding to requests and behavioral limits. *Rewarding the patient's efforts will increase positive behaviors and help with the development of self-control.*
5. Allow the patient to question the requests or limits within reason. Give a simple, understandable rationale for requests or limits. *Discussion allows the patient to maintain some sense of autonomy and power. The rationale is tailored to the developmental age and promotes socialization.*
6. Use medication if indicated to reduce anxiety, rage, and aggression and to stabilize mood. *A variety of medications are effective in children who experience behavioral and emotional lack of control.*
7. When feasible, negotiate an agreement on the expected behaviors. Avoid bribes or allowing the patient to manipulate the situation. *An agreement on expected behavior will result in improved compliance. However, constant negotiations can result in increased manipulation and testing of limits.*

Impaired Socialization

Related to
- Neurological dysfunction
- Lack of appropriate role models
- Poor impulse control, frustration tolerance, or empathy for others
- Disturbed relationship with parents or caregivers
- Identification with aggressive/abusive models
- Loss of friendships due to disruptions in family life and living situation

Desired Outcome The patient will demonstrate improved socialization.

Assessment/Interventions and *Rationales*
1. Use the one-to-one relationship to engage the patient in a working relationship. *The patient needs positive role models for healthy identification.*
2. Monitor for negative behaviors and identify maladaptive interaction patterns. *Negative behaviors are identified and targeted for replacement with age-appropriate social skills.*

3. Intervene early to give feedback and alternative ways to handle the situation. *Children learn from feedback. Early intervention prevents rejection by peers and provides immediate ways to cope.*
4. Use therapeutic play to teach social skills such as sharing, cooperation, realistic competition, and manners. *Learning new ways to interact with others through play allows the development of satisfying friendships and improved self-esteem.*
5. Use role-playing, stories, and therapeutic games to practice skills. *Enjoyable activities support the practice of new skills in a safe environment.*
6. Help the patient find and develop a special friend and set up one-on-one play situations. Be available to problem solve peer relationship conflicts and role model social skills. *The abilities to reality test, problem solve, and resolve conflicts in peer relationships are important interpersonal skills.*
7. Help the patient develop peer relationships with honest and appropriate expression of feelings and needs. *When patients can identify personal feelings and needs, they are better prepared to use more direct communication rather than manipulation and/or intimidation.*

Chronic Low Self-Esteem
Related to
- Perceived lack of belonging
- Perceived lack of respect from others
- Lack of success in role functioning
- Disturbed relationship with parent or caregiver
- Bullied by peers

Desired Outcomes The patient will demonstrate an improved self-esteem:
- Describe self in positive ways.
- Fulfill personally significant roles.
- Engage in meaningful interaction with others.

Assessment/Interventions and *Rationales*
1. Give unconditional positive regard without reinforcing negative behaviors. *Demonstrating basic acceptance and respect of a person regardless of what they say or do is essential for healthy development.*

2. Reinforce the patient's self-worth with time and attention. *Giving one-to-one time or attention supports the patient's self-worth.*
3. Help the patient identify positive qualities and accomplishments. *An accurate appraisal of accomplishments can help reduce unrealistic expectations.*
4. Help the patient identify behaviors needing change and set realistic goals. *To change, the patient needs goals and knowledge of new behaviors.*
5. Use a behavior modification program that rewards the patient for practicing new behaviors and evaluates results. *Rewarding the patient's efforts will increase the positive behaviors and foster the development of increased self-esteem.*

Impaired Family Process
Related to
- Neurological dysfunction
- Disruptive symptoms of ADHD in the child
- Limited understanding of ADHD (e.g., biological origins and treatment)
- Role strain or overload
- Relationship disturbance in the caregivers
- Disability in the parent(s)
- History of being abused or history of being abusive
- Lack of parent or caregiver fit with the child

Desired Outcome The family will demonstrate improved family processes.

Assessment/Interventions and *Rationales*
1. Explore the impact of ADHD on the life of the family. *Helps the nurse understand the parent or caregiver situation. Feeling understood and supported can reinforce the development of a therapeutic relationship.*
2. Assess the parent's or caregiver's knowledge of childhood growth and development and parenting skills. *Problem identification and analysis of learning needs are necessary before intervention begins.*
3. Assess the parent's or caregiver's understanding of the child's diagnosis and treatment. *Knowledge will increase parental or caregiver participation, motivation, and satisfaction.*

4. Help the parent or caregiver identify the child's physical, emotional, and social needs. *Adequate parenting involves being able to identify the child's age-appropriate needs.*
5. Involve the parent or caregiver in identifying a realistic plan for how these needs will be met. *Parents or caregivers have the opportunity to learn the skills necessary to meet the child's needs.*
6. Work with the parent or caregiver to set realistic behavioral goals. *Mutually setting goals provides continuity and prevents the child from using splitting or manipulation to sabotage treatment.*
7. Teach behavioral principles and give the parent or caregiver support in using them and evaluating the effectiveness. Positive reinforcement for good behavior and logical consequences for negative behavior are basic behavioral principles. *Education and follow-up support are key to a successful treatment program.*
8. Assess the parent or caregiver support system. Use referrals to establish additional supports. *Self-help groups and special programs such as respite care can increase the caregiver's ability to cope.*
9. Provide information on legal rights and available resources that can assist in advocating for services for the child. *The parent or caregiver commonly lacks information on how to secure services for the child.*

TREATMENT FOR ATTENTION-DEFICIT/ HYPERACTIVITY DISORDER

Biological Treatments

Pharmacotherapy

Psychostimulants are used to treat ADHD to improve the sluggish frontal lobe that is believed to be involved in this disorder. See Chapter 21 for medications used in the treatment of ADHD. To control severely aggressive behaviors, other pharmacological agents—including stimulants, mood stabilizers, alpha-adrenergic agonists, and antipsychotics—are used.

Psychological Therapies

Treatment for ADHD includes behavior modification, special education programs for academic difficulties, and psychotherapy and play therapy for concurrent emotional problems. Cognitive–behavioral therapy (CBT) is used to change patterns of impulsivity by fostering the development of internal control. Mindfulness meditation may also help individuals with ADHD to self-observe and to develop different responses to stressful experiences. Chapter 29 provides more information on these treatment modalities.

AUTISM SPECTRUM DISORDER

ASD is a complex neurobiological and developmental disability that typically appears during the first 3 years of life. ASD affects the normal development of social interaction and communication skills. It ranges in severity from mild to moderate to severe.

Symptoms associated with ASD include deficits in social relatedness with deficits in developing and maintaining relationships. Other behaviors include stereotypical repetitive speech, obsessive focus on specific objects, rigid adherence to routines or rituals, hyperreactivity or hyporeactivity to sensory input, and resistance to change. The symptoms first occur in childhood and cause impairments in everyday functioning.

Epidemiology

The prevalence of ASD is 1 in 68 children (Christensen et al., 2016). The prevalence is significantly higher in boys. ASD has no racial, ethnic, or social boundaries and is not influenced by family income, educational levels, or lifestyles.

Risk Factors

There is a genetic component to autism. The concordance rate for monozygotic (identical) twins is 70% to 90%, meaning that most of the time if one twin is affected, the other is as well.

ASSESSMENT GUIDELINES
AUTISM SPECTRUM DISORDER

1. Assess for developmental delays, uneven development, or loss of acquired abilities. Use baby books and diaries, photographs, videotapes, or anecdotal reports from nonfamily caregivers.

2. Assess the child's verbal and nonverbal communication, sensory, social, and behavioral skills including the presence of any aggressive or self-injurious behaviors.
3. Assess the parent–child relationship for evidence of bonding, anxiety, tension, and fit of temperaments.
4. Assess for physical and emotional signs of possible abuse since children with behavioral and developmental problems are at increased risk for abuse.
5. Ensure that screening for comorbid intellectual disability has been completed.
6. Assess the need for community programs with support services for parents and children, including parent education, counseling, and after-school programs.

Nursing Diagnoses

Several ICNP (ICN, 2019) nursing diagnoses are applicable for ASD. In ASD, the severity of the impairment is demonstrated by the child's lack of responsiveness to or interest in others, a deficiency of empathy or sharing with peers, and little or no cooperative or imaginative play with peers. Therefore *impaired socialization* is always present. Language delay or absence of language and the unusual stereotyped or repetitive use of language are other areas for nursing, making *impaired communication* a useful focus. Stereotyped and repetitive motor movements can include behaviors such as head banging, face slapping, and hand biting. The child's apparent indifference to pain can result in serious self-injury, so *risk for injury* can become a priority. Individuals with ASD often lack an interest in activities outside of self, and they frequently disregard bodily needs. These deficiencies interfere with the development of a personal identity, so *disturbed personal identity* might also be the focus for care.

Nursing Care for Autism Spectrum Disorders
Impaired Socialization
Related to
• Neurological dysfunction
• Self-concept disturbance (e.g., immaturity or developmental deviation)
• Absence of available significant others or peers

- Disturbed thought processes
- Disturbance in response to external stimuli
- Disturbance in attachment or bonding with the parent or caregiver

Desired Outcomes The patient will demonstrate improved socialization.

Assessment/Interventions and *Rationales*

1. Use one-to-one interaction to engage the patient in a therapeutic relationship. *Assigning the same primary nurse can promote attachment.*
2. Monitor for signs of anxiety or distress. Intervene early to provide comfort. *Anticipating the need for assistance in managing stress will enhance the patient's feelings of security.*
3. Provide emotional support and guidance for activities of daily living (ADLs) and other activities. Use a system of rewards for attempts and successes. *Behavior change occurs through meaningful social interactions involving imitation, modeling, feedback, and reinforcement.*
4. Set up social interactions beginning with parallel play and moving toward cooperative play. *Learning to play with peers is sequential.*
5. Help the patient find a special friend. *A connection with one other person may lead to connections with others.*
6. Role model social interaction skills (e.g., interest, empathy, sharing, and taking turns speaking). *Role modeling facilitates the development of necessary social and emotional skills.*
7. Reward attempts to interact and play with peers and the use of appropriate emotional expressions. *Behaviors that are rewarded are repeated.*
8. Role-play situations that involve conflicts in social interactions to teach reality testing, cause and effect, and problem solving. *These cognitive skills are needed for successful social and emotional reciprocity.*

Impaired Communication
Related to
- Neurological dysfunction
- Physiological conditions and/or emotional conditions
- Disturbance in attachment or bonding with the parent or caregiver

Desired Outcome The patient will demonstrate improved communication.

Assessment/Interventions *Rationales*

1. Use one-to-one interaction to engage the patient in nonverbal play. *The nurse enters the patient's world using a nonthreatening interaction to form a trusting relationship.*
2. Recognize subtle cues indicating the patient is paying attention or attempting to communicate. *Cues are often difficult to recognize (e.g., glancing out of the corner of the eye).*
3. Describe to the patient what is happening and put into words what the patient might be experiencing. *Naming objects and describing actions, thoughts, and feelings help the patient to use symbolic language.*
4. Encourage vocalizations with sound games and songs. *Children learn through play and enjoyable activities.*
5. Identify desired behaviors and reward them with hugs (if tolerated or accepted), treats, tokens, points, or food. *Behaviors that are rewarded will increase in frequency. The desire for food is a powerful incentive in modifying behavior.*
6. Use names frequently, and encourage the use of correct pronouns (e.g., I, me, he). *Problems with self-identification and pronoun reversal are common.*
7. Encourage verbal communication with peers during play activities using role modeling, feedback, and reinforcement. *Play is the normal medium for learning in a child's development.*
8. Increase verbal interaction with parents and siblings by teaching them how to facilitate language development. *Education and emotional support help parents and siblings become more therapeutic in their interactions with the patient.*

Risk for Injury
Related to
- Neurological dysfunction
- History of self-directed violence (e.g., head banging, biting, scratching, hair pulling when frustrated or angry)
- Reduction of tension by self-mutilation
- Unable to express self verbally
- Lack of impulse control
- Self-injurious behavior in response to change

Desired Outcome The patient will be free of self-inflicted injury.

Assessment/Interventions *Rationales*
1. Monitor the patient's behavior for signs of increasing anxiety. *Behavioral cues signal increasing anxiety and the potential for injury.*
2. Determine emotional and situational triggers. *Knowledge of triggers is used in planning ways to prevent or manage outbursts.*
3. Intervene early with verbal comments or limits or removal from the situation. *Potential outbursts can be defused through early recognition, verbal interventions, or removal.*
4. Give plenty of notice when having to change routines or rituals or end pleasurable activities. *These children often have catastrophic reactions to change and need time to adjust.*
5. Provide support for the recognition of feelings, reality testing, and impulse control. *These competencies are often underdeveloped in this population.*
6. Help the patient connect feelings and anxiety to self-injurious behaviors. *Self-control is enhanced through understanding the relationship between feelings and behaviors.*
7. Help the patient develop ways to express feelings and reduce anxiety verbally and through play activities. Use various types of motor and imaginative play (e.g., swinging, tumbling, role-playing, drawing, and singing). *Methods for regulating the expression of emotions and anxiety are necessary in order to control destructive impulses.*

Disturbed Personal Identity
Related to
- Neurological dysfunction
- Failure to develop attachment behaviors
- Biochemical imbalance
- Interrupted or incomplete separation and individuation process

Desired Outcome The patient will demonstrate an increase in self-awareness and other awareness.

Assessment/Interventions and *Rationales*

1. Use one-to-one interaction to engage the patient in a safe relationship with the nurse or caregiver. *Interpersonal consistency provides for the development of trust needed for a sense of safety and security.*

2. Use names and descriptions of others to reinforce their separateness. *Consistent reinforcement will help connect the patient to others.*

3. Draw the patient's attention to the activities of others and events that are happening in the environment. *Interrupts the patient's self-absorption and stimulates outside interests.*

4. Limit self-stimulating and ritualistic behaviors by providing alternative play activities or by providing comfort when stressed. *Redirecting the patient's attention to favorite or new activities increases interaction and personal identity.*

5. Foster self-concept development. Reinforce identity and body boundaries through drawing, stories, and play activities. *Learning body parts helps to establish self-identity and a differentiation from others.*

6. Help the patient distinguish body sensations and how to meet bodily needs by picking up on cues and using ADLs to teach self-care. *The lack of self-awareness contributes to problems with self-care, especially toileting.*

7. Provide play opportunities for the patient to identify the feelings of others (e.g., stories, puppet play, and peer interactions). *Consistent feedback about the feelings of others helps with self-differentiation and the development of empathy.*

TREATMENT FOR AUTISM SPECTRUM DISORDERS

Biological Treatments

Pharmacotherapy

Medications are used to target specific symptoms. They may be used to improve relatedness and decrease anxiety, compulsive behaviors, or agitation. The second-generation antipsychotics risperidone (Risperdal) and aripiprazole (Abilify) have US Food and Drug Administration approval for treating children with ASD beginning at 5 and 6 years of age, respectively. See Chapter 22 for more information on these drugs.

Stimulant medications may be used to target hyperactivity, impulsivity, or inattention (see Chapter 21). Selective serotonin reuptake inhibitors (SSRIs) are used for people with ASD to improve mood and reduce anxiety (see Chapter 24).

Psychological Therapies

Behavioral intervention strategies focus on social communication skill development, especially when the child would naturally be gaining these skills. In higher functioning individuals, CBT may be helpful in addressing the anxiety associated with ASD. See Chapter 29 for behavioral therapy and CBT. For some children, occupational and speech therapy may be useful.

Applied Behavior Analysis (ABA) encourages positive behaviors and discourages negative behaviors. The Early Intensive Behavioral Intervention (EIBI) is a long-term, intensive approach that improves language and cognitive skills. The Early Start Denver Model (ESDM) is also evidence based in the treatment of individuals with ASD.

 ## Nurse, Patient, and Family Resources

American Academy of Child and Adolescent Psychiatry
www.aacap.org

American Psychiatric Nurses Association (search child)
www.apna.org

Asperger/Autism Network
www.aane.org

Autism Resources
www.autism-resources.com

Autism Society
www.autism-society.org

Children and Adults With Attention-Deficit/Hyperactivity Disorder
www.chadd.org

CHAPTER 5

Schizophrenia Spectrum Disorders

Schizophrenia spectrum disorders are disorders that share features with schizophrenia. These disorders are characterized by psychosis, which refers to disorganized thinking, delusions (false thoughts), and hallucinations (false sensory input).

DELUSIONAL DISORDER

Delusional disorder is characterized by delusions that have lasted 1 month or longer. The delusions tend to be grandiose, persecutory, somatic, and referential (these terms are defined in later paragraphs). The delusions in delusional disorder are not usually severe enough to impair functioning.

BRIEF PSYCHOTIC DISORDER

Brief psychotic disorder involves the sudden onset of at least one of the following: delusions, hallucinations, disorganized speech, and disorganized or catatonic (severely decreased motor activity) behavior. The symptoms must last longer than 1 day but no longer than 1 month, with the expectation of a return to normal functioning.

SCHIZOPHRENIFORM DISORDER

The essential features of schizophreniform disorder are exactly like those of schizophrenia, except that the symptoms last less than 6 months. Also, impaired social or occupational functioning may not be apparent. Some individuals return to their previous level of functioning, whereas others develop a persistent or recurrent psychosis.

SCHIZOAFFECTIVE DISORDER

Schizoaffective disorder involves a major depressive, manic, or mixed episode concurrent with symptoms that meet the criteria for schizophrenia. The symptoms are not be caused by any substance use or a general medical condition.

SUBSTANCE-INDUCED PSYCHOTIC DISORDER AND PSYCHOTIC DISORDER RELATED TO ANOTHER MEDICAL CONDITION

Illicit drugs, alcohol, medications, or toxins can induce delusions or hallucinations. Delusions or hallucinations can also be caused by a general medical condition such as delirium, neurological problems, and hepatic or renal diseases. Substance use and medical conditions are ruled out prior to making a primary diagnosis of schizophrenia or other psychotic disorder.

SCHIZOPHRENIA

Schizophrenia is a potentially devastating brain disorder. It is often considered the cancer of mental illness. Schizophrenia affects more than 1% of adults (3.2 million people in the United States) and can be among the most disruptive and disabling of psychiatric disorders. Schizophrenia often first appears in people in their teens or early 20s at the beginning of their productive lives. Age of onset is typically 15-25 years of age for males and 25-35 years of age for females.

Schizophrenia may be the result of multiple inherited genetic abnormalities in combination with other factors. Viral infections, birth injuries, environmental stressors, prenatal malnutrition, and trauma have been associated with this disorder. Abnormal neural pruning that alters brain development or function has also been associated with schizophrenia.

Some people with schizophrenia can function well with the aid of medications and social support. Others are more disabled and need a higher level of assistance in terms of housing, health maintenance, financial aid, and daily functioning. A large percentage of people with schizophrenia are homeless. The longer the psychoses remains untreated, the poorer the prognosis. About 95% of affected individuals experience the disorder throughout their lifetime. People who develop paranoid features usually have a later age of onset. Although schizophrenia is a biologically based illness, stressful life events can trigger an exacerbation or relapse of the illness.

Phases of Schizophrenia

Schizophrenia usually progresses through predictable phases, although the presenting symptoms during a given phase and the length of the phase may vary. The phases are as follows:

- **Prodromal:** Before acute symptoms of schizophrenia occur, people may experience mild changes in thinking, reality testing, and mood. Speech and thoughts may be odd, and anxiety, obsessive thoughts, and compulsive behaviors may be present. The person may feel "not right" or that "something strange" is happening. Symptoms typically appear 1 to 12 months before the first full episode of schizophrenia.

- **Acute:** Symptoms vary, from few and mild to many and disabling. Hallucinations, delusions, apathy, social withdrawal, diminished affect, anhedonia, disorganized behavior, and impaired judgment and cognition result in functional impairment. The person can have difficulty coping, and symptoms become apparent to others. This phase can last several months, even with treatment. Increased support and additional treatment or hospitalization may be required.

- **Stabilization:** In this phase, symptoms are stabilizing and diminishing, and there is movement toward a previous level of functioning. This phase can last for months. Care in an outpatient mental health center or a partial hospitalization program may be needed. The person may receive care in a residential crisis center (similar to a mental health unit but based in the community) or a staff-supervised residential group home or apartment.

- **Maintenance or residual:** In this phase, the condition has stabilized and a new baseline may be established. Positive symptoms are usually significantly diminished or absent, but negative and cognitive symptoms continue to be a concern. Ideally, recovery with few or no residual symptoms will occur, and the patient is again able to live independently or with family.

KEY FEATURES OF SCHIZOPHRENIA

Positive Symptoms

Positive symptoms of schizophrenia occur suddenly. The term positive refers to symptoms that are present that should *not* be present. Positive symptoms include hallucinations, delusions, and disorganized thinking.

Hallucinations

Hallucinations occur when a person perceives a sensory experience in the absence of an external source. Auditory hallucinations, or hearing voices, are the most common hallucination in psychosis. The voices may seem like they are coming from inside the person's head or outside. This can make it hard to tell what is real and what is not. The content of the auditory hallucination may be degrading (e.g., calling the person worthless), persecutory (e.g., telling the person the doctor will kill self), or commanding (e.g., instructing the person to kill self or hurt others). Other less common types of hallucinations include visual, olfactory (smelling odors), gustatory (experiencing tastes), and tactile (feeling bodily sensations). Hallucinations and delusions can be frightening to the patient. They also can be frightening to nurses and other health care team members, as well as family and friends.

Delusions

Delusions are false beliefs that are held despite a lack of evidence to support them. There are several types of delusions. The most common delusions include:

- Grandiose delusions center on feeling special, being exceptionally talented, or being extremely important (e.g., "I have a personal relationship with the US President").

- Persecutory delusions result in feeling singled out for harm by others (e.g., "People break into my house when I am not there and read my email").

- Somatic delusions are obsessions with the health and functioning of specific bodily organs (e.g., "My heart has mold growing on it").

- Referential delusions are a belief that events going on in the environment or with other people are personally directed (e.g., "The newscaster commented about sunshine because she knows about my golf plans").

Disorganized Thinking

Disorganized thinking is manifested in disorganized speech. Poverty of thought, poor problem solving, poor decision making, and illogical thinking most profoundly affect the individual's ability to engage in normal social and occupational experiences. One unusual speech pattern, associative looseness or looseness of association, results from haphazard and illogical thinking where concentration is poor and thoughts are only loosely connected.

Negative Symptoms

Positive symptoms are obvious to others and can make treatment seem more urgent than negative symptoms do. However, negative symptoms are quite severe and debilitating. Negative refers to the absence of essential human qualities that should be present but are not. The following negative symptoms are known as the five A's of schizophrenia:
- Affective blunting—facial expression with diminished or absent emotion
- Alogia—lack of verbalization, also known as poverty of speech
- Avolition/apathy—lack of motivation
- Anhedonia/asociality—an inability to experience joy or pleasure; lack of interest in interaction
- Attentional impairment—an inability to maintain the attention necessary to focus on important details

Cognitive Symptoms

Cognitive symptoms are perhaps the most crucial because they interfere with the person's ability to function in all areas of life (e.g., learn, hold a job, have friends). Cognitive symptoms that are altered in schizophrenia include:
- Working memory
- Attention and vigilance
- Verbal learning and memory

- Reasoning and problem solving
- Speed of processing
- Social learning and cognition

Affective Symptoms

Affective symptoms involve an altered experience and expression of emotions. Mood may be unstable, erratic, labile (changing rapidly and easily), or incongruent (not what would be expected for the circumstances). Co-occurring major depressive disorder is a common complication in people with schizophrenia, as are substance use disorders, both of which alter affect.

ASSESSMENT GUIDELINES
POSITIVE SYMPTOMS

1. Assess for command hallucinations (e.g., voices telling the person to harm self or another). If present, ask the following:
   a. Do you plan to follow the command?
   b. Do you believe the voices are real?
2. Assess for delusions. Determine whether the patient has a fragmented, poorly organized, well-organized, systematized, or extensive system of beliefs that are not supported by reality. If so, follow-up is necessary.
   a. Assess whether delusions have to do with someone trying to harm the patient and whether the patient is planning to retaliate against a person or organization.
   b. Assess whether precautions need to be taken.
   c. Assess for suspiciousness about everyone and their actions (paranoia)—for example, whether the patient is:
      i. On guard, hyperalert, vigilant
      ii. Blaming others for consequences of own behavior
      iii. Hostile, argumentative, or threatening in verbalization or behavior.

NEGATIVE SYMPTOMS

Assess for negative symptoms of schizophrenia (that is, affective blunting, alogia, avolition/apathy, anhedonia/asociality, attentional impairment).

COGNITIVE SYMPTOMS
1. Assess the severity of the cognitive symptoms.
2. Assess how the cognitive symptoms interfere with the patient's functioning.

AFFECTIVE SYMPTOMS
1. Assess for the depressive symptoms and the potential for self-harm.
2. Assess for anger and agitation and the potential for harm to others.

Mood is an essential component of any nursing assessment, particularly due to the potential for self-harm with depressive symptoms and the potential for other-directed violence with angry or aggressive symptoms. What makes the affective symptoms particularly problematic with schizophrenia is their combination with altered judgment and the possibility of persecutory delusions.

Nursing Diagnoses

Communicating with people with schizophrenia can be a challenge, especially in the acute phase. The diagnosis *impaired verbal communication* addresses this challenge. Another related nursing diagnosis pertaining to interacting and social skills is addressed with *impaired socialization*. Hearing voices that seem to originate either inside or outside of the person is addressed with the diagnosis of *hallucinations*. Because of delusions and disorganized thinking, *distorted thinking* is a focus. Due to uncomfortable and often intolerable side effects, coupled with the belief that medication is unnecessary, the diagnosis *nonadherence to medication regime* provides direction for useful interventions. Finally, *impaired family process* addresses the exhaustive needs of families dealing with symptoms of schizophrenia.

Nursing Care for Schizophrenia

Impaired Verbal Communication
Related to
- Biochemical alterations in the brain
- Negative symptoms (i.e., alogia, attentional impairment)
- Positive symptoms (i.e., delusions, hallucination, disorganized thought)

- Medication side effects (i.e., alogia, incoherence, extrapyramidal side effects)

Desired Outcomes The patient will demonstrate improved communication.

Assessment/Interventions and *Rationales*

1. Assess whether incoherence in speech is chronic or is the result of a current acute episode with an exacerbation of symptoms. *Establishing a baseline facilitates the development of realistic goals, the cornerstone for planning effective care.*
2. Determine if and how long the patient has been on antipsychotic medication. *Therapeutic levels of an antipsychotic medication can help clear thinking and improve communication.*
3. Plan short, frequent meeting periods with the patient throughout the day. *Short periods are less stressful, and periodic meetings give the patient a chance to develop familiarity and safety.*
4. Use simple words and keep directions simple. *The patient might have difficulty processing and responding to even simple sentences.*
5. Keep your voice low and speak slowly. *A high-pitched or loud tone of voice can raise anxiety levels. Slow speaking improves understanding.*
6. When you do not understand a patient, ask for clarification (e.g., "I want to understand what you are saying, but I am having difficulty"). *Pretending to understand when you do not may limit your credibility, decrease the potential for trust, and result in missing important information.*
7. Use therapeutic techniques to try to understand the patient's concerns (e.g., "Are you saying…?" "You mentioned demons. Are you feeling frightened?"). *Even if the words are hard to understand, try getting to the feelings behind them.*
8. Focus on and direct the patient's attention to concrete aspects of the environment. *Helps draw focus away from delusions and focus on an objective reality.*
9. Keep the environment quiet and as free of stimuli as possible. *Helps to prevent anxiety from escalating and may reduce confusion, hallucinations, and delusions.*
10. Use simple, concrete, and literal explanations. *Minimizes the patient misunderstanding and incorporating those misunderstandings into delusional systems.*

11. Encourage methods to lower anxiety and minimize voices and "worrying" thoughts. Take time out, read out loud, seek out another supportive person, listen to music, replace irrational thoughts with rational statements, replace negative thoughts with constructive thoughts, and practice deep breathing. *Help the patient use tactics to lowers anxiety, which can enhance functional speech.*

Impaired Socialization
Related to
- Negative symptoms (i.e., alogia, avolition/apathy, anhedonia/asociality, attentional impairment)
- Positive symptoms (i.e., hallucinations, delusions, disorganized thought)
- Negative self-concept
- Inappropriate or inadequate emotional responses
- Feeling threatened in social situations

Desired Outcomes The patient will demonstrate improved socialization.

Assessment/Interventions and *Rationales*
1. Structure times each day to include brief interactions and activities with the patient on a one-on-one basis. *Helps to develop a sense of connection to another and eventual connection with peers.*
2. Communicate the expectation that the patient stays in shared areas rather than the patient's room during most of the day. *Patients often find it easiest to isolate in their rooms, thereby eliminating the potential for interaction with others.*
3. Encourage attendance at group meetings, educational groups, and therapies. You may even suggest, "How about I walk with you to the next meeting?" *Even if the patient does not participate in group activities, simply being with others is a good first step toward socialization.*
4. Review the patient's evaluation of the group experience and the patient's participation in the group. *Reviewing the patient's perception of the group allows for debriefing, support for concerns, and positive reinforcement for participation.*
5. Administer antipsychotic medication as ordered. *Antipsychotic medication helps to reduce psychotic symptoms, thereby supporting interaction with others.*

6. Engage other patients and significant others in social interaction and activities with the patient (e.g., card games, ping-pong, singing, group outings) at the patient's level. *External support helps the patient to feel safe and competent in a graduated hierarchy of interactions.*
7. Provide social skills training to learn adaptive skills such as using good eye contact, appropriate personal space, and a moderate voice tone. *Social skills training helps the patient adapt and function at a higher level in society and increases the patient's quality of life. These simple skills might take time for a patient with schizophrenia but can increase both self-confidence and positive responses from others.*
8. Recognize and acknowledge positive steps the patient takes in increasing social skills and appropriate interactions with others. *Recognition and acknowledgment go a long way toward sustaining and increasing a specific behavior.*

Hallucinations

A change in the amount or patterning of incoming stimuli accompanied by a diminished, exaggerated, distorted, or impaired response to such stimuli.

Related to
- Biochemical alterations in the brain
- Positive symptom of schizophrenia
- Environmental stressors

Desired Outcome
The patient will report a cessation of auditory hallucinations.
or
The patient will manage auditory hallucinations effectively.

Assessment/Interventions and *Rationales*
1. If auditory hallucinations are suspected, ask the patient directly about hearing something that you cannot hear. *Because hearing voices is a subjective experience and not measurable, directly asking about hallucinations is necessary.*
2. Assess the nature of the hallucinations: Is the content of the hallucination affirmative (e.g., providing reassurance or praise) or destructive (e.g., degrading, insulting, or angry)? *Gaining an understanding of the patient's internal world will help to address the resulting emotions.*

3. Assess whether the voices are commanding the patient to engage in self-harm or to harm others. *Understanding the impact of hallucinations on the patient's feeling of safety or the safety of others is essential in planning precautions.*
4. Let the patient know that although the voices seem real, that you cannot hear them. *Instilling reasonable doubt as to the reality of the voices is supportive when carefully presented.*
5. Explore methods of distraction to reduce the voices. Methods include singing, listening to music, reading, or a hobby such as gardening. *Distraction is an important part of managing auditory hallucinations.*
6. Teach thought-stopping techniques such as simply using the word "Stop!" until the voice(s) subsides. *Self-help methods such as thought-stopping can give the patient a sense of control. Using the word "stop" can be a distraction from the hallucination.*
7. Help the patient identify the times that the hallucinations are most prevalent and frightening. Keeping a diary of the voices and exploring the impact of stressors on their frequency may help some patients. *Anxiety has been implicated in provoking auditory hallucinations. Identifying triggers provides points of intervention.*
8. Decrease environmental stimuli when possible. *Reduces the potential for anxiety that might trigger hallucinations.*
9. Encourage the patient to test reality by validating hallucinations with trusted others. *Validation provides reassurance and grounding.*
10. Discuss medication management. Identify potential adherence issues and encourage the patient to take on the role of self-advocate in this treatment. *Medication adherence is an essential part of reducing auditory hallucinations. Ownership of the illness, its symptoms, and its treatment is essential for recovery.*
11. Educate family and significant others about ways to deal with a patient who is experiencing hallucinations. *Educating others in the patient's environment provides an additional level of safety and security for the patient.*

Distorted Thinking

A disruption in mental activities in which a person experiences disturbances in thinking, reality orientation, problem solving, and judgment.

Related to
- Neurological dysfunction
- Positive symptoms of schizophrenia
- Environmental stressors

Desired Outcome The patient will demonstrate improved thinking, as evidenced by an accurate interpretation of the environment, an intact reality orientation, and communicating clearly with others.

Assessment/Interventions and *Rationales*
1. Initiate safety measures to protect the patient and others if the patient feels threatened by others. *During the acute phase of psychosis, delusional thinking might put others at risk. External controls may be needed.*
2. Attempt to understand the significance of false beliefs to the patient. *Important clues to underlying fears and issues can be found in the patient's seemingly illogical delusions.*
3. Be aware that delusions represent the way that the patient experiences reality. *Identifying the patient's experience allows the nurse to understand the patient's feelings.*
4. Identify feelings related to delusions. *When patients feel understood, anxiety might lessen.*
5. Do not argue with the patient's beliefs or try to correct false beliefs using facts. *Arguing will reinforce false beliefs. This will result in the patient feeling even more isolated and misunderstood.*
6. Do not touch the patient unless necessary for care activities (e.g., blood pressure). *A person with psychosis might misinterpret touch as threatening. Patients with altered thought need increased personal space.*
7. Use distraction to minimize the focus on delusional thoughts. For example, attempt to engage the patient in cards, simple board games, and arts and crafts projects. *When thinking is focused on reality-based activities, the patient is free from delusional thinking during that time. This helps focus attention externally.*
8. Encourage healthy habits to optimize functioning, such as maintaining a regular sleep pattern, abstaining from alcohol and drug use, maintaining self-care, and adhering to the medication regimen. *Psychotic illness interferes with sleep, results in self-medication, reduces the completion of activities of daily living (ADLs), and reduces medication adherence.*

9. Teach the patient coping skills that minimize troubling thoughts, including talking to a trusted person, phoning a helpline, going to a gym, and using thought-stopping techniques. *Self-care strategies promote recovery.*

Nonadherence to Medication Regime
Lack of follow-through with an agreed-upon medication regimen

Related to
- Neurological dysfunction
- Side effects of medication
- Inability to acquire medication (e.g., transportation, lack of access)
- Financial limitations
- Disagreement with medication regimen

Desired Outcome   The patient will demonstrate adherence to medication regime.

Assessment/Interventions and *Rationales*
1. Evaluate the medication response and side effects. *Identify drugs and dosages that have increased therapeutic value and decreased side effects.*
2. Convey empathy and support while providing education about how to manage side effects so that they are less disruptive. *Reduces distress and resulting resistance caused by side effects, increasing the patient's sense of control.*
3. Explore the benefits of medications in meeting goals (e.g., eliminate or decrease hallucinations). *Seeing that medication helps the patient to achieve goals will increase the motivation for treatment.*
4. Include the patient as a partner in planning for the medication regime. *The most important person in the treatment plan is the patient. If medication choices, doses, and dosing are unacceptable, there is a strong possibility for nonadherence.*
5. Discuss the possibility of long-acting injectables to eliminate the need for remembering to take medication or to remember if they have already taken it. *Patients may unintentionally not adhere to the medication regimen because they forget to take medications or forget whether they have already taken them.*

6. Explore using technology such as electronic reminders and monitoring systems linked to electronic medication dispensers to enhance adherence. *Technology may support individuals who are unintentionally nonadherent in remembering to take medication.*

7. Discuss your recommendations regarding potential medication changes with the patient's prescriber to promote adherence and improve quality of life. *Patient advocacy and functioning as part of a team are primary nurse roles. Nurses usually have more interaction with patients and are aware of medication benefits and side effects.*

8. Explore social services and community support in securing medication if access and transportation are problems. *Barriers to access to medication can be addressed by social supports to improve adherence.*

Impaired Family Process
Related to
- Neurological dysfunction in a family member
- Deterioration of the health status of a family member
- Situational crisis or transition
- Developmental crisis or transition

Desired Outcome The family will demonstrate an improved family process.

Assessment/Interventions and *Rationales*

1. Assess the family's ability to cope (e.g., experience of loss, caregiver burden, needed supports). *The family's needs must be addressed to stabilize the family unit.*

2. Provide an opportunity for the family to discuss feelings and identify their immediate concerns. *Nurses and staff can best intervene when they understand the family's experience and needs.*

3. Assess the family's current knowledge about schizophrenia and medications used for treatment. *The family might have misconceptions and misinformation about schizophrenia and treatment, or little knowledge at all.*

4. Provide information regarding schizophrenia and treatment strategies at the family's level of knowledge. *Gear teaching strategies based on the family's level of understanding and readiness to learn.*

5. Provide teaching in understandable terms verbally and in written form. Topics include: the purpose of medication therapy, the dose, the importance of a schedule and adherence, managing side effects, and monitoring for potential

serious side effects. *Understanding the disorder and its treatment encourages greater family support and patient adherence.*
6. Provide information on patient and family community resources after discharge, such as support groups, organizations, day treatment programs, educational programs, and respite centers. *Schizophrenia is an overwhelming disorder for both the patient and family. Patient and family community resources can help.*
7. Teach the patient and family the warning symptoms of relapse including insomnia, social withdrawal, difficulty concentrating, loss of interests, increasing paranoia, and hallucinations. *Recognizing relapse symptoms and getting help early can help prevent a more severe episode.*

TREATMENT FOR SCHIZOPHRENIA SPECTRUM DISORDERS

Biological Treatments

Pharmacotherapy

Antipsychotic medications are used to treat psychotic disorders such as schizophrenia. The first of these medications became available in the 1950s. Until the late 1960s, patients with schizophrenia usually spent months or years in state or private hospitals, resulting in great emotional and financial costs to patients, families, and society. A combination of antipsychotic medications along with psychosocial support provide symptom control and allow most people with these disorders to live and be treated in the community. See Chapter 22 for information about antipsychotic medications.

Psychological Therapies

Advanced practice mental health professionals are qualified to provide individual and group psychotherapy (e.g., cognitive–behavioral therapy [CBT]). Cognitive symptoms can be addressed with cognitive remediation or enhancement therapy. These therapies enhance recall, attention, and other skills to reduce cognitive impairment, thereby improving functioning and quality of life.

Family therapy is also important. Families often experience considerable distress related to living with individuals who have acute or residual symptoms of schizophrenia. Direct caregivers and caregivers who are subjected to hostility are in special need of outside support. In family therapy sessions, fears, faulty communication patterns, and distortions are identified. Communication, symptom management, and problem-solving skills are taught, healthier alternatives to conflict are explored, and guilt and anxiety can be lessened. In some cases, therapists may recommend alternate living arrangements such as a group home or assisted living.

The Recovery Model

The recovery model is supported by the National Alliance on Mental Illness (NAMI), the leading mental health consumer support and advocacy organization in the United States. Nurses are encouraged to provide care with the goal of recovery. Patients with schizophrenia or other serious mental illness will benefit by this type of care and also as they adopt the model as a way of life for themselves.

Important aspects of the recovery model include:

- Emphasizes the person and the future rather than the illness and the present
- Involves an active partnership between the individual (also known as the mental health consumer) and care providers
- Focuses on strengths and abilities rather than dysfunction and disability
- Encourages independence and self-determination.
- Focuses on achieving goals of the individual's choosing rather than care providers' choosing
- Emphasizes staff working collaboratively with clients, building on strengths to help consumers achieve the highest possible quality of life
- Aims for increasingly productive and meaningful lives for individuals with serious mental illness (SMI)

 NURSE, PATIENT, AND FAMILY RESOURCES

Brain and Behavior Research Foundation
www.bbrfoundation.org

National Alliance on Mental Illness (NAMI)
www.nami.org

Overcoming Schizophrenia Blog Spot
https://overcomingschizophrenia.blogspot.com/

Schizophrenia and Related Disorders Alliance of America (SARDAA)
https://sardaa.org

Schizophrenia.com
www.schizophrenia.com

Schizophrenic.com
www.schizophrenic.com

SCZ Now – Contemporary Perspectives in Schizophrenia Care
www.scznow.com/

CHAPTER 6

Bipolar Disorders

Bipolar spectrum disorders are among the most serious of the psychiatric disorders. The extreme symptoms may result in the loss of partners, families, friendships, employment, and financial security.

Bipolar disorders consist of diagnoses that are characterized by one or more episodes of mania or hypomania and usually one or more depressive episodes.

- Mania is a period of intense mood disturbance with persistent elevation, expansiveness, irritability, and extreme goal-directed activity or energy. These periods last at least 1 week for most of the day, every day. An acute manic phase usually requires hospitalization to protect and stabilize the patient.
- Hypomania refers to a low-level and less dramatic mania. The hypomania of bipolar II disorder tends to be euphoric and often increases functioning. Psychosis is never present in hypomania, and hospitalization is rarely necessary. Table 6.1 contrasts the differences between mania and hypomania.
- A major depressive episode is a sustained (2 weeks or more) depressed mood and/or a loss of interest or pleasure in everyday activities. Concentration and decision making are usually impaired. People with depression feel empty, hopeless, anxious, worthless, guilty, and/or irritable. The depression in people with a bipolar disorder can be profound and dangerous because of suicidal ideation and the potential for psychotic symptoms.

The lifetime risk, or the percent of the population who experiences bipolar disorder sometime in their lives, is 4.4% for adults and 2.9% for adolescents (Merikangas et al., 2010). Many factors increase the risk for bipolar disorder, including a genetic predisposition. Other

Table 6.1 **Characteristics of Hypomania and Acute Mania**

Hypomania	Acute Mania
Communication	
1. Talks and jokes incessantly, life of the party, gets irritated when not center of attention.	1. Mood is labile—may change suddenly from elation to anger or sadness.
2. Far more outgoing and sociable than usual.	2. Inappropriate demands of people's attention, intrusive.
3. Talk is often sexual and can be obscene; inappropriate propositions to strangers.	3. Speech may contain profanities and crude sexual remarks.
4. Jumps from one topic to the next, pressured speech.	4. Flight of ideas, jumps from topic to topic, complains of racing thoughts.
Affect and Thinking	
1. Full of energy and humor, feelings of euphoria, sociability.	1. Humor gives way to irritability, hostility, and short-lived periods of rage, especially when not getting the patient's way or when limits are set for behaviors. Mood may shift from hostile to calm.
2. Increase in goal-directed activity and planning, may be more creative.	2. Delusional thinking may result in grandiose plans and schemes or paranoid plans for protection.
3. Judgment often poor, but usually not severe enough for hospitalization.	3. Judgment is so poor that hospitalization is often necessary.
4. May write large quantities of mail or make calls to famous people regarding schemes.	4. May attempt to contact famous people. Severe mania may interfere with planning.
5. Decreased attention span to internal and external cues.	5. Decreased attention span and distractibility are intensified.
Physical Behavior	
1. Overactive, distractible, buoyant, occupied with grandiose plans, goes from one activity to the next.	1. Extremely restless and chaotic. May have outbursts such as throwing things. May be dangerous, disoriented, and agitated.

Continued

Table 6.1 **Characteristics of Hypomania and Acute Mania—cont'd**

Hypomania	Acute Mania
2. Hypersexual, desire, sexually irresponsible, indiscreet. Unplanned pregnancies in females with hypomania women. Sexually transmitted disease may be contracted.	2. No time for sex—too busy. Poor concentration. Distractibility and restlessness are severe.
3. May have voracious appetite, eat on the run, or gobble food during brief periods.	3. Too distracted and disorganized to eat.
4. May go without sleeping or feel rested after 3 hours of sleep. However, may be able to take short naps.	4. No time for sleep— Psychomotor activity too high to sleep.
5. Financially extravagant, goes on spending sprees, gives money and gifts away freely, can easily go into debt.	5. Same as in hypomania, but in the extreme.

risk factors include an imbalance in neurotransmitters; neurological dysfunction in regions such as prefrontal cortex, hippocampus, and hypothalamic-pituitary-thyroid-adrenal (HPTA) axis; and environmental stress and adverse experiences.

The bipolar spectrum consists of three main disorders: (1) bipolar I, (2) bipolar II, and (3) cyclothymic disorder. Separate diagnostic categories categorize bipolar disorders that are caused by other factors such as substances, medications, and other medical conditions.

BIPOLAR I

Bipolar I is the most severe bipolar disorder. Individuals with bipolar I disorder have experienced at least one manic episode. Prior to or following the manic episode, individuals may experience a hypomanic or major depressive episode. In order to be diagnosed with bipolar I, the manic episode must last for at least 1 week for most of the day, every day. Some individuals with manic episodes may also experience psychosis, which includes disorganized thinking, false beliefs, and/or hallucinations.

Considerable impairment in social, occupational, and interpersonal functioning exists with bipolar I. Symptoms of mania are so severe that this state may be a psychiatric emergency. Hospitalization is often required to protect the person from the consequences of poor judgment and hyperactivity.

BIPOLAR II

Individuals with bipolar II disorder have experienced at least one hypomanic episode *and* at least one major depressive episode. Psychosis is never present in hypomania but may be a feature of the depressive episode. The hypomanic episode lasts at least 4 days, while the major depressive episode lasts at least 2 weeks.

CYCLOTHYMIC DISORDER

In cyclothymic disorder, symptoms of hypomania alternate with symptoms of mild to moderate depression for at least 2 years in adults and 1 year in children. Hypomanic and depressive symptoms do not meet the criteria for either bipolar II or major depressive disorder, yet the symptoms are disturbing enough to cause social and occupational impairment.

PHASES OF BIPOLAR DISORDER

Bipolar I disorder symptoms are categorized by acute and maintenance phases:
1. The acute phase begins with the onset of a new manic or hypomanic episode. Hospitalization is usually indicated for patients in the acute manic phase of bipolar disorder. Hospitalization protects patients from harm (e.g., exhaustion, financial loss) and allows time for medication stabilization.
2. During the maintenance phase, the most acute symptoms have been controlled. The longer-term maintenance phase begins after the resolution of an acute episode. The goal now is the prevention of future cycles of mania or hypomania.

Many of the interventions discussed in this chapter address the acute phase, because this phase often requires hospitalization along with immediate and complex nursing care. Interventions addressing the major depressive episodes associated with the bipolar disorders are available in Chapter 7.

ASSESSMENT

Signs and Symptoms

- Euphoric mood (i.e., intense feelings of well-being, overly joyous mood)
- Periods of hyperactivity (e.g., pacing, restlessness, accelerated actions)
- Overconfident, exaggerated view of own abilities
- Decreased need for sleep, no acknowledgment of fatigue, increased energy
- Poor social judgment, engages in reckless and self-destructive activities (e.g., risky business ventures, hypersexuality, spending sprees)
- Rapid speech, pressured speech, loud talking, rhyming, punning
- Brief attention span, easily distractible, flight of ideas, loose associations
- Expansive, irritable, paranoid behaviors
- Impatient, uncooperative, abusive, sexually crude, manipulative

ASSESSMENT TOOLS

The Altman Self-Rating Mania Scale (ASRM) is a five-item scale to assess the presence or severity of symptoms of mania over the past 7 days. The individual can complete the scale or, if the patient is too impaired to complete the form, a knowledgeable friend, family member, or clinician can do so. See Table 6.2 for the rating scale.

ASSESSMENT GUIDELINES

MANIC PHASE

1. Assess whether the patient is a danger to self or others
   - Patients with mania can exhaust themselves.
   - The patient might not eat or sleep for days at a time.
   - Poor impulse control might result in harm to self or others.

Table 6.2 **Altman Self-Rating Mania Scale**

Choose the one statement in each group that best describes the way you (the individual receiving care) have been feeling for **the past week**.	
Points	**Score**
	Question 1
1	I do not feel happier or more cheerful than usual.
2	I occasionally feel happier or more cheerful than usual.
3	I often feel happier or more cheerful than usual.
4	I feel happier or more cheerful than usual most of the time.
5	I feel happier or more cheerful than usual all of the time.
	Question 2
1	I do not feel more self-confident than usual.
2	I occasionally feel more self-confident than usual.
3	I often feel more self-confident than usual.
4	I frequently feel more self-confident than usual.
5	I feel extremely self-confident all of the time.
	Question 3
1	I do not need less sleep than usual.
2	I occasionally need less sleep than usual.
3	I often need less sleep than usual.
4	I frequently need less sleep than usual.
5	I can go all day and all night without any sleep and still not feel tired.
	Question 4
1	I do not talk more than usual.
2	I occasionally talk more than usual.
3	I often talk more than usual.
4	I frequently talk more than usual.
5	I talk constantly and cannot be interrupted.
	Question 5
1	I have not been more active (either socially, sexually, at work, home, or school) than usual.
2	I have occasionally been more active than usual.
3	I have often been more active than usual.
4	I have frequently been more active than usual.
5	I am constantly more active or on the go all the time.

Reprinted by permission of Elsevier from Altman, E. G., Hedeker, D., Peterson, J. L., & Davis, J. M. (1997). The Altman Self-Rating Mania Scale. *Biological Psychiatry, 42*, 948–955.

2. Assess for the need for hospitalization to safeguard and stabilize the patient.
3. Assess the patient's medical status. A thorough physical examination helps determine whether mania is primary (i.e., part of bipolar I) or secondary. Mania can be secondary to:
   • A general medical condition
   • A substance such as a drug, medication, or toxin exposure
4. Assess the patient's and family's understanding of bipolar disorder and knowledge of medications, support groups, and organizations that provide information on bipolar disorder.

Nursing Diagnoses

Because of the patient's poor judgment, excessive and constant motor activity, probable dehydration, and difficulty evaluating reality, *risk for injury* is a likely and appropriate diagnosis. Because disinhibition and aggression may occur in mania, *risk for violence* is an essential nursing diagnosis.

Grandiose thinking, extremely poor judgment, and hyperactivity makes *impaired impulse control* useful in guiding care. Disturbed thinking and impaired reality testing make *distorted thinking* an essential part of the plan of care. Patients have limited ability to engage in social activities, making *impaired socialization* an appropriate focus of nursing care. Diminished levels of self-care in hygiene, dressing, feeding, and toileting due to mania are addressed with the nursing diagnosis of *self-care deficit*.

INTERVENTION GUIDELINES

Overall guidelines that are effective for patients during periods of mania include the following:
1. Use a firm and calm approach.
2. Use short, concise explanations or statements.
3. Remain neutral and avoid power struggles.
4. Provide a consistent and structured environment.
5. Firmly redirect energy into appropriate and non-destructive channels.
6. Decrease environmental stimulation whenever possible.

7. Provide structured solitary activities. Tasks that take minimal concentration are best. Avoid groups and stimulating activities until the patient can tolerate that level of activity.
8. Avoid groups and stimulating activities until the patient can tolerate that level of activity.
9. Spend time with the patient if psychosis or anxiety is present. Consider providing staff for one-on-one observation.
10. Provide frequent rest periods.
11. Provide high-calorie fluids and finger foods frequently throughout the day.
12. Monitor the following:
    - Sleep pattern
    - Food intake
    - Elimination (constipation is a common problem)
13. Provide the patient and family with education about the illness, and give the patient and family with written information regarding the illness and medications.
14. Provide the patient and family with information on supportive services in their community for further information and support.

Nursing Care for Mania

The following sections identify primary nursing diagnoses for use with a patient who is experiencing mania, particularly in the acute and severe manic phases of the illness.

Risk for Injury
Related to
- Neurological dysfunction
- Cognitive, affective, and psychomotor factors
- Alteration in cognitive functioning
- Alteration in psychomotor functioning
- Compromised nutrition
- Malnutrition
- Alteration in affective orientation

Desired Outcome   The patient will be free from injury.

Assessment/Interventions and *Rationales*
1. Maintain a low level of stimuli in the patient's environment (e.g., away from loud noises, bright lights, and people). *Helps decrease the escalation of anxiety.*

2. Provide structured solitary activities with a nurse or an aide. *Structure provides security and focus.*
3. Provide frequent high-calorie fluids. *Nutritional status may be compromised due to lack of interest in food and liquids. Regularly offering fluids increases the success of acceptance.*
4. Provide frequent rest periods in a darkened room even if sleep is not possible. *Prevents exhaustion.*
5. Redirect aggressive behavior and encourage exercise. *Physical exercise can decrease tension and provide focus.*
6. Provide prescribed and as-needed medications. *Exhaustion, dehydration, lack of sleep, and increased confusion are the result of constant physical activity. Medication will reduce this activity.*
7. Observe for signs of lithium toxicity (if applicable). *There is a narrow margin of safety between therapeutic and toxic doses.*
8. Hold valuables in the hospital safe or send them home. *Protect the patient from giving away money and possessions.*

Risk for Violence
Related to
- Neurological dysfunction
- Alteration in cognitive functioning
- Impulsiveness
- Excessive energy and agitation
- Delusional thinking

Desired Outcome The patient will refrain from assaultive, combative, or destructive behaviors toward others.

Assessment/Interventions and *Rationales*
1. Use a calm and firm approach. *Provides structure and control for a patient who is out of control.*
2. Use short and concise explanations or statements. *A short attention span limits comprehension to small bits of information.*
3. Maintain a consistent approach, employ consistent expectations, and provide a structured environment. *Clear and consistent limits and expectations minimize the potential for the patient to manipulate the staff.*
4. Remain neutral: avoid power struggles and value judgments. *The patient can use inconsistencies and value judgments as justification for arguing which may result in escalating mania.*

5. Decrease environmental stimuli (e.g., keep away from loud music and noises, people, and bright lights). *A calm environment decreases the escalation of anxiety and manic symptoms.*
6. Assess the patient's behavior frequently (e.g., every 15 minutes) for signs of increased agitation and hyper-activity. *Early detection and intervention of escalating mania might help prevent harm to the patient or others and decrease the need for seclusion.*
7. Redirect agitation with physical outlets in areas of low stimulation (e.g., punching bag, exercise bike). *Relieves agitation and muscle tension.*
8. Alert staff if the potential for restraint or seclusion appears imminent. The usual priority of interventions is (1) setting limits, (2) encouraging time out, (3) offering as-needed medication, and (4) restraint or seclusion. *A team approach to aggression is essential. Always use the least restrictive intervention when intervening a patient with potentially violent behavior.*
9. Document the patient behaviors, interventions, what seemed to escalate agitation, what helped to calm agitation, if and when as-needed medications were given and their effect, and what proved most helpful. *Documentation provides staff with guidelines for future interventions.*

Impaired Impulse Control
Related to
- Neurological dysfunction
- Alteration in cognitive functioning
- Mania

Desired Outcome The patient will demonstrate self-restraint of impulsive behaviors.

Assessment/Interventions *(Rationales)*
1. Administer prescribed and as-needed medications, as ordered, and evaluate for efficacy, side effects, and toxic effects. *Bipolar spectrum disorders are caused by biochemical imbalances in the brain. Medication is effective in stabilizing dysregulated mood.*
2. Observe for destructive behavior toward self or others. Intervene in the early phases of escalation of manic behavior. *Hostile verbal behaviors, poor impulse control, and violent acting out against others or property are seen in acute*

mania. Early detection and intervention can prevent harm to the patient or others in the environment.

3. Send valuables, credit cards, and cash home with family or put in the hospital safe until the patient is discharged. *During manic episodes, individuals may give away valuables and money indiscriminately to strangers, often leaving themselves in debt.*

4. Maintain a firm, calm, and neutral approach at all times. Avoid power struggles and arguing. *Professional behavior by the staff will reduce the chance for conflict and escalation.*

5. Provide hospital legal service when and if a patient is involved in making or signing important legal documents during an acute manic phase. *Judgment and reality testing are both impaired during acute mania. Patients might need legal advice and protection against making important decisions that are not in their best interest.*

6. Assess and recognize early signs of manipulative behavior and intervene appropriately. *Consistently setting limits is important when intervening in manipulative behaviors.*

Distorted Thinking
Related to
- Neurological dysfunction
- Mania
- Disruption in cognitive operations and activities
- Sleep deprivation
- Biochemical alterations

Desired Outcomes The patient will experience reduced distortion in thinking processes.
or
The patient will experience clarity in thinking processes.

Assessment/Interventions and *Rationales*
1. Meet with the patient for short periods each day. *Short, consistent meetings help establish contact and decrease anxiety.*

2. Convey acceptance of the patient's need for a false belief. At the same time, let the patient know that you do not share the belief. *Acceptance will help to develop rapport and support the patient. Expressing reasonable doubt is a good first step in challenging delusions.*

3. Explore the content of hallucinations. *Understanding the content of auditory hallucinations helps to determine whether they are dangerous [e.g., command hallucinations telling the patient to harm someone].*
4. Decrease environmental stimuli if possible. Respond to cues of increased agitation by removing stimuli. A private room may be helpful. *Disturbed thought processes are challenging enough for the patient. Reducing a stressful environment will help to decrease agitation and confusion.*
5. Reinforce reality by talking about actual events and topics such as unit activities. *Engaging the patient into reality and present issues can increase a here-and-now focus.*

Impaired Socialization
Related to
- Neurological dysfunction
- Disturbance in thought processes
- Biochemical disturbances in the brain
- Excessive hyperactivity and agitation
- Mania

Desired Outcome The patient will demonstrate improved socialization.

Assessment/Interventions and *Rationales*

1. When possible, provide an environment with minimal stimuli (e.g., quiet, soft music; dim lighting). *Reduction in stimuli lessens distractibility.*
2. Initially, suggest solitary activities that require a short attention span with mild physical exertion (e.g., writing, painting [finger painting, murals], woodworking, or walks with staff). *Solitary activities minimize stimuli. Mild physical activities release tension constructively.*
3. When mania lessens encourage the patient to join one or two other patients in quiet, nonstimulating activities (e.g., board games, drawing, cards). Avoid competitive games. *As mania subsides, involvement in activities that provide focus and social contact becomes more appropriate. Competitive games can stimulate aggression and increase psychomotor activity.*

Self-Care Deficit
Related to
- Neurological dysfunction
- Alteration in cognitive functioning
- Hyperactivity

Desired Outcome The patient will conduct optimal self-care activities based on personal abilities.

Assessment/Interventions and *Rationales*
Insufficient Nutritional Intake.
1. Monitor intake and output. *Minimizes dehydration and supports interventions for adequate fluid and caloric intake.*
2. Encourage frequent high-calorie protein drinks and finger foods (e.g., sandwiches, fruit, milkshakes). *Constant fluid and calorie replacement are needed. The patient might be too active to sit at meals. Finger foods allow for "eating on the run."*
3. Frequently remind the patient to eat (e.g., "Tom, finish your milkshake." "Sally, eat this banana."). *The patient is unaware of bodily needs, is easily distracted, and requires supervision to eat.*

Sleep Pattern Disturbance.
4. Encourage frequent rest periods during the day. *Lack of sleep can lead to exhaustion and worsen manic symptoms.*
5. Keep the patient in areas of low stimulation. *Promotes relaxation and reduces manic behavior.*
6. At night, encourage warm baths, soothing music, and medication when indicated. Avoid giving the patient caffeine. *Promotes relaxation, rest, and sleep.*

Dressing or Grooming Problems.
7. If necessary, supervise the choice of clothes. Minimize bizarre dress and sexually suggestive clothing. *Lessens the potential for inappropriate attention, which can increase level of mania, or ridicule, which lowers self-esteem. Assists patient in maintaining dignity.*
8. Give simple step-by-step reminders for hygiene and dress (e.g., "Here is your razor. Shave the left side … now the right side." "Here is your toothbrush. Put the

toothpaste on the brush."). *Distractibility and poor concentration are countered by simple, concrete instructions.*

Constipation.
9. Monitor bowel habits. Offer fluids and foods that are high in fiber. Evaluate the need for a laxative. Encourage the patient to go to the bathroom. *Promotes regular toileting. Prevents fecal impaction resulting from dehydration and decreased peristalsis.*

TREATMENT FOR BIPOLAR DISORDERS

Biological Treatments

Pharmacotherapy

Patients with bipolar disorder often resist medication. Many patients want to maintain the higher level of energy, creativity, and confidence. Unfortunately, if left untreated, the high progresses into a more disastrous mania or painful depression. Chapter 23 provides an overview of mood stabilizers along with treatment for bipolar depression.

Brain Stimulation Therapy

Electroconvulsive therapy (ECT) is useful when a patient is unable to wait until a medication starts to become effective, cannot tolerate one of the first-line medications, or does not respond to the first-line medications. ECT is most commonly used with patients who have bipolar disorder with severe depressive episodes. ECT may also be considered for mania, mixed, and depressed states of bipolar disorder, as well as in maintenance treatment.

Transcranial magnetic stimulation (TMS) and repetitive transcranial magnetic stimulation (rTMS) are noninvasive neuromodulation techniques. They work through repeated magnetic pulses targeting hypoactive or hyperactive cortical areas. In 2020 the first TMS device received a Food and Drug Administration (FDA) breakthrough device designation for bipolar depression. This designation specifies its use to adult patients with bipolar I or II disorders with treatment-resistant depression. See Chapter 30 for more information about brain stimulation therapies.

Psychological Therapies

Many patients with bipolar disorder have strained interpersonal relationships, marriage and family problems, academic and occupational problems, and legal or other social difficulties. Psychotherapy provided by an advanced practice professional can help them work through these difficulties, decrease some of the psychic distress, and increase self-esteem. Psychotherapy can also help patients improve their functioning between episodes and attempt to decrease the frequency of future episodes.

A number of psychological therapies along with pharmacotherapy can reduce the morbidity and mortality associated with bipolar disorder. Cognitive–behavioral therapy (CBT) is typically used as an adjunct to pharmacotherapy in many psychiatric disorders. Depression and manic-type states impair a person's ability to interact with others. Interpersonal and social rhythm therapy can be helpful for this. Family-focused therapy helps improve communication among family members. See Chapter 29 for descriptions of these psychological treatments.

 ## Nurse, Patient, and Family Resources

Bipolar Disorder Guide
www.bipolar.about.com

Bipolar Disorder Page
www.mentalhelp.net (search Bipolar)

Depression and Bipolar Support Alliance
www.dbsalliance.org

National Alliance on Mental Illness (NAMI)
www.nami.org

National Institute of Mental Health
www.nimh.nih.gov

CHAPTER 7

Depressive Disorders

Disappointment and unhappiness are appropriate responses to life events. However, when sadness, grief, or hopelessness is extremely intense and the low mood is prolonged, a depressive disorder may be the cause.

Depressive symptoms often coexist in people with alcohol or substance use. Depressive symptoms are common in people who have other psychiatric disorders such as anxiety disorders, eating disorders, personality disorders, and schizophrenia. Major depressive disorder is highly comorbid in individuals who have been abused (e.g., physically, psychologicallyy, sexually). Depression might also be a critical symptom of another medical disorder or condition such as hepatitis, mononucleosis, multiple sclerosis, dementia, cancer, diabetes, or chronic pain.

The two depressive disorders discussed here are major depressive disorder and persistent depressive disorder (dysthymia) (American Psychiatric Association, 2013).

MAJOR DEPRESSIVE DISORDER

In major depressive disorder, a severely depressed mood, usually recurrent, causes clinically significant distress or impairment in social, occupational, or other important areas of the person's life. The depressed mood can be distinguished from the person's usual functioning and might occur suddenly or gradually.

People with major depressive disorder may have other problems, such as the following:
- Anxious distress: feeling tense, restless, fearful (e.g., something bad might happen, loss of control), worrying, poor concentration
- Psychotic features: delusions or hallucinations

- Catatonia: peculiarities of voluntary movement, motor immobility, purposeless motor activity, echolalia, or echopraxia
- Melancholic features: severe symptoms, loss of feelings of pleasure, exacerbation (i.e., worsening) in the morning, early morning awakening, significant weight loss, excessive feelings of guilt
- Peripartum onset: during pregnancy or within 4 weeks of delivery
- Seasonal pattern: most prominent during certain seasons (e.g., winter or summer). More prevalent in climates with longer periods of darkness in a 24-hour cycle

Epidemiology

Major depressive disorder is a leading cause of disability worldwide (World Health Organization [WHO], 2019). In the United States, about 17 million adults had at least one major depressive episode in 2017 (Substance Abuse and Mental Health Services Administration [SAMHSA], 2018). This number represents about 7% of all US adults. In 2017 about 3 million adolescents aged 12 to 17 in the United States had at least one major depressive episode (SAMHSA, 2018).

About 1% to 5% of older adults who live in the community have depression. This statistic rises to 11.5% of hospitalized older adults and 13.5% for those requiring home care (National Institute of Mental Health, 2012). A disproportionate number of older adults with depression are likely to die by suicide.

The length of a major depressive episode may be 5 to 6 months (Parikh et al., 2019). About 20% of cases become chronic (i.e., lasting more than 2 years). While depression begins with a single occurrence, most people experience recurrent episodes. People experience a recurrence within the first year about 50% of the time and within a lifetime up to 85% of the time.

The high variability in symptom manifestation, response to treatment, and course of the illness supports the belief that major depressive disorder is the result of a complex interaction of causes. For example, genetic predisposition to depression combined with childhood stress may lead to significant neurochemical changes that result in depression. Risk factors for major depressive disorder are listed in Box 7.1.

> ### Box 7.1 **Primary Risk Factors for Major Depressive Disorder**
>
> - Female
> - Adverse childhood experiences
> - Stressful life events
> - First-degree family members with major depressive disorder
> - Neuroticism (i.e., a negative personality trait characterized by anxiety, fear, moodiness, worry, envy, frustration, jealousy, and loneliness)
> - Psychiatric disorders (e.g., substance use, anxiety, personality disorders)
> - Chronic or disabling physical conditions

PERSISTENT DEPRESSIVE DISORDER (DYSTHYMIA)

Persistent depressive disorder, formerly known as dysthymia (dys = bad + thymia = mood), is diagnosed when low-level depression occurs most of the day, for the majority of days. These depressive feelings last at least 2 years in adults and 1 year in children and adolescents.

While the symptoms are difficult for the patient to live with, they are usually not severe enough to require hospitalization. Because the onset of persistent depressive disorder is usually in the teens, patients will frequently express that they have "always felt this way."

The prevalence of persistent depressive disorder ranges from 1.5% to 3.3% (Vandeleur et al., 2017). Persistent depressive disorder tends to have an early onset and, as the name suggests, it is a chronic illness. It is more common among women.

Assessment
Signs and Symptoms
- Mood of sadness, despair, emptiness
- Diminished interest or pleasure in almost all activities (anhedonia)
- Vegetative signs: over eating, over sleeping, low activity level (fatigue), and decreased libido
- Agitated symptoms: loss of appetite, difficulty sleeping, anger, irritability, rumination (i.e., overthinking things), pacing

- Feelings of worthlessness or guilt
- Difficulty with concentration, memory, and making decisions
- Recurrent thoughts of death or self-harm
- Apathy, low motivation, and social withdrawal
- Excessive emotional sensitivity
- Possible complaints of pain, such as backache or headache, that do not seem to have a physical cause

Assessment Tools

Numerous standardized depression screening tools that help assess the type and severity of depression are available. Common screening tools are the Beck Depression Inventory, the Hamilton Depression Scale, and the Geriatric Depression Scale. The Patient Health Questionnaire-9 (PHQ-9) is a short inventory that highlights predominant symptoms seen in depression. It is presented here due to of its ease of use and popularity (Fig. 7.1) in primary care and community settings. Administering these tools at baseline and then again periodically allows clinicians to follow changes in the patient's symptoms and depression severity over time.

Assessment Guidelines

A. A thorough physical and neurological examination helps determine whether the depression is primary or secondary to another disorder. Depression is a mood that can be secondary to many medical or other psychiatric disorders, as well as drugs or medications. Essentially, the nurse evaluates whether the following are evident:
  1. The patient is experiencing a psychosis.
  2. The patient has ingested drugs or alcohol.
  3. Physical conditions are present.
  4. Always evaluate the patient's risk for harm to self or others. Overt hostility is highly correlated with suicide.

Nursing Diagnoses

Depression can drastically affect many areas of a person's life. Due to the potential for lethal consequences, *risk for suicide* is the first priority for assessment and intervention. Poor concentration, lack of judgment, and difficulties

Over the last two weeks, how often have you been bothered by any of the following problems?

	Not at all	Several days	More than half the days	Nearly every day
Little interest or pleasure in doing things?	0	1	2	3
Feeling down, depressed, or hopeless?	0	1	2	3
Trouble falling or staying asleep, or sleeping too much?	0	1	2	3
Feeling tired or having little energy?	0	1	2	3
Poor appetite or overeating?	0	1	2	3
Feeling bad about yourself — or that you are a failure or have let yourself or your family down?	0	1	2	3
Trouble concentrating on things, such as reading the newspaper or watching television?	0	1	2	3
Moving or speaking so slowly that other people could have noticed? Or the opposite — being so fidgety or restless that you have been moving around a lot more than usual?	0	1	2	3
Thoughts that you would be better off dead, or of hurting yourself in some way?	0	1	2	3
Total = ____ /27				

Depression severity:
0–4 none, 5–9 mild, 10–14 moderate, 15–19 moderately severe, 20–27 severe.

Fig. 7.1 Patient Health Questionnaire-9 (PHQ-9).

with memory can all affect a person's ability to cope with confused thoughts and profound feelings of despair. Therefore *impaired coping* is almost always present. Feelings of self-worth plummet, resulting in *chronic low self-esteem.* The inability to gain strength from usual spiritual support and religious activities may result in *spiritual distress.*

Feelings of hopelessness are common. Most noticeably, the ability to interact and gain support from others is markedly reduced, making *impaired socialization* a valuable focus. Depression can also lead to physical complications such as changes in sleep, eating patterns, and elimination resulting in a *self-care deficit.*

Intervention Guidelines

A. Convey caring, and empathy by spending time with the patient, even in silence, and anticipating the patient's needs.
B. Recognize that the instillation of hope is a key tool for recovery.
C. Enhance the patient's sense of self by highlighting past accomplishments and strengths.
D. Whether in the hospital or in the community, the following are important:
   1. Assess the patient's needs for self-care, and offer support when appropriate.
   2. Monitor and intervene to maintain adequate nutrition, hydration, and elimination.
   3. Monitor and intervene to maintain adequate balance of rest, sleep, and activity.
   4. Monitor and record increases and decreases in symptoms and which nursing interventions are effective.
   5. Identify and involve the patient's support system, and explore community support.
E. Encourage the patient to replace the negative thinking associated with major depressive disorder with more realistic positive thoughts.
F. Continually assess for suicidal thoughts and ideation.
G. Provide verbal and written education about the specific medications the patient is taking.
H. Assess the needs of the family and significant others for teaching, counseling, support groups, and community resources.

Nursing Care Plans for Major Depressive Disorder

Risk for Suicide

Related to
- Neurological dysfunction
- Physical health problems
- Hopelessness
- Helplessness
- Loss
- Suicidal ideation
- Suicide plan
- Lack of personal resources (e.g., coping skills, insight, judgment)
- Lack of social resources (e.g., socially isolated, unresponsive family)
- Conflictual interpersonal relationships

Desired Outcome. The patient will be free from self-harm.

Assessment/Interventions and *Rationales*

1. Continuously monitor patients with active suicidal thoughts *Place patients with active suicidal thoughts, particularly with a plan, on 1:1 observation.*
2. Determine the level of suicide precautions needed. If high, does the patient need hospitalization? If low, will the patient be safe to go home with supervision from a friend or family member? *A high-risk patient will need constant supervision and a safe environment.*
3. Depending on the medication, determine whether the patient has more than 1 week's supply of medication. *Most commonly prescribed antidepressants, such as the selective serotonin reuptake inhibitors [SSRIs], are rarely fatal in overdose. Other medications, such as the tricyclics, are more dangerous. Limiting supplies of more lethal medications is essential.*
4. Encourage expression of feelings such as anger and disappointment, and explore alternative ways to handle anger and frustration. *The patient can learn alternative coping methods for dealing with overwhelming emotions and gain a sense of control.*

5. Develop a safety plan for dealing with feelings of intense hopelessness and despair. *Reinforces actions the patient can take when having suicidal thoughts.*
6. Contact the patient's family and arrange for crisis counseling. Activate links to self-help groups. *Patients need a network of resources to decrease feelings of worthlessness, isolation, and helplessness.*

Impaired Coping
Related to
- Neurological dysfunction
- Inability to deal with stressors
- Inadequate resources
- Overwhelming life circumstances
- Prolonged grief reaction
- Extreme fatigue, lack of motivation
- Inadequate social support

Desired Outcome The patient will demonstrate improved coping.

Assessment/Interventions and *Rationales*
1. Identify the patient's previous level of cognitive functioning from the patient, family, friends, and medical records. *Establishing a baseline of ability allows for evaluation of the patient's progress.*
2. Encourage postponing important major life decisions. *Major life decisions require optimal functioning.*
3. Minimize the patient's responsibilities during episodes of severe depression. *This will decrease feelings of pressure and anxiety and minimize feelings of guilt.*
4. Use simple, concrete words. *Slowed thinking and difficulty concentrating may impair comprehension.*
5. Allow the patient plenty of time to think and respond. *Slowed thinking requires time to formulate a response.*
6. Help the patient and significant others to reestablish routines during a major depressive episode. *A routine that is fairly repetitive and nondemanding is easier to both follow and remember.*
7. Allow more time than usual for the patient to finish activities of daily living, such as dressing and eating. *The usual tasks might take a long time. Rushing the patient increases anxiety and slows the patient's ability to think clearly.*

8. Teach the patient to recognize negative thoughts and to challenge and replace them with more realistic appraisals. *Negative thinking is part of the cycle of depression and these thoughts often do not reflect true circumstances. Intervening in this process aids in a healthier and more useful outlook.*

Chronic Low Self-Esteem
Related to
- Neurological dysfunction
- Past failures
- Negative reinforcement from others
- Lack of social support
- Lack of family support
- Negative self-appraisal
- Unrealistic expectations of self

Desired Outcome The patient will report and demonstrate an improved self-esteem.

Assessment/Interventions and *Rationales*
1. Work with the patient to identify cognitive distortions that encourage negative self-appraisal. These distortions include overgeneralization, self-blame, mind reading, and discounting positive attributes. *Cognitive distortions reinforce a negative, inaccurate perception of the self and the world by taking one fact or event and making a general rule of it ["He always," "I never"], assuming others "do not like me," without evidence that assumptions are correct, or focusing on negative qualities.*
2. Teach visualization techniques that help the patient replace negative self-images with more positive thoughts and images. *Promotes a healthier and more realistic self-image by helping the patient choose more positive actions and thoughts.*
3. Work with the patient on areas to improve using problem-solving skills. Evaluate the need for more teaching in this area. *Feelings of low self-esteem can interfere with the usual problem-solving abilities.*
4. Evaluate the need for assertiveness training to pursue goals. Arrange for training through resources such as community-based programs, personal counseling, and literature. *People with low self-esteem often feel unworthy and have difficulty asking appropriately for what they need and want.*

5. Encourage participation in a support group or group therapy where others are experiencing similar thoughts, feelings, and situations. *Participation in such a group can decrease feelings of isolation and provide an atmosphere where positive feedback and a more realistic appraisal of self are available.*

Spiritual Distress
Related to
- Isolation
- Death or dying of self or others
- Chronic illness of self or others
- Life changes
- Pain
- Lack of purpose and meaning in life
- Ambivalence regarding prior religious beliefs

Desired Outcome The patient will demonstrate decreased spiritual distress.

Assessment/Interventions and *Rationales*
1. Assess what spiritual practices have provided comfort and meaning to the patient's life prior to the depressive episode. *This assessment will evaluate neglected areas in patient's life that, if reactivated, might add comfort and meaning during a painful depression.*
2. Discuss what has given meaning and comfort to the patient in the past. *Patients experiencing depression often struggle for meaning in life and reasons to go on when feeling hopeless and despondent.*
3. Encourage the patient to keep a written or electronic journal on a daily basis to express thoughts, reflections, and feelings. *Journaling can help the patient to identify patterns and emotional triggers while tracking improvement from depressive symptoms.*
4. If the patient is unable or unwilling to journal, encourage audio recording and playing back. *Speaking aloud often helps the patient clarify thinking and explore issues.*
5. Provide information on referrals (if interested and receptive) for religious or spiritual information (e.g., printed material, online sources, community resources). *Recommendations from a healthcare professional narrow down important resources in an often-overwhelming environment of information.*

6. Determine whether the patient is interested in a visit from the hospital chaplain or receiving pastoral care. *Spiritual advisors in an institution or community [i.e., priests, clergy, rabbis, the spiritual advisors congruent with the individual's lifestyle] are familiar with spiritual distress and may provide comfort to the patient.*

Impaired Socialization
Related to
- Neurological dysfunction
- Negative view of self
- Absence of significant others or peers
- Disturbed thought processes
- Feelings of worthlessness
- Self-concept disturbance
- Fear of rejection
- Anergia (lack of energy) and avolition (lack of motivation)

Desired Outcome The patient will report and demonstrate improved socialization.

Assessment/Interventions and *Rationales*
1. During severe depression, involve the patient in a one-to-one activity. *One-to-one activities can maximize the potential for interactions while minimizing anxiety.*
2. Engage the patient in gross-motor activities that call for limited concentration (e.g., walking). *Physical activities can help relieve tension and provide stimulation.*
3. Initially, provide activities that require little concentration (e.g., playing simple card games, looking through a magazine, or drawing). *Concentration and memory are poor in people with major depressive disorder. Activities that have no "right or wrong" or "winners or losers" minimize opportunities for negative self-evaluation.*
4. Increase the patient's contacts with others gradually (e.g., first one other, then two others). *Contact with others distracts the patient from self-preoccupation.*
5. Encourage attendance in group activities (e.g., meals, art therapy, group therapy). *Socialization decreases feelings of isolation. Genuine regard for others can increase self-worth.*
6. Refer both the patient and family to support groups and educational groups within the community. *Both the patient and family can gain tremendous support and insight from people through sharing their experiences and learning more about the disorder.*

Self-Care Deficit
Related to
- Neurological dysfunction
- Perceptual or cognitive impairment
- Decreased or lack of energy (anergia)
- Lack of motivation (avolition)
- Fatigue
- Severe preoccupation
- Severe anxiety

Desired Outcome The patient will demonstrate improved self-care.

Assessment/Interventions and *Rationales*
Insufficient Nutritional Intake
1. Encourage small, high-calorie, high-protein snacks and fluids frequently throughout the day and evening if weight loss is a concern. *Minimizes weight loss, dehydration, and constipation.*
2. Encourage eating with others. *Eating with others increases socialization and decreases the focus on food.*
3. Help the patient to select foods or drinks. *Patients may lack motivation to select menu choices. Including the patient in the selection will improve consumption because people are more likely to eat foods they like.*
4. Weigh the patient weekly, and observe the patient's eating patterns. *Weighing provides objective information needed for revising the plan of care.*

Sleep Pattern Disturbance
5. Encourage rest periods after activities. *Fatigue can intensify feelings of depression.*
6. Encourage the patient to get up and dress and to stay out of bed during the day. *Restricting sleep during the day increases the likelihood of sleep at night.*
7. Encourage relaxation measures in the evening (e.g., back massage, warm bath, or warm milk). *Relaxation measures induce relaxation and sleep.*
8. Reduce environmental and physical stimulation in the evening; discourage electronic activities and provide caffeine-free drinks, soft lights, soft music, and quiet activities. *Sleep hygiene measures promote sleep.*
9. Teach relaxation exercises such as progressive muscle relaxation and guided imagery. *Besides deeply relaxing the body, relaxation exercises often lead to sleep.*

Bathing or Hygiene Inattention

10. Encourage the use of a toothbrush, washcloth, soap, makeup, shaving equipment, and other grooming items. *Being clean and well-groomed supports a positive self-esteem and interaction with others.*
11. Give step-by-step reminders, such as "Wash the right side of your face, now the left." *Slowed rate of thinking and difficulty concentrating make organizing simple tasks difficult.*

Constipation

12. Monitor intake and output, especially bowel movements. *People with depression are often constipated. If this condition is not addressed, fecal impaction can occur.*
13. Suggest foods that are high in fiber and encourage exercise. *Fiber intake and regular exercise stimulate peristalsis and support regularity.*
14. Encourage the intake of fluids (6–8 glasses per day). *Hydration results in less water being withdrawn from the colon, making stool easier to pass.*
15. Evaluate the need for laxatives and enemas. *These temporary measures reduce the occurrence of fecal impaction and promote regularity.*

TREATMENT FOR MAJOR DEPRESSIVE DISORDERS

Biological Treatments

Pharmacotherapy

Major depressive disorder is a recurring condition, and most people will go on to have multiple episodes. However, antidepressants result in depression being one of the most treatable disorders. Medication can improve poor self-concept, degree of withdrawal, vegetative signs of depression, and activity level. Refer to Chapter 24 for a discussion of pharmacotherapy used in the treatment of major depressive disorder.

Brain Stimulation Therapy

Prior to 2008, there was only one brain stimulation therapy, electroconvulsive therapy (ECT). ECT has US Food and Drug Administration (FDA) approval for depressive symptoms associated with major depressive disorder or bipolar disorder in patients aged 13 years and older. In 2008 and

2009, respectively, repetitive transcranial magnetic stimulation (rTMS) and vagus nerve stimulation (VNS) were approved for use in patients with treatment-resistant depression. Magnet seizure therapy (MST) is also being used off-label. Chapter 30 provides more information regarding brain stimulation therapies.

Integrative Therapies

Light therapy is the first-line treatment for the seasonal variety of depression known as seasonal affective disorder (SAD) with or without medication. Full-spectrum wavelength light is the specific type of light used. People with SAD often live in climates with marked seasonal differences in the amount of daylight. Seasonal variations in mood disorders in the Southern Hemisphere are the reverse of those in the Northern Hemisphere. Light therapy also may be useful as an adjunct to medications in treating chronic major depressive disorder or dysthymia with seasonal exacerbations.

Non–FDA-approved integrative pharmacological approaches are also used in the treatment of major depressive disorder. Herbal therapies such as St. John's wort and S-adenosylmethionine (SAMe) are commonly used over-the-counter drugs. Refer to Appendix B for integrative therapies used in the treatment of major depressive disorder.

Exercise is a healthy and extremely useful approach to reducing depressive symptoms. It has biological, social, and psychological effects on symptoms of depression.

Psychological Therapies

Cognitive–behavioral therapy (CBT), interpersonal therapy (IPT), time-limited focused psychotherapy, and behavioral therapy are especially effective in the treatment of depression. However, only CBT and IPT demonstrate superiority in the maintenance phase. CBT helps people reconstruct their negative thought patterns and behaviors, leading to lasting mood improvements, whereas IPT focuses on working through personal relationships that may contribute to depression. Group therapy is a widespread modality for the treatment of depression and provides many benefits, particularly in helping individuals to feel "not alone" with their symptoms. See Chapter 29 for more information about psychological models of therapy.

Nurse, Patient, and Family Resources

Depressed Anonymous
www.depressedanon.com

Depression and Bipolar Support Alliance
www.dbsalliance.org

Depression Central
www.psycom.net/depression.central

Internet Mental Health
www.mentalhealth.com

National Alliance on Mental Illness (NAMI)
www.nami.org

National Foundation for Depressive Illness
www.depression.org

National Institute of Mental Health (NIMH): Depression
www.nimh.nih.gov/publicat/depression.cfm

CHAPTER 8

Anxiety and Obsessive–Compulsive Disorders

In this chapter, two groups of psychiatric disorders that are accompanied by a significant level of anxiety are addressed. We begin by defining the concept of anxiety and its manifestation on a continuum of mild to severe. Specific anxiety disorders and specific obsessive–compulsive disorders (OCDs) are then described. The nursing process and suggestions for nursing care are provided.

ANXIETY

Anxiety is a universal human experience and is among the most basic of emotions. Anxiety is a feeling of apprehension, uncertainty, or dread resulting from a real or perceived threat. Normal anxiety is a healthy reaction that is a necessary evolutionary strategy for survival.

LEVELS OF ANXIETY

Peplau (1968) developed a useful model of anxiety that consists of four levels: mild, moderate, severe, and panic. The boundaries between these levels are not distinct, and the behaviors and characteristics of individuals experiencing anxiety may and often do overlap. Identification of a general level of anxiety is helpful in selecting appropriate nursing interventions.

Mild Anxiety

Mild anxiety occurs in the normal experience of everyday living allowing the individual to perceive reality in sharp focus. A person experiencing a mild level of anxiety sees, hears, and grasps more information making problem solving more effective. Physical symptoms of mild anxiety may include slight discomfort, restlessness, or mild tension-relieving behaviors (e.g., nail biting, foot or finger tapping, fidgeting).

Moderate Anxiety

As anxiety increases, the perceptual field narrows, and some details are excluded from attention. The person sees, hears, and grasps less information and may demonstrate selective inattention, where only certain aspects of the environment are observed unless they are pointed out. The ability to think clearly is hampered, but suboptimal learning and problem solving can still take place. Sympathetic nervous system symptoms begin to kick in, resulting in an increased pulse, increased respiratory rates, and perspiration. Mild somatic symptoms such as gastric discomfort, headache, and urinary urgency are also common in moderate anxiety.

Severe Anxiety

A person experiencing severe anxiety experiences a greatly reduced perceptual field. At this level, the focus is on one particular detail or on many scattered details. Other environmental stimuli are disregarded, even when another person points them out. Learning and problem solving are not possible. In this state, behavior is automatic and aimed at reducing or relieving anxiety. Trembling and a pounding heart are common, and the person may hyperventilate and feel a sense of impending doom or dread. Somatic symptoms such as headache, nausea, and dizziness often increase.

Panic Anxiety

Panic is the most extreme level of anxiety and results in markedly dysregulated behavior. Someone in a state of panic is unable to process what is going on in the environment and may lose touch with reality. Behaviors range from pacing, running, or screaming to complete withdrawal. Patients report a sense of impending doom or danger or feelings of unreality or detachment. Physical symptoms include a racing heart, sweating, chills, hot flashes, trembling, shortness of breath, weakness or dizziness, and tingly or numb hands. Other somatic symptoms include headache, nausea, abdominal cramping, and chest pain.

ANXIETY DISORDERS

Anxiety disorders are among the most common of all psychiatric conditions. Individuals with these disorders experience anxiety to such a degree that it interferes with personal, occupational, or social functioning. Anxiety disorders include:

- Separation anxiety disorder
- Specific phobia
- Social anxiety disorder
- Panic disorder
- Agoraphobia
- Generalized anxiety disorder

Separation Anxiety Disorder

Separation anxiety is a normal part of infant development that begins around 8 months of age, peaks at about 18 months, and then begins to decline. People with separation anxiety disorder exhibit developmentally inappropriate levels of concern over being away from a significant other. There may also be fear that something horrible will happen to the other person and that it will result in permanent separation. The anxiety is so intense that it interferes with normal activities and causes sleep disruptions and nightmares. The separation anxiety is often manifested in physical symptoms, such as gastrointestinal disturbances and headaches.

Although this disorder is most often associated with children, This disorder results in harm avoidance, worry, shyness, uncertainty, fatigability, and a lack of self-direction. Fear of separation from a significant other (e.g., parent or spouse) is accompanied by a significant level of discomfort and disability that impairs educational, social, and occupational functioning.

Separation anxiety disorder is typically diagnosed before the age of 18, after about a month of symptoms. Lifetime prevalence rates in children and adults are 4.1% and 6.6%, respectively (Shear et al., 2006). Approximately one-third (about 36%) of childhood cases persist into adulthood, while the majority (78%) of adult cases have onsets in adulthood. It is the most common anxiety disorder in children. Females are more likely to be affected.

Specific Phobia

A specific phobia is a persistent irrational fear of a specific object, activity, or situation. This fear leads to a desire to avoid or actual avoidance of the object, activity, or situation. Phobias compromise a person's daily functioning, since people with phobias are consumed with avoiding the feared object or situation.

We may, in fact, be hardwired for phobias as a protective evolutionary measure. Common, and potentially protective phobias include arachnophobia (fear of spiders and other arachnids), ophidiophobia (fear of snakes), acrophobia (fear of heights), and cynophobia (fear of dogs).

Twelve-month prevalence rate for specific phobias is 5.5%, with higher rates in females (7.7%) than in males (3.3%) (Wardenaar et al, 2017). Phobic reactions tend to run in families. Having a first-degree relative with a specific phobia puts one at greater risk for having the same specific phobia. Negative and traumatic experiences with the feared objects or situations often precede the phobia.

Social Anxiety Disorder

Social anxiety disorder, formerly called social phobia, is characterized by severe anxiety or fear. This response is provoked by social or performance situations that have the potential for negative evaluations by others. Social anxiety triggers include the fear of saying the wrong thing in a public setting, eating or drinking in front of others, or by public speaking. These fears lead to extreme avoidance of these situations. If unable to avoid them, individuals endure the situation with intense anxiety and emotional distress. Fear of public speaking is the most common manifestation of social anxiety disorder.

Young children with this disorder may be mute and nervous and may hide behind their parents. Older children and adolescents may be paralyzed by fear of speaking in class due to worry of saying the wrong thing or being criticized. Conversely, younger people may act out to compensate for this fear, making an accurate diagnosis more difficult. Physical complaints are often used to avoid social situations, particularly school.

The 12-month prevalence of social anxiety disorder is 2.4% (Stein et al., 2017). Females are more likely to be affected. Risk factors for social anxiety disorder include childhood mistreatment and adverse childhood experiences. Since the trait of shyness is strongly heritable, having parents who are shy carries a double risk of genetic transmission and parental modeling.

Panic Disorder

Panic attacks are the key feature of panic disorder. A panic attack is the sudden onset of extreme apprehension or fear, usually associated with feelings of impending doom. During a panic attack, normal functioning is suspended, the perceptual field is severely limited, and misinterpretation of reality may occur. People feel like they are losing their minds or are having a heart attack. Typically, panic attacks come on suddenly, last a matter of minutes, and then subside. A secondary disability occurs when people who experience these attacks begin to "fear the fear" and become so preoccupied with the possibility of future episodes that they avoid what could be pleasurable activities.

Panic disorder also occurs in children and adolescents. During the attack, the young person is less able to articulate feelings such as fear. They may become avoidant of situations where help is not available, may develop feelings of hopelessness in controlling these attacks, and may become depressed. Alcohol or substance use is common among adolescents with this disorder.

The 12-month prevalence for panic disorder is fairly low—about 2% to 3% in adolescents and adults (American Psychiatric Association [APA], 2013). Panic disorder is likely to be genetically transmitted.

Agoraphobia

The term agoraphobia is derived from the Greek agora ("open space") and phobia ("fear"). This term refers to excessive anxiety or fear about being in places or situations from which escape might be difficult or embarrassing or where help might not be available. The feared places or situations are avoided in an effort to control anxiety. People with agoraphobia often have a fear of being alone, traveling (e.g., in a car, bus, or airplane), being on a bridge, and riding in an elevator.

These situations may be more tolerable when accompanied by another person.

Nearly 2% of adolescents and adults experience agoraphobia in a given year (APA, 2013). Some children may experience agoraphobia, but it typically begins in late adolescence or early adulthood. The ratio of females to males with agoraphobia is 2:1.

Generalized Anxiety Disorder

The key pathological feature of generalized anxiety disorder is excessive worry. Children, teens, and adults may experience this worry, which is out of proportion to the true impact of events or situations.

Common concerns in generalized anxiety disorder are inadequacy in interpersonal relationships, job responsibilities, finances, and health of family members. Because of this worry, huge amounts of time are spent in preparing for activities. Putting things off and avoidance are key symptoms, which may result in lateness or absence from school or employment and overall social isolation. Family members and friends are overtaxed as the person seeks constant reassurance and perseverates about meaningless details.

Sleep disturbances are common due to worrying about the day's real or imagined mistakes, reviewing past problems, and anticipating future difficulties. Fatigue is a side effect of this sleep deprivation.

The 12-month prevalence rate of generalized anxiety disorder is nearly 1% in adolescents and nearly 3% in adults (APA, 2013). Over a lifetime, the risk of this disorder is 9%. The ratio of affected females to males is 2:1.

Parental overprotection and adverse experiences are associated with anxiety disorders. Genetics accounts for about a of the risk of developing generalized anxiety disorder.

OBSESSIVE–COMPULSIVE DISORDERS

OCDs are a group of anxiety related disorders that all have obsessive–compulsive characteristics. Obsessions are thoughts, impulses, or images that persist and recur. They cannot be dismissed even though the individual attempts to do so. Obsessions often seem senseless to the individual who experiences them (referred to as egodystonic), and their presence causes severe anxiety.

Compulsions are ritualistic behaviors individuals feel driven to perform as the result of obsessions. They are an attempt to reduce anxiety or prevent an imagined calamity. Performing the compulsive act temporarily reduces anxiety, but because the relief is only temporary, the compulsive act must be repeated again and again.

OCDs include the following:

- Obsessive–compulsive disorder
- Body dysmorphic disorder
- Hoarding disorder
- Trichotillomania (hair-pulling) disorder
- Excoriation (skin-picking) disorder

Obsessive–Compulsive Disorder

Obsessive–compulsive behavior exists along a continuum. Most of us experience mild obsessive–compulsive symptoms, such as nagging doubts as to whether a door is locked or if the stove is turned off. These doubts may compel us to go back to check the door or stove. Mild obsessions with timeliness, orderliness, and reliability are actually valued traits in US society.

At the pathological end of the continuum is OCD, with symptoms that occur on a daily basis and may involve issues of sexuality, violence, contamination, illness, or death. One form of OCD is scrupulosity where individuals are overly concerned that something they thought or did might be a sin or other violation of religious or moral doctrine. Pathological obsessions or compulsions cause marked distressing feelings such as humiliation and shame. Rituals are time-consuming and interfere with normal routines, social activities, and relationships. Severe OCD occupies so much of the individual's mental process that cognition is impaired.

The 12-month prevalence of OCD is 1.2% (APA, 2013). Females are slightly more affected, but males have an earlier age of onset (about 25% before age 10). Onset after age 35 is rare.

Sexual and physical abuse or trauma in childhood increases the risk of this disorder. Some children develop OCD as a postinfectious autoimmune syndrome. Genetics are strongly associated with this disorder. First-degree relatives have twice the risk. Early-onset OCD results in a 10 times greater risk of the disorder appearing in first-degree relatives.

Body Dysmorphic Disorder

Individuals with body dysmorphic disorder are commonly seen in psychiatric, cosmetic surgery, and dermatological settings. Although these individuals tend to have a normal appearance, their preoccupation with an imagined flaw results in obsessional thinking and compulsive behavior such as mirror checking and camouflaging. People may be aware that their thoughts are distorted, or they may be convinced of the existence of the defect.

The prevalence of body dysmorphic disorder is slightly higher in females (2.5%) than in males (2.2%) (APA, 2013). The incidence is higher among individuals seeking cosmetic surgery, dermatology treatment, adult orthodontia, and oral/maxillofacial surgery.

Risk factors for this disorder are backgrounds of abuse and neglect. Body dysmorphic disorder seems to be related to OCD with first-degree relatives often sharing these conditions.

Hoarding Disorder

Hoarding disorder results in the over accumulation of belongings with little or no value. This hoarding interferes with everyday functioning. Belongings may cover every available surface and fill every drawer, cupboard, and closet. Animal hoarding is particularly insidious and may result in disease, starvation, and death of the pets.

Usually family and other guests are reluctant to or will not visit. Hoarding behaviors may progress to the point where the home is nearly uninhabitable due to unsafe and unsanitary conditions. Individuals who hoard may or may not be aware of the problem and how collecting has consumed their lives and alienated others.

Hoarding disorder occurs in an estimated 2% to 6% of the population (APA, 2013). This disorder may be more common in males than in females. Three times as many older adults aged 55 to 94 years are affected by hoarding disorder when compared with adults aged 34 to 44 years old.

Stressful life events seem to precede the onset of symptoms. The disorder is strongly heritable, with a twin concordance rate (i.e., the rate of probability that one twin will be affected when the other one is) of 50%.

Trichotillomania Disorder and Excoriation Disorder

Two of the OCDs are referred to as body-focused repetitive behaviors-trichotillomania (hair–pulling disorder) and excoriation disorder (skin-picking disorder). These disorders are distressing problems that may result in varying degrees of disability, social stigma, and altered appearance. The compulsions are egodystonic, and affected individuals usually try to conceal them.

The phrase "I was so annoyed that I wanted to pull my hair out" attests to the anxiety–related component of trichotillomania (tricho·til·lo·ma·nia). Typically, head hair is pulled, but it may be hair anywhere, including eyebrows, eyelashes, pubic areas, axillae, and limbs. The amount of hair removed ranges from small patches to completely bare skin. For some, the pain brought on by hair pulling reduces their anxiety, as in the case of those who engage in cutting, another form of self-injurious behavior. Individuals may not be aware of the behavior until they notice a nearby wad of hair.

The disorder seems to run in families. People with relatives who have OCD tend to have higher rates of trichotillomania.

The 12-month prevalence of trichotillomania in adolescents and adults is 1% to 2% (APA, 2013). Females are more commonly affected with a ratio of 10:1. Infants who pull their hair out generally grow out of this practice. The usual period of onset is puberty, and commonly results in a chronic, long-term condition. Genetics may play a role in this disorder.

It is often accompanied by OCD and their first-degree relatives.

Skin-picking or excoriation (ex·co·ri·ay·shun) disorder may be used to relieve anxiety, whereas others may pick their skin without thinking about it. Fingers and fingernails are the usual implements, but nail cutters, tweezers, and teeth may also be used. The most common areas of focus are the face, head, cuticles, back, arms and legs, and hands and feet. Complications include pain, sores, scars, and infections.

The lifetime prevalence of this usually chronic problem is 1.4% (APA, 2013). About 75% of those affected are female. The onset is in adolescence and frequently begins with conditions such as acne.

ASSESSMENT

People with anxiety disorders rarely need hospitalization unless they have suicidal thoughts or have behaviors with the potential for injury (e.g., severe avoidance and dangerous hoarding). Most individuals with anxiety and OCD disorders are encountered incidentally in a variety of community settings. A common example is someone being seen in the emergency department to rule out a myocardial infarction when in fact the individual is actually experiencing a panic attack.

Signs and Symptoms

- Narrowed perceptual field, difficulty concentrating, ineffective problem solving
- Increased vital signs (e.g., blood pressure, pulse, respirations), increased muscle tension, activated sweat glands, dilated pupils
- Palpitations, urinary urgency or frequency, nausea, tightening of the throat, unsteady voice
- Complaints of fatigue, difficulty sleeping, irritability, disorganization
- Panic attacks, obsessions, compulsions, phobias, compulsive hoarding, free-floating anxiety interfering with the ability to function at optimal levels
- A sense of impending doom or the feeling of dying

Assessment Tools

Objectively, a variety of scales are available to measure anxiety and anxiety-related symptoms. There are specific measures for phobias, panic symptoms, and obsessive thoughts and behaviors. The Severity Measure for Generalized Anxiety Disorder in Adults is a popular tool for measuring anxiety (Fig. 8.1). High scores may indicate generalized anxiety disorder or panic disorder, although it is important to note that high anxiety scores may also indicate major depressive disorder. Another measure, with identical assessment items, is available for people 11 to 17 years of age.

ASSESSMENT GUIDELINES

It is essential to determine whether anxiety is the primary problem, as in an anxiety disorder, or secondary to another cause, such as physical condition or substance use.

PROMIS Emotional Distress—Anxiety—Short Form

	In the past SEVEN (7) DAYS....	Never	Rarely	Sometimes	Often	Always	Use Item Score
1.	I felt fearful.	☐ 1	☐ 2	☐ 3	☐ 4	☐ 5	
2.	I felt anxious.	☐ 1	☐ 2	☐ 3	☐ 4	☐ 5	
3.	I felt worried.	☐ 1	☐ 2	☐ 3	☐ 4	☐ 5	
4.	I found it hard to focus on anything other than my anxiety.	☐ 1	☐ 2	☐ 3	☐ 4	☐ 5	
5.	I felt nervous.	☐ 1	☐ 2	☐ 3	☐ 4	☐ 5	
6.	I felt uneasy.	☐ 1	☐ 2	☐ 3	☐ 4	☐ 5	
7.	I felt tense.	☐ 1	☐ 2	☐ 3	☐ 4	☐ 5	
						Total Score	

2008-2012 PROMIS Health Organization (PHO) and PROMIS Cooperative Group.
This material can be reproduced without permission by clinicians for use with their patients.
Any other use, including electronic use, requires written permission of the PHO.

Fig. 8.1 Severity Measure for Generalized Anxiety Disorder in Adults.

A. Assess for a history of childhood abuse.
B. Assess for the potential for self-harm. Severe anxiety disorder is associated with suicide as well as overuse of medications or illicit drugs.
C. Assess the patient's community for clinics, groups, and counselors who offer anxiety-reduction techniques.
D. Be aware that differences in culture can affect how anxiety is manifested.

Nursing Diagnoses

Not surprisingly, the nursing diagnosis *anxiety* is most often used to address these disorders. When focusing on this diagnosis, the nurse needs to clarify the level of anxiety, because different levels call for different intervention strategies. *Impaired coping* is another common nursing diagnosis, because high levels of anxiety lead to interference in ability to work, disruptions in relationships, and changes in one's ability to interact satisfactorily with others.

The nursing diagnosis *lack of knowledge of treatment regime* indicates that there is a need for increased knowledge regarding the anxiety disorder, its symptoms, and symptom management. People with anxiety often have difficulty falling asleep, difficulty maintaining sleep, and early-morning awakening. Sleep disruptions can lead to impaired functioning at work, at school, and in social situations. Therefore the problem of *impaired sleep* is essential when caring for this population.

INTERVENTION GUIDELINES

When medications are used in conjunction with therapy, patients and their significant others can benefit from thorough teaching. Give written information and instructions to the patient and family.

A. Use counseling, milieu therapy, promotion of self-care activities, pharmacotherapy, biological, and health teaching interventions.

B. Guide patients through relaxation techniques such as progressive muscle relaxation.

C. Identify community resources that can offer the patient specialized treatment proven to be highly effective for people with a variety of anxiety disorders.

D. Identify community support groups for people with specific anxiety disorders and their families.

Nursing Care for Anxiety and Obsessive–Compulsive Disorders

Anxiety

Related to
- Neurological dysfunction
- External stressors (e.g., economic, job loss, housing problems)
- Internal stressors (e.g., illness, altered self-concept)
- Deficient resources
- Substance use
- Crisis (situational, maturational, adventitious)
- Exposure to phobic object or situation
- Ritualistic behavior
- Fear of panic attack
- Intrusive, unwanted thoughts

Desired Outcome The patient will experience decreased anxiety.

Assessment/Interventions and *Rationales*

1. Promote as calm environment by reducing environmental stimuli. *Stimulating environments increase anxiety.*

2. Provide reassurance that you will help the patient reduce anxiety. *When people feel fearful and vulnerable, a sense of support with someone can reduce anxiety.*

3. Help the patient to reduce anxiety from severe or panic to mild or moderate through slow, deep breathing or medication if prescribed. *Reducing anxiety to mild or moderate is necessary for subsequent learning to take place.*

4. Encourage the patient to talk about feelings and concerns. *When concerns are stated out loud, problems can be discussed, and feelings of isolation decreased.*

5. Reframe the problem in a way that is solvable. Provide a new perspective and correct distorted perceptions. *Correcting distortions increases the possibility of finding workable solutions to a realistically defined problem.*

6. Identify thoughts or feelings before the onset of anxiety: "What were you doing/thinking right before you started to feel anxious?" *Identifies triggers for escalating anxiety and a chance to understand why these triggers are so frightening to the patient.*

7. Teach relaxation techniques (e.g., deep breathing exercises, meditation, progressive muscle relaxation). *When patients learn to lower their levels of anxiety, their ability to assess a situation and use their own problem-solving skills are improved.*

8. Identify negative self-talk or messages (e.g., "I'll never be able to do this right." "This means I'll never succeed in anything."). *Cognitive skills can be used to help the patient to reframe thinking so that problems can be solved.*

9. Refer the patient and significant others to support groups, self-help programs, or advocacy groups when appropriate. *Patients with specific problems are known to greatly benefit from being around others who are grappling with similar issues. This provides the patient with information and support and decreases feelings of isolation in stressful and difficult situations.*

10. Administer medications or obtain an order for medications when appropriate. *Use the least restrictive interventions to decrease anxiety.*

Impaired Coping
Related to
- Severe to panic levels of anxiety—panic attack, generalized anxiety disorder
- Excessive negative beliefs about self
- Presence of obsessions and compulsions
- Avoidance behavior
- Compulsive hoarding

Desired Outcome The patient will verbally demonstrate the ability to cope effectively with anxiety.

Assessment/Interventions and *Rationales*
1. Monitor and reinforce the patient's use of positive coping skills. *Identifies what does and does not work for the patient. The patient learns to build upon strengths.*
2. Explore new coping skills to substitute for ineffective ones. *Provides more adaptive options.*
3. At the patient's level of understanding, explain the fight-or-flight response and the relaxation response of the autonomic nervous system. Address how breathing can be used to bring about the relaxation response. *Understanding the physiological aspects of anxiety and that people have some degree of control over their physiological responses gives patients hope and a sense of control in their lives. Such knowledge aids them in learning relaxation techniques.*
4. When the patient's level of anxiety is mild to moderate, teach proper breathing techniques, and practice breathing with the patient. *Learning occurs at mild to moderate anxiety. Breathing techniques can prevent anxiety from escalating. Practice reinforces learning and a sense of mastery of the technique.*
5. When the patient's level of anxiety is mild to moderate, teach the patient relaxation techniques such as imaging or visualization. *Help the patient gain some control over switching the autonomic nervous system from the fight-or-flight response to the relaxation response.*
6. Use a cognitive approach. *Helps the patient recognize that thoughts and beliefs can cause anxiety.*
7. Teach the patient proven behavioral techniques. The patient can become desensitized to a feared object or situation over time. *Behavioral techniques are extremely effective interventions for treating anxiety disorders. Once*

they are learned, patients can draw upon these skills for the rest of their lives.

8. Encourage the patient to Keep focus on manageable problems, defining them simply and concretely. *Concrete, well-defined problems lend themselves to intervention.*

9. Use role-play to practice responding to stressful situations. *Determination of previous effective or new coping strategies, along with practice, increases potential for success.*

10. Explore using biofeedback through a smart phone application or other wearable device to monitor and reduce anxiety through relaxation techniques. *Biofeedback is an evidence-based approach to relaxation by monitoring physiological processes such as heart rate, blood pressure, skin temperature, and muscle tension and addressing them through relaxation techniques.*

11. Provide verbal and written education, including the medication's purpose, onset of action and therapeutic effect, side effects, and adverse responses. *Understanding medications supports the therapeutic regimen and the patient's role as self-advocate.*

Lack of Knowledge of Treatment Regime

Related to
- Unfamiliarity with the psychiatric disorder and its symptoms
- Unfamiliarity with relaxation techniques, cognitive techniques, and journaling
- Unawareness regarding community resources

Desired Outcomes The patient will demonstrate improved knowledge of treatment regime.

Assessment/Interventions and *Rationales*

1. Provide verbal and written teaching regarding the patient's psychiatric diagnosis including symptoms, potential etiology, and treatment modalities, *In order to self-advocate and manage symptoms, the patient needs to first understand the disorder and its treatment.*

2. Link the patient's relief behaviors to thoughts and feelings. *The patient becomes aware of how anxiety can be the result of thoughts and realizes that with practice, people*

can have some control over their thoughts and therefore their anxiety levels.

3. Teach cognitive principles. Anxiety is the result of dysfunctional appraisal of a situation and automatic thinking. *Reinforces that the patient has some control over thoughts and feelings. This also instills hope and stimulates trying new ways of thinking.*

4. Teach some cognitive techniques that the patient can try out right away. *Increases self-awareness while distancing the patient from anxiety.*

5. Teach behavioral techniques such as thought stopping (i.e., actually saying "stop" to intrusive thoughts) that can interrupt unwanted thoughts. *While clinicians disagree with this method, many individuals find thought stopping techniques to be useful in stopping unwanted thoughts.*

6. Role-play and rehearse alternative coping strategies that can be used in threatening or anxiety-provoking situations. *Gives the patient a chance to be proactive, giving the patient a choice of alternatives instead of the patient using the usual unsatisfactory automatic reactions.*

7. Encourage the patient to keep a daily journal of thoughts and situations that seem to precede anxiety and the coping strategies used. *Allows the patient to monitor triggers and evaluate coping strategies over time.*

8. Teach the patient to rate anxiety levels on a scale from 1 to 10, where 1 is the least and 10 the highest. Encourage the patient to record situations and anxiety levels in a journal. *Allows the patient to evaluate the effectiveness of coping strategies and monitor the decrease in anxiety levels over time.*

9. Review the journal and identify which strategies worked and which did not work. *Helps the patient to see what seems to be working and what does not, and encourages adherence when going through periods of feeling discouraged.*

10. Review progress made and give credit for the patient's hard work. *Positive feedback helps to reinforce learning.*

11. Review stress-reduction techniques with the patient, family, and significant others during family and patient teaching. Encourage the patient and family members to practice relaxation techniques. *Anxiety is communicated interpersonally. Sometimes simple steps*

make big differences in people's lives. Printed information reinforces learning.

12. Refer the patient to support groups in the community in which people are dealing with similar issues. *Groups can foster a sense of belonging and diminish feelings of isolation and alienation. Positive feedback from others helps foster adherence and enhances self-esteem.*

13. Refer family members and significant others to resources in the community such as family therapy, couples counseling, financial counseling, support groups, or relaxation classes. *Family and others close to the patient might need support and may benefit from learning new coping strategies.*

Impaired Sleep
Related to Provide written material.
- Neurological dysfunction
- Fear
- Anxiety
- Inadequate sleep hygiene
- Obsessive thoughts

Desired Outcome The patient will report satisfaction with falling asleep, maintaining sleep, and time upon awakening.

Assessment/Interventions and *Rationales*

1. Assess the patient's usual sleep patterns, changes that have occurred, and whether there was a precipitating event around the onset of the sleep problem or whether it is chronic. *Understanding the baseline sleep pattern provides direction for addressing the impaired sleep.*

2. Identify the patient's usual sleep patterns, including bedtime rituals, time of retiring, time of rising, use of alcohol or caffeine before bedtime, and use of sleep aids (prescribed or over-the-counter medications.) *Establishing a baseline helps to determine useful interventions.*

3. Develop a sleep relaxation routine (e.g., self-hypnosis, progressive muscle relaxation, imagery). *Using both physical and mental relaxation can help minimize anxiety and promote sleep.*

4. Demonstrate and rehearse relaxation techniques until the patient is able to practice them at bedtime. *Practicing new skills increases the likelihood for success in their use.*

5. Suggest the use of online relaxation recordings. *Relaxation recordings provide external support for reducing anxiety.*
6. Encourage the patient to avoid caffeine six hours before bedtime; limit fluid intake 3 to 5 hours before bedtime; increase physical activity during the day, even if fatigued; avoid daytime naps; establish regular times of retiring and waking. *These simple measures promote sleep hygiene.*
7. Help the patient to establish a sleep program that incorporates the elements of good sleep hygiene and relaxation tools. *The plan is more likely to be followed if the patient is actively involved in it.*
8. Suggest that if after 20 minutes of being in bed, but not sleeping, the patient should get up and engage in a quiet activity that is "boring"—*not* stimulating. *Waiting for sleep that will not come can increase anxiety and frustration. Doing something monotonous at bedtime might help the patient become drowsy.*
9. Encourage the patient to practice the agreed-upon bedtime routine for 2 weeks, even if there does not seem to be a benefit. *It might take 2 weeks or longer for habits to settle in.*
10. Encourage the patient to simultaneously identify issues that might be adversely affecting sleep (e.g., anxiety, social or personal problems, job-related issues, interpersonal difficulties). Offer referrals when appropriate. *Disturbances in sleep are often secondary to other issues, either emotional or physical and need to be addressed.*

TREATMENT FOR ANXIETY AND OBSESSIVE–COMPULSIVE DISORDERS

Biological Treatments

Pharmacotherapy

Several classes of medications have been found to be effective in the treatment of anxiety disorders. Antidepressants are typically a first line of defense when treating anxiety as well as major depressive disorders.

Most FDA approved OCD medications are SSRIs including fluoxetine (Prozac), fluvoxamine (Luvox), paroxetine

(Paxil), and sertraline (Zoloft). Another approved drug, clomipramine (Anafranil), is a tricyclic antidepressant. For children and adolescents with OCD, fluoxetine (Prozac) is approved for ages 7 to 17, fluvoxamine (Luvox) for ages 8 to 17, sertraline (Zoloft) for ages 6 to 17, and clomipramine (Anafranil) for ages 10 to 17.

There are no FDA approved medications for body dysmorphic disorder, hoarding disorder, trichotillomania, or excoriation disorder. However, the same medications used for OCD – the SSRIs – are used. See Chapter 24 for a discussion of antidepressants. Chapter 25 provides an overview of antianxiety agents.

Brain Stimulation Therapies

A reversible surgical treatment used for OCD is deep brain stimulation (DBS). The Food and Drug Administration (FDA) approved DBS as an adjunct to medications in treatment-resistant OCD in adults who have failed at least three selective serotonin reuptake inhibitor (SSRI) trials. In DBS, electrodes are surgically placed bilaterally in the subthalamic nucleus of the brain. Then an implanted pulse generator in the chest activates a low-dose current for a specified period of time (several months in some cases). Chapter 30 discusses brain stimulation therapies in more depth.

Integrative Care

Appendix B identifies a number of complementary practices or integrative therapies that people use to cope with anxiety.

Psychological Therapies

Psychiatric–mental health advanced practice registered nurses, like other advanced practice psychiatric professionals, are qualified to conduct individual and group psychotherapy. Two important forms of therapy for anxiety disorders are behavioral therapy and cognitive–behavioral therapy. Examples of these types of therapies include:
- Cognitive restructuring
- Breath restraining and muscle relaxation
- Modeling techniques
- Systematic desensitization or graduated exposure
- Flooding (implosion therapy)

- Teaching of self-monitoring for panic and other symptoms
- In vivo (real life) exposure to feared objects or situations
  Nonpharmacologic therapies seem to be particularly useful for OCDs. They include:
- Exposure and response prevention
- Flooding
  See Chapter 29 for more discussion on psychotherapeutic models.

NURSE, PATIENT, AND FAMILY RESOURCES

Anxiety and Depression Association of America
www.adaa.org

Body Dysmorphic Disorder Foundation
www.bddfoundation.org/

International OCD Foundation
www.iocdf.org

Mental Help Net
www.mentalhelp.net

Panic Disorder
www.nlm.nih.gov/medlineplus/panicdisorder.html

Panic/Anxiety Disorders Guide
www.panicdisorder.about.com

TLC Foundation for Body-Focused Repetitive Behavior
www.bfrb.org/

CHAPTER 9

Trauma-Related Disorders

Traumatic life events are associated with a wide range of psychiatric and physical disorders. Traumatic events includes witnessing frightening or distressing events, interpersonal trauma, sexual abuse, physical abuse, severe neglect, emotional abuse, repeated abandonment, or sudden and traumatic loss in childhood, adolescence, or adulthood.

Understanding of the long-term physiological and psychological effects of trauma has grown, and effective treatments are available. Trauma-informed care is a treatment framework that involves recognizing and responding to the effects of all types of trauma. Integrating trauma-informed care into health care settings can reduce the pervasive and damaging effects of trauma.

The American Psychiatric Association (APA, 2013) identifies trauma- and stressor-related disorders as disorders in which exposure to trauma is an explicit diagnostic criterion. The disorders included in the trauma disorders chapter in the *Diagnostic and Statistical Manual of Mental Disorders* (APA, 2013) include the following:

- Reactive attachment disorder in children whose trauma leaves them unable to respond emotionally to caregivers.
- Disinhibited social engagement disorder in children whose trauma leads them to superficially and indiscriminately bond to unfamiliar adults.
- Adjustment disorder occurs when emotional or behavioral symptoms in response to stress are out of proportion to the stress.

Two other trauma-related disorders that are the focus of care in this chapter are acute stress disorder (ASD) and posttraumatic stress disorder (PTSD). Both disorders follow exposure to an extremely traumatic event, usually outside the range of normal experience. The main difference between ASD and PTSD is timing. ASD symptoms occur within 1 month of the traumatic event and resolve within that month. If symptoms last longer than 1 month, the diagnosis is changed from ASD to PTSD.

ACUTE STRESS DISORDER

ASD may develop after exposure to a highly traumatic event within 3 days to 1 month after the traumatic event.

Examples of ASD-inducing events include:

- Military combat, prisoner-of-war experience, or being taken hostage
- Crime-related events such as bombing, assault, mugging, or rape
- Natural disasters such as floods, tornadoes, and earthquakes
- Human disasters such as automobile, airline, and train accidents

An often-overlooked cause of ASD is being diagnosed with a life-threatening illness or being treated for a serious illness, particularly in the intensive care unit.

To be diagnosed with ASD, the individual must display 8 out of the following 13 symptoms either during or after the traumatic event:

- A subjective sense of numbing
- Derealization (i.e., a sense of unreality related to the environment)
- Inability to remember at least one important aspect of the event
- Intrusive distressing memories of the event
- Recurrent disturbing dreams
- Feeling as if the event is recurring
- Intense prolonged distress or physiological reactivity
- Avoidance of thoughts or feelings about the event
- Sleep disturbances
- Hypervigilance
- Irritable, angry, or aggressive behavior
- Exaggerated startle response
- Agitation or restlessness

POSTTRAUMATIC STRESS DISORDER

PTSD in children older than 6 years and adults is characterized by persistent reexperiencing of a highly traumatic event. This event typically involves actual or threatened death or serious injury to self or others. Responses of intense fear, helplessness, or horror are felt. PTSD may occur after any traumatic event that is outside the range of usual experience such as those listed in the prior section on ASD. PTSD is diagnosed after a month of symptoms, yet it is not uncommon for a delay of symptoms for months or years after the event.

In both adults and children, the major features of PTSD include the following:

1. Reexperiencing the trauma through recurrent intrusive recollections of the event or dreams about the event.
2. Dissociative experiences (e.g., flashbacks) during which the event is relived.
3. Avoidance of stimuli associated with the trauma, causing the individual to avoid talking about the event or avoid activities, people, or places that arouse memories of the trauma. This avoidance is accompanied by feelings of detachment, emptiness, and numbing.
4. Persistent symptoms of increased arousal, as evidenced by irritability, difficulty sleeping, difficulty concentrating, hypervigilance, or exaggerated startle response.
5. Alterations in mood, such as chronic depression, negative outlook, and lack of interest in previously pleasurable activities (APA, 2013).

The APA (2013) makes a distinction in diagnostic criteria for PTSD in children 6 years or younger. A primary symptom in preschool children may manifest as a reduction in play. Other symptoms include aspects of the traumatic event, social withdrawal, and negative emotions such as fear, guilt, anger, horror, sadness, shame, or confusion. Children may blame themselves for the traumatic event. In addition, there may be a feeling of detachment or estrangement from others and diminished interest or participation in significant activities.

Epidemiology

About 60% of men and 50% of women have at least one trauma in their lifetime (US Department of Veterans Affairs, 2018). Men are more likely to have experienced physical assaults, accidents, disasters, combat, and witnessed injury or death. Women are more like to experience sexual abuse as children and be victims of sexual assault. Approximately 8% of the population have PTSD at some time in their lives.

Not everyone who experiences trauma will develop PTSD. An individual's response to a disturbing event is highly individual, depending on factors such as the person's age, developmental stage, coping skills, support system, cognitive deficits, and preexisting neural physiology.

Assessment

Assessment includes the onset, frequency, course, and severity of symptoms. It is also important to determine level of distress, and degree of functional impairment. Additional assessment includes suicidal or violent thoughts, family and social supports, insomnia, social withdrawal, current life stressors, medication, past medical and psychiatric history, and a mental status exam.

A popular screening tool for PTSD in adults is the Primary Care PTSD Screen for DSM-5 (PC-PTSD-5) (Prins et al., 2015). See Box 9.1.

Nursing Care for Trauma-Related Disorders

After a comprehensive trauma assessment, priority nursing diagnoses are identified (International Council of Nurses [ICN], 2019). The most common nursing diagnosis for both children and adults is *posttrauma response*, which directly addresses both ASD and PTSD. *Anxiety* is another essential nursing diagnosis for this population. *Anxiety* levels may be levels of moderate, severe, and panic and are impacted by intrusive memories, distressing dreams, and flashbacks. Anxiety also causes symptoms such as avoidance, hypervigilance, and an exaggerated startle response.

Posttrauma Response
Related to
- Neurological dysfunction
- Physical, psychological, and sexual abuse
- Neglect
- Assault and violence
- Man-made and natural disasters
- Motor vehicle and industrial accidents
- Terrorism, military combat, being a prisoner of war, torture
- Near-death medical experiences

Box 9.1 **Primary Care PTSD Screen for DSM-5**

Sometimes things happen to people that are unusually or especially frightening, horrible, or traumatic. For example:

- A serious accident or fire
- A physical or sexual assault or abuse
- An earthquake or flood
- A war
- Seeing someone be killed or seriously injured
- Having a loved one die through homicide or suicide

Have you ever experienced this kind of event?
If no, screen total = 0. Please stop here
If yes, please answer the questions below.
In the past month, have you:

1. Had nightmares about the event(s) or thought about the event(s) when you did not want to?
   Yes   No
2. Tried hard not to think about the event(s) or went out of your way to avoid situations that reminded you of the event(s)?
   Yes   No
3. Been constantly on guard, watchful, or easily startled?
   Yes   No
4. Felt numb or detached from people, activities, or your surroundings?
   Yes   No
5. Felt guilty or unable to stop blaming yourself or others for the event(s) or any problems the event(s) may have caused?
   Yes   No

Scoring: Patients screen positive if they answer "yes" to three or more items and should receive further evaluation for PTSD.

PTSD, Posttraumatic stress disorder.
(From Prins, A., Bovin, M. J., Kimerling, R., Kaloupek, D. G, Marx, B. P., Pless Kaiser, A., & Schnurr, P. P. (2015). *The primary care PTSD screen for DSM-5 (PC-PTSD-5)*. http://www.ptsd.va.gov/professional/assessment/screens/pc-ptsd.asp.)

- Witnessing traumatic event(s)
- Learning about trauma in family and friends
- Repeated or extreme exposure to details of trauma

Desired Outcome The patient will report and demonstrate a return to the pre-trauma level of functioning.

Assessment/Interventions and *Rationales*

1. Assess for suicidal or homicidal thoughts. *The priority concern and nursing measures are for the safety of the patient and others.*

2. Assess the patient's anxiety level. *Identify what level of intervention might be needed to minimize escalation of anxiety.*

3. Assess for alcohol or drug use. If the patient is using alcohol or drugs, assess readiness for substance use therapies (e.g., support groups, counseling). Offer referrals if the patient is ready. *Patients cannot effectively participate in learning coping skills, reliving traumatic memories, and making positive changes while impaired.*

4. Identify the patient's symptoms and clarify that they are anxiety related and not the result of a physical condition (e.g., chest tightness, headaches, dizziness, numbness). *Physical causes of symptoms are ruled out before assumptions of psychiatric causes are made (e.g., a patient might have PTSD and also a cardiac problem that need to be addressed).*

5. Identify and document psychiatric symptoms (e.g., shock, anger, withdrawal, panic, confusion, psychosis, emotional instability, nightmares, flashbacks). *There are a variety of psychiatric symptoms, which require specific intervention strategies.*

6. Identify and refer the patient to support groups with others who deal with similar traumatic issues. *Support groups made up of people with similar experiences, allow for expressing similar feelings in a safe and healing environment.*

7. Spend time with the patient, allowing the patient to set the pace when describing present or past traumatic events. *Feelings and memories of trauma are often buried. It takes time and trust for a person to open up to a stranger or discuss a topic that has not been shared with anyone before.*

8. Monitor your own feelings in response to the individual's experience. *Background stories are upsetting and may trigger personal reactions.*

9. Avoid interrupting, minimizing the painfulness of events, or over-identifying with events.

10. Therapeutic communication is important when working with patients who have experienced significant trauma. Remain nonjudgmental in your interactions

with patients who have experienced trauma. *Patients who have experienced trauma often blame themselves and feel guilt and are extremely sensitive to disapproval. Nurses are most supportive when they monitor their responses and avoid reinforcing blame, shame, and guilt.*

11. Listen attentively to the patient's description of traumatic events. *Although it might be difficult to listen to the trauma, sharing the pain with others may be the beginning of healing.*

12. Encourage expression of feelings through talking, writing, crying, role-playing, or other ways in which the patient is comfortable. *The description of the events and the expression of feelings associated with the event are essential to the healing process.*

13. Teach cognitive and behavioral strategies to manage symptoms of emotional and physical reactivity. These strategies include deep breathing, relaxation exercises, cognitive techniques, desensitization, assertive behavior, thought-stopping techniques, and stress-reduction techniques. *Once repressed areas are addressed, accompanying, unexpressed feelings will emerge thereby inceasing anxiety.*

14. Assess the family and social support system. Is there a need for family interventions or counseling? *Often family and friends are confused, afraid, hurt, angry, or feel hopeless. They have been coping with intense emotions and distressing symptoms behaviors and will benefit from external support.*

15. Provide education for the patient and family on signs and symptoms of PTSD. *Often when actions and behaviors that seem chaotic and unrelated are viewed in terms of an identifiable syndrome, relief is experienced, especially when treatment is available.*

Anxiety (Moderate or Severe)

Related to
- Neurological dysfunction
- Dysregulation of the hypothalamic-pituitary-adrenal (HPA) axis
- Traumatic event
- Intrusive recurrent memories
- Flashbacks
- Recurrent distressing dreams
- Exaggerated negative beliefs
- Sleep disturbance

Desired Outcome   The patient will report decreased anxiety.

Assessment/Interventions and *Rationales*
1. Spend time with the patient and provide a calm presence. *Spending time with another provides reassurance.*
2. Be conscious of the patient's need for increased personal space, particularly when hypervigilance is experienced. *During periods of high anxiety, patients might feel threatened. You can gauge the amount of space an individual requires with nonverbal cues such as leaning back or backing away as you get closer.*
3. Acknowledge the patient's anxiety with a statement such as, "I understand that you have been going through a rough time and that you've been anxious. How would you describe your level of anxiety now?" *Discussing anxiety symptoms out loud and identifying the level of anxiety provide empathy to the patient and help guide interventions.*
4. Encourage the use of a quiet environment such as the patient's room during periods of acute anxiety. *External stimuli and unit noise increase anxiety levels.*
5. If the patient is agitated or restless, offer to walk together with him or her as you talk. *Sitting in a quiet room could actually make anxiety worse. Walking will help to reduce excess energy.*
6. Provide immediate guidance if anxiety is severe, especially if the anxiety seems to be escalating. "Molly, take a deep breath in through your nose… now out through your mouth [repeat]." *As anxiety levels increase to severe, measures such as slow deep breathing not only reduce the stress response, but they also provide a focus.*
7. If guidance does not help to reduce the level of anxiety, offer as-needed medication if ordered. If none is available, discuss this option with the care provider. *When patients are experiencing an acute exacerbation of a psychiatric illness, medication may provide them with much-needed relief from anxiety. Once anxiety is reduced, other non-pharmacological interventions may be used.*
8. Ask the patient what calming measures have worked in the past. "What usually helps you feel less anxious?" *Supporting successful past measures at reducing*

anxiety provides external reassurance for known coping methods.

9. As anxiety decreases ask what was happening immediately prior to the onset of anxiety symptoms. *Understanding triggers for anxiety is the first step in addressing the problem. The patient may be unaware of thoughts, feelings, or events that set the anxious feelings in motion.*

10. When the patient's anxiety is reduced to moderate or mild, explore behavioral (e.g., progressive muscle relaxation) and cognitive methods (e.g., challenging exaggerated, negative thoughts) to interrupt or reduce anxiety in the future. *Identifying relaxation skills can be used when anxiety begins to help prevent episodes from escalating.*

TREATMENT FOR TRAUMA-RELATED DISORDERS

Biological Approaches

Pharmacotherapy

While the primary treatment for PTSD is trauma-focused psychotherapy, there are some medications used for this condition. Antidepressants can help with symptoms of depression and anxiety. They also help with sleep problems and concentration. The selective serotonin reuptake inhibitors (SSRIs) sertraline (Zoloft) and paroxetine (Paxil) are Food and Drug Administration (FDA) approved for the treatment of PTSD. Other antidepressants that are prescribed off-label include fluoxetine (Prozac) and venlafaxine (Effexor). Nefazodone (Serzone), imipramine (Tofranil), and phenelzine (Nardil) are suggested if other medications are ineffective (US Department of Veterans Affairs and Department of Defense, 2017). See Chapter 24 for more information on antidepressants.

Psychological Therapies

Advanced practice psychiatric professionals including advanced practice psychiatric–mental health registered nurses are qualified to conduct individual and group psychotherapy. International guidelines recommend the use of cognitive-behavioral therapy (CBT) for PTSD as a first-line intervention in the treatment of PTSD. In CBT, patients are encouraged to reevaluate their thinking patterns and identify unhelpful patterns or distortions.

Another first-line treatment is eye movement desensitization and reprocessing (EMDR) therapy. In EMDR, the patient is encouraged to briefly focus on the trauma while engaging in stimulation or sensory input, such as side-to-side eye movements or hand tapping. See Chapter 29 for more information on these psychological therapies.

Nurse, Patient, and Family Resources

International Society for Traumatic Stress Studies
www.istss.org

National Alliance on Mental Illness [PTSD]
www.nami.org

National Center for PTSD
www.ptsd.va.gov

David Baldwin's Trauma Information Pages
www.trauma-pages.com

Trauma Survivors Network
https://www.traumasurvivorsnetwork.org

CHAPTER 10

Eating Disorders

Eating disorders result in a severe disruption in normal eating patterns and the perception of body shape and weight. Eating disorders can be severe and disabling, and successful treatment requires long-term care and follow-up. As compared to most other psychiatric conditions, these disorders can cause substantial physical damage and disability and may even be fatal.

The focus of this chapter is anorexia nervosa, bulimia nervosa, and binge-eating disorder. Three additional feeding problems—pica, rumination disorder, and avoidant/restrictive food intake disorder—are first briefly described.

PICA

Pica is the persistent ingestion of substances that have no nutritional value, such as dirt or paint. Eating nonfood items may interfere with eating nutritional items and can also be dangerous. For example, paint may contain lead that can lead to brain damage. Objects such as stones may cause intestinal blockage. Sharp objects, such as tacks or open paper clips, may result in intestinal laceration. Bacteria from dirt or other soiled objects, may be the source of tooth decay or serious systemic infection. Maternal pica may result in intrauterine toxicity.

Pica usually begins in early childhood or during pregnancy and spontaneously disappears. However, pica that is associated with intellectual disability and development disorders such as autism may persist for years.

Patient education regarding the consequences of ingesting nonnutritive substances is essential with this condition. In children, monitoring eating behavior is obviously an important aspect of treating this problem. Behavioral interventions such as rewarding healthy eating are helpful.

RUMINATION DISORDER

Rumination disorder is characterized by bringing food back up from the stomach (regurgitating) and then rechewing, reswallowing, or spitting the food out. Rumination symptoms tend to occur after some triggering event such as a viral illness or a stressful event. Once the illness or event is over, the regurgitation continues after most meals. The symptoms tend to spontaneously remit but may become habitual and result in esophageal erosion, malnutrition, and even death. Intellectual disability is associated with rumination, as is neglect.

This rare disorder typically occurs in infants between the ages of 3 and 12 months. In individuals with intellectual disability disorder, the onset can occur at any age but typically occurs around age 6. Interventions include repositioning infants and small children during feeding. Improving the interaction between the caregiver and child and making mealtimes a pleasant experience often reduce rumination. Distracting the child when rumination begins is also helpful. Behavioral therapy may be useful for individuals with intellectual disability. Family therapy may provide additional support.

AVOIDANT/RESTRICTIVE FOOD INTAKE DISORDER

A lack of interest in food and an aversion to the sensory experience of eating are symptoms of avoidant/restrictive food intake disorder. Unlike anorexia nervosa, there are no concerns with body shape or weight. This disorder may result in nutritional deficiencies, weight loss, growth retardation, and interference with emotional and social functioning.

Avoidant/restrictive food intake disorder commonly begins in infancy or early childhood and may continue into adulthood. This disorder is more common in adults who focus on specialized diet trends that eliminate one or more food groups from the diet. Anxiety, depression, and obsessive–compulsive characteristics are risk factors. A history of gastrointestinal problems such as reflux is also associated with this feeding disorder.

Children may fail to meet their nutritional or energy needs and may fall off the normal growth curve.

Therefore, they will require aggressive treatment. Family-based therapy focuses on lifting blame, providing compassion for the patient, and empowering parents to focus on the goal of weight gain. Detailed food diaries and the use of weekly weight graphs are helpful in illustrating improvement.

Cognitive–behavioral therapy (CBT) is useful in uncovering unrealistic automatic thoughts and replacing them with realistic responses. Anxiety and depressive symptoms may be treated off-label with second-generation antipsychotics (e.g., olanzapine) and selective serotonin reuptake inhibitors (SSRIs) (e.g., fluoxetine). Appetite stimulants such as cyproheptadine (Periactin), an antihistamine, have also been used for treating this disorder.

ANOREXIA NERVOSA

Individuals with anorexia nervosa have an intense fear of gaining weight. Often there is a misperception that individuals with anorexia refuse to eat despite being hungry. However, evidence suggests that people with anorexia experience significant differences in sensation of taste, appetite, and satiety, which help to perpetuate the disorder (Kerr et al., 2016).

Individuals with anorexia may engage in compensatory behaviors to make up for the effects of eating or to mitigate previous intake (National Eating Disorder Association, 2018). Purging is a type of compensatory behavior that refers to ridding the body of food in order to prevent weight gain. Self-induced vomiting, laxative abuse, diuretic abuse, enemas, and excessive exercise are common purging behaviors.

Anorexia nervosa is difficult to treat. Even when remission is achieved, the 1-year relapse rate is approximately 50%. Even after 4 years, up to 40% of patients continue to meet some criteria for anorexia (Harrington et al., 2015). Recovery is evaluated as a stage in the process rather than a fixed event. Factors that influence the stage of recovery include the percentage of weight restoration, extent to which self-worth is defined by shape and weight, and functional impairment in the patient's personal life.

Epidemiology

The estimated lifetime prevalence of anorexia nervosa is 0.5%, with a median age of onset of 18 years (Hudson et al., 2007). Actual prevalence must be higher, as individuals may conceal symptoms. In fact, research indicates that less than half of individuals with anorexia seek help for the disorder (Rosenvinge & Petterson, 2015). Anorexia nervosa commonly begins during adolescence or in young adults. It is unusual for this disorder to occur before puberty or after age 40.

Risk Factors

The relationship between a lack of tryptophan and its impact on serotonin, anxiety, and dysphoria is implicated. Individuals with anorexia nervosa have less gray and white matter in the central nervous system (Zipfel et al., 2015). They exhibit decreases in the size and/or function of portions of the hypothalamus, basal ganglia, and somatosensory cortex. Regions of the insula, amygdala, and dorsolateral prefrontal cortex appear larger or experience greater activation in comparison to observations in healthy controls (Brownell & Walsh, 2017).

Anxious and perfectionistic temperaments are associated with a need for control and an unrealistic ideal of thinness. Culture also exerts an influence on the development of self-concept and satisfaction with body size. Anorexia nervosa is associated with cultures that value thinness.

Assessment

Signs and Symptoms
Psychological
- Fear of gaining weight
- Poor social adjustment
- Preoccupation with thoughts of food
- Self-image is based on weight
- Mood and/or sleep disturbances
- Obsessive focus on food
- Views self as fat even when emaciated
- Perfectionistic

Behavioral
- Compulsive food behaviors
- Food restriction

- Calorie counting
- Excessive exercise
- Binge-eating
- Purging (e.g., laxatives, diuretics, enemas)
- Chewing then spitting out food
- Hiding or throwing away food
- Drinking water prior to being weighed
- Complaining about weight
- Avoiding eating in public
- Food rituals (e.g., arrangement of food on plates, order of eating food in a certain order, cutting food into tiny pieces, eating slowly)
- Constant mirror checking

Physiological
- Body mass index (BMI): 17+ (mild), 16–17 (moderate), 15–16 (severe), <15 (extreme)
- Cardiovascular abnormalities (hypotension, bradycardia, heart failure)
- Abnormal laboratory test values (low triiodothyronine, thyroxine levels)
- Abnormal computed tomography (CT) scans, electroencephalographic changes
- Impaired renal function
- Glucose <60 mg/dL
- Cold extremities
- Hypokalemia (<3.5 mEq/L)
- Electrolyte imbalance
- Dehydration
- Peripheral edema
- Muscle weakening
- Dry, yellowish skin
- Amenorrhea (loss of menstruation)
- Lanugo (downy hair on face, chest, shoulders, arms)
- Constipation

ASSESSMENT GUIDELINES

1. Determine the patient's perception of the problem and a verbatim chief complaint.
2. Perform a complete nursing assessment, including orthostatic vital signs, review of systems, and general appearance.
3. Gather a psychosocial history, including screening for suicide or self-harm behaviors.

4. Assess nutritional pattern and fluid intake.
5. Assess daily activities, including exercise.
6. Review laboratory testing, including the following:
   a. Electrolyte levels
   b. Glucose level
   c. Thyroid function tests
   d. Complete blood count
   e. Electrocardiogram (EKG)
   f. Dual-energy x-ray absorptiometry (DEXA) to measure bone density
   g. Erythrocyte sedimentation rate (ESR)
   h. Creatine phosphokinase (CPK)
7. Determine the patient's goals of treatment.

Nursing Diagnoses

The main characteristic of anorexia is a low BMI, making *impaired low nutritional intake* a top safety priority. Individuals with anorexia nervosa also tend to view themselves as fat even while emaciated. The nursing diagnosis *disturbed body image* is an important focus.

INTERVENTION GUIDELINES

1. Acknowledge the patient's desire for thinness and control.
2. Do a self-assessment and be aware of reactions that might limit your ability to help the patient. Some nurses might experience the following:
   • Feeling shock or disgust for the patient's behavior or appearance
   • Resenting the patient, believing that the disorder is self-inflicted
   • Feeling helpless to change the patient's behavior, leading to anger and frustration
   • Becoming overwhelmed by the patient's problems, leading to feelings of hopelessness
   • Engaging in power struggles with the patient, which result in angry feelings in the nurse toward the patient
3. Limit discussions of food.
4. Monitor laboratory values and report abnormal values to the care provider.

Nursing Care for Anorexia Nervosa

Impaired Low Nutritional Intake

Related to

- Neurological dysfunction
- Psychological factors
- Restricting caloric intake or refusing to eat
- Excessive fear of weight gain
- Excessive physical exertion
- Self-induced vomiting
- Laxative, diuretic, or enema use

Desired Outcome By discharge (inpatient) or after 2 weeks (outpatient) the patient's nutritional intake will be sufficient.

Assessment/Interventions and *Rationales*

Severely Malnourished Patients: Nutritional Rehabilitation

1. When severely malnourished and refusing nourishment, the patient may require tube feedings, either alone or in conjunction with oral or parenteral nutrition. *Tube feedings may be the only means available to maintain the patient's life. The patient may not tolerate solid foods at first. The use of nasogastric tube feedings decreases the chance of vomiting.*

2. Tube feedings or parenteral nutrition is often given at night. *Nighttime administration helps diminish drawing attention or sympathy from other patients and allows the patient to participate more fully in daytime activities.*

3. After completion of nasogastric tube feeding, supervise the patient for 90 minutes initially, and gradually reduce the time to 30 minutes. *Helps minimize the patient's chance of vomiting or siphoning off feedings.*

4. Assess vital signs at least three times daily until stable, and then daily. Regularly review electrocardiogram (EKG) and laboratory tests (electrolytes, acid–base balance, liver enzymes, albumin, and others). *As the patient's weight begins to increase, cardiovascular status improves to within normal range, and less frequent monitoring is needed.*

5. Administer tube feedings in a matter-of-fact, nonpunishing manner. Tube feedings are not to be used as threats, nor are they to be bargained about. *Tube*

*feedings are medical treatments, not a punishment or bar-
gaining chip. Being consistent and enforcing limits lower
the chance of manipulation and chance of power struggles.*

6. Give the patient the opportunity to take foods or liquid
   supplements orally, and supplement insufficient intake
   through tube feedings. *Allows the patient some control
   over the need for tube feedings.*
7. Weigh the patient weekly or biweekly at the same time
   of day each week. Use the following guidelines:
   a. Before the morning meal
   b. After the patient has voided
   c. In a hospital gown and undergarment only
   *Patients are terrified about gaining weight. Staff members
   monitor for strategies such as drinking excess water, having
   a full bladder, or putting heavy objects in their pockets or on
   their person before being weighed.*
8. Remain neutral, neither approving nor disapproving.
   *Keep issues of approval and disapproval separate from issues
   of health. Weight gain and loss is a health matter,
   not an area that has to do with the staff's pleasure or
   disapproval.*

   Less Severely Malnourished Patients: Nutritional
   Maintenance
1. When possible, set up a contract with the patient
   regarding treatment goals and outcome criteria. *When
   the patient agrees to take part in establishing goals, there is a
   greater chance of achieving them.*
2. Provide a pleasant, calm atmosphere at mealtimes.
   Structure mealtimes. Tell the patient the specific time
   and duration of a meal (e.g., 30 minutes). *Mealtimes
   become episodes of high anxiety, and knowledge of regula-
   tions decreases tension in the milieu, particularly when
   the patient has given up so much control by entering
   treatment.*
3. Observe the patient during meals to prevent hiding
   or throwing away food. Accompany the patient to the
   bathroom if purging is suspected. Observe the patient
   for at least 1 hour after meals and snacks to prevent
   purging. *These behaviors are difficult for the patient to stop.
   External control will help until the patient develops more
   internal resources.*
4. Observe the patient closely for the use of physical
   activity to control weight. *Patients are discouraged from
   engaging in exercise until their weight reaches 85% of ideal
   body weight.*

5. Closely monitor and record the following:
   a. Fluid and food intake
   b. Vital signs
   c. Elimination pattern (discourage the use of laxatives, enemas, or suppositories)
   Fluid and electrolyte balance are crucial to the patient's well-being and safety. Abnormal data should alert staff to potential physical crises.
6. Continue to weigh the patient as described previously. *Objectively monitors progress.*
7. As the patient approaches the target weight, gradually encourage personal choices for menu selection. *Fosters a sense of control and promotes recovery.*
8. Privileges are based on weight gain (or loss) when setting limits. When weight loss occurs, decrease privileges. Use this time to focus on circumstances surrounding the weight loss and the feelings of the patient. *By not focusing on eating, physical activity, and calorie counts, there is more emphasis on the patient's feelings and perceptions.*
9. When weight gain occurs, increase privileges. *The patient receives positive reinforcement for healthy outcomes and behaviors.*

Nutritionally Stabilized Patients: Maintenance of Recovery

1. Continue to provide a supportive and empathetic approach as the patient continues to meet target weight. *For patients with anorexia, eating regularly, even within the framework of restoring health, is extremely difficult.*
2. The weight maintenance phase of treatment challenges the patient. This is the ideal time to address more of the issues underlying the patient's attitude toward weight and shape. *At a healthier weight, the patient is cognitively better prepared to examine emotional conflicts and themes.*
3. Use a cognitive–behavioral approach to the patient's expressed fears regarding weight gain. Identify dysfunctional thoughts such as, "If I gain weight, I am a failure." *Confronting dysfunctional thoughts and beliefs is crucial to changing eating behaviors.*
4. Emphasize the social nature of eating. Encourage conversation that does not have the theme of food during mealtimes. *Eating is a social activity and participating in conversation serves both as a distraction from obsessional preoccupation and as a pleasurable event.*

5. Focus on the patient's strengths, including progress in normalizing weight and eating habits. *The patient has achieved a major accomplishment. Explore activities unrelated to eating as sources of gratification.*

6. Encourage the patient to apply all the knowledge, skills, and gains made from the various individual, family, and group therapy sessions. *Intensive therapy (cognitive–behavioral) and education provide tools and techniques useful for maintaining healthy eating and living behaviors.*

7. Teach and role model assertiveness. *The patient learns to get needs met appropriately, which helps reduce anxiety and acting-out behaviors.*

Stabilized Patients: Follow-Up Care

1. Involve the patient's family and significant others with teaching, treatment, and discharge and follow-up plans. Teaching includes nutrition, medication, and the dynamics of the illness. *Family involvement is a key factor to patient success. Family dynamics are often a significant factor in the patient's illness and distress.*

2. Plan for follow-up therapy for both the patient and family. *Follow-up therapy for both the patient and family is key to relapse prevention.*

3. Offer referrals to the patient and family for in-person and/or virtual support groups. (See the list at the end of the chapter for suggestions.) *Support groups offer emotional encouragement, resources, and important information; help minimize feelings of isolation; and encourage healthier coping strategies.*

Disturbed Body Image

Related to
- Neurological dysfunction
- Cognitive and perceptual factors
- Psychosocial factors
- Negative perception of body
- Morbid fear of obesity
- Low self-esteem

Desired Outcome By discharge (inpatient) or within 2 weeks (outpatient), the patient will verbalize a report of a positive body image.

Assessment/Interventions and *Rationales*

1. Establish a therapeutic alliance with the patient. *Patients with anorexia are highly resistant to giving up*

unhealthy eating behaviors. A trusting relationship with a nurse is a first step toward recovery.

2. Give the patient feedback about the low weight and resultant impaired health. Do not argue or challenge the patient's perceptions. *Focuses on health and the benefits of increased energy. Arguments or power struggles will increase the patient's need to control.*

3. Recognize that the distorted image is real to the patient. Avoid minimizing the patient's perceptions while, at the same time, challenging distortions (e.g., "I understand you see yourself as fat. I do not see you that way.") *This recognition acknowledges the patient's perceptions, and the patient feels understood even though your perception is different. This kind of feedback is easier to hear than negation of the patient's beliefs.*

4. Encourage expression of feelings regarding how the patient thinks and feels about self and body. *Promotes a clear understanding of the patient's perceptions and lays the groundwork for future interventions.*

5. Assist the patient to distinguish between thoughts and feelings. Statements such as "I feel fat" should be challenged and reframed. *It is important for the patient to distinguish between feelings and facts. The patient often speaks of feelings as though they are reality.*

6. Use a cognitive–behavioral approach to encourage the patient to keep a journal of thoughts and feelings and teach how to identify and challenge irrational beliefs. *Cognitive–behavioral approaches can be effective in helping the patient challenge irrational beliefs about self and body image. Journaling allows the patient to reflect on thoughts, feelings, and behaviors and facilitates sharing with the nurse.*

7. Encourage the patient to identify positive aspects of personal appearance. *Helps the patient refocus on strengths and actual physical and other attributes. Disrupts negative rumination.*

8. Educate the family regarding the patient's illness and encourage attendance at family sessions. *The reactions of family members may be triggers of emotional responses and distorted perceptions.*

9. Encourage family therapy for family and significant others. *Families and significant others need assistance in learning how to communicate with and relate to a patient who has anorexia.*

TREATMENT MODALITIES

Treatment for anorexia may occur in inpatient, day treatment programs, and outpatient environments. Regardless of setting, treatment will consist of psychosocial interventions, pharmacotherapy, psychotherapy, nutrition, and medical intervention.

Biological Treatments

Pharmacotherapy

There are no drugs approved by the US Food and Drug Administration (FDA) for the treatment of anorexia nervosa. Research does not support the use of pharmacological agents to treat the core symptoms (Harrington et al., 2015). Consequently, pharmacotherapy is used to treat associated symptoms of co-occurring disorders. These medications include SSRIs, antianxiety agents, second-generation antipsychotics, and mood stabilizers.

Integrative Care

Individuals with anorexia nervosa may benefit from integrative approaches that can be used in conjunction with traditional eating disorder treatment. These approaches include yoga, massage, acupuncture, or light therapy.

Psychological Therapies

There is no empirical evidence to support any specific psychotherapy model in adults with anorexia nervosa. However, in adolescent patients with anorexia, there is evidence to support insight-oriented individual therapy, where patients are encouraged to learn more about themselves (Lock, 2015). Family approaches, especially family-based treatment (F-BT), have been demonstrated to be more effective than individual therapy.

Young people with anorexia nervosa may also benefit from adolescent-focused therapy (AFT). This model focuses on self-monitoring of eating and weight gain that is supported by the therapeutic relationship with the advanced practice nurse or other therapist. CBT, which helps to identify automatic negative thoughts and to challenge them, has also been used with success in this population. See Chapter 29 for more information on psychological therapies.

BULIMIA NERVOSA

Individuals with bulimia nervosa engage in repeated episodes of binge eating at least once a week for 3 months. Binge eating is eating an amount of food that is larger than what most people would eat in a certain period of time (e.g., 2 hours). The binge eating is followed by compensatory behaviors such as self-induced vomiting; misuse of laxatives, diuretics, or other medications; fasting; or excessive exercise. This disorder is characterized by a significant disturbance in the perception of body shape and weight. A sense of being out of control accompanies the consumption of large amounts of food. Binge eating is usually done alone and in secret. After a binge, individuals experience tremendous guilt, depression, or disgust with themselves.

Epidemiology

The 12-month prevalence of bulimia nervosa among young women is 1% to 1.5%. The lifetime incidence of bulimia nervosa for women is 2.3%, and the lifetime incidence for men is 0.5% (Rosenvinge & Petterson, 2015). Bulimia commonly begins in later adolescence, when the prevalence peaks, up to young adulthood. Onset of bulimia nervosa is rare in children younger than 12 years of age and adults over the age of 40.

Risk Factors

Increased frequency of bulimia nervosa is found in first-degree relatives of people with this disorder. Cycles of binging and purging may have an association with neurotransmitters, specifically serotonin and dopamine.

Corticostriatal circuits in individuals with bulimia nervosa, as compared with those in healthy controls, do not function normally. These circuits include the orbitofrontal, prefrontal, and insular cortices (Donnelly et al., 2018).

The psychological roots of bulimia nervosa have been explained by some theorists as poor early attachment with parents and later problems with attachment in friendships and intimate relationships. Parents of affected offspring were described as negative and unsupportive of independence in their offspring.

Internalization of a thin body ideal increases the risk for weight worries, which in turn increase the risk for bulimia nervosa. There is also some connection between the disorder and childhood sexual or physical abuse. In some cases, traumatic events and environmental stress may be contributing factors.

Assessment

Signs and Symptoms
Psychological
- Obsessive thinking about food
- Feels out of control during binges
- Evaluates self based on body shape and weight
- Dissatisfied with body
- Feelings of dissociation during binges
- Ashamed of eating habits and attempts to conceal the behavior
- Binges are preceded by negative feelings and negative self-evaluation

Behavioral
- Compulsive food behaviors
- Binge eating large amounts of food in a discrete period of time (e.g., 2 hours) at least once a week for 3 months
- Eating to the point of discomfort
- Compensatory behavior (e.g., self-induced vomiting; use of laxatives, diuretics, enemas; fasting; excessive exercising)
- Disappearing after meals
- Eating in isolation and secrecy

Physiological
- Normal to slightly low body weight
- Parotid swelling
- Dental caries, tooth erosion
- Scars on knuckles (Russell's sign) from self-induced vomiting
- Chronic hoarseness, chronic sore throat
- Cardiovascular abnormalities
- Gastric rupture
- Electrolyte imbalance (e.g., hypokalemia, hypochloremia, hyponatremia)
- Seizure

ASSESSMENT GUIDELINES

1. Determine the patient's perception of the problem and a verbatim chief complaint.
2. Perform a complete nursing assessment, including vital signs, review of systems, and general appearance.
3. Gather a psychosocial history.
4. Assess the patient's nutritional pattern and fluid intake.
5. Assess the patient's binging and purging patterns with direct questions.
6. Assess the patient's daily activities, including exercise.
7. Review the patient's laboratory tests, including the following:
   a. Electrolyte levels
   b. Glucose level
   c. Thyroid function tests
   d. Complete blood count
   e. EKG
8. Determine the patient's goals for treatment.

Nursing Diagnoses

Nursing diagnoses that relate to the disordered eating and weight-control behaviors in bulimia nervosa. The most applicable nursing diagnosis is *compulsive eating behavior* (International Council of Nurses, 2019). This bulimia-specific diagnosis is defined as behaviors related to insatiable craving for food, excessive appetite, and episodes of binge eating followed by self-induced vomiting, associated with depression and self-deprivation. Also, given the out-of-control symptoms that individuals with bulimia nervosa experience, *powerlessness* is an essential nursing diagnosis with which to frame nursing care.

Disturbed body image is another priority focus. Interventions previously identified with anorexia nervosa may be modified in the care of individuals with bulimia nervosa.

INTERVENTION GUIDELINES

1. Coexisting disorders such as major depressive disorder, substance use, personality disorders often complicate the clinical picture. These problems require additional treatment and interventions.
2. Cognitive–behavioral techniques have been shown to be useful.

3. Group therapy with other individuals who have bulimia is often part of successful therapy.
4. Because anxiety and feelings of stress often precede binging, alternative ways of dealing with anxiety and alternative coping strategies to lessen anxiety are useful tools.
5. Family therapy is helpful and encouraged.

Nursing Care for Bulimia Nervosa

Compulsive Eating Behavior

Related to
- Neurological dysfunction
- Uncontrollable binge–purge cycles
- Inadequate coping mechanisms to deal with anxiety and stress
- Poor impulse control

Desired Outcome By discharge (inpatient) or within 2 weeks (outpatient), the patient will report and demonstrate regulated eating behavior.

Assessment/Interventions and *Rationales*
1. Assess for suicidal thoughts and other self-destructive behaviors. Patients with bulimia feel out of control and have a negative self-evaluation. *Maintaining physical safety is the priority nursing intervention.*
2. Educate the patient regarding the negative effects of self-induced vomiting (i.e., dental erosion, low potassium level, cardiac problems). *Health teaching is crucial for the patient to understand the insidious and unseen effects of purging behavior.*
3. Educate the patient about the binge–purge cycle and its self-perpetuating nature. *The compulsive nature of the binge–purge cycle is maintained by repeated restricting, hunger, binging, and then purging accompanied by feelings of guilt.*
4. Identify triggers that produce compulsive eating and purging behaviors. *Being aware of triggers helps the patient to substitute healthier coping when triggers occur.*
5. Explore dysfunctional thoughts that precede the binge–purge cycle. Teach the patient to challenge these thoughts and reframe them in healthier ways. *Cognitive–behavioral techniques can balance and combat distorted thinking. More rational thinking can lead to healthier behaviors, improved self-esteem, body image, and self-worth.*

6. Encourage the patient to record thoughts, feelings, and behaviors in a journal and share it with the nurse. *Journaling helps to clarify thoughts and feelings and leads to increased self-awareness, problem solving, and healing. Sharing journal content provides the patient with a sounding board for feedback.*

7. Work with the patient to identify problems and mutually establish short- and long-term goals. *The patient needs to develop tools for dealing with personal problems rather than turning to automatic binge–purge behaviors. Goals support hope and provide direction.*

8. Assess and teach problem-solving skills. *Alternative methods of relieving stress and getting needs met are vital in helping individuals to substitute healthy behaviors for binge-eating behaviors.*

9. Arrange for the patient to learn ways to increase interpersonal communication, socialization, and assertiveness skills. *Individuals with bulimia are often isolated, self-isolate from close relationships, and lack appropriate skills for getting their needs met.*

10. Encourage attendance at support groups, recovery groups, or therapy groups with other individuals with bulimia. Provide information for family members as well. *Eating disorders are chronic diseases, and long-term follow-up therapy and support are critical for success.*

Powerlessness

Related to

- Unsatisfying interpersonal interactions
- Lifestyle of helplessness
- Inability to control binge eating
- Distortion of body image
- Feelings of low self-worth
- Impulsivity
- Insufficient coping skills

Desired Outcome By discharge (inpatient) or within 2 weeks (outpatient), the patient will verbalize decreased powerlessness.

Assessment/Interventions and *Rationales*

1. Explore the patient's experience of out-of-control eating behavior. *Listening in an empathetic, nonjudgmental manner helps the patient feel that someone understands the patient's experience.*

2. Encourage the patient to keep a journal of thoughts and feelings associated with binge–purge behaviors. *Automatic thoughts and beliefs maintain the binge–purge cycle. A journal is an excellent way to identify these dysfunctional thoughts and underlying assumptions.*
3. Teach the patient how to challenge negative and self-defeating thoughts and beliefs in a systematic manner. *These automatic dysfunctional thoughts must be examined and challenged if a change in patient thinking and behavior is to occur.*
4. Explore the kinds of cognitive distortions that affect feelings, beliefs, and behaviors. *Cognitive distortions reinforce unrealistic views of the self in terms of strengths and future potential. Realistic self-views promote healing and growth.*
5. Encourage the patient's participation in decisions and responsibility related to care and to the future. *Self-advocacy helps the patient gain a sense of control over his or her life and recognizing options for making important changes.*
6. Teach the patient alternative stress-reduction techniques and visualization skills to improve self-confidence and feelings of self-worth. *Visualizing a positive self-image and positive outcomes for life goals stimulates problem solving toward desired goals.*
7. Encourage the patient to role-play new skills in counseling sessions and in group therapy to practice communications with others, particularly family. *Role-play allows an opportunity for the patient to become comfortable with new and different ways of relating and responding to others in a safe environment.*
8. Teach the patient that one lapse is not a relapse. One slip of control does not eliminate all positive accomplishments. *At the time of the lapse, it is helpful to examine what led to the lapse, knowing that one lapse does not eliminate all positive accomplishments.*

TREATMENT MODALITIES

Biological Treatments

Pharmacotherapy

Fluoxetine (Prozac), an SSRI antidepressant, is the only FDA-approved medication for the treatment of bulimia nervosa in adult patients. This drug can be helpful for people with bulimia even in the absence of depressive symptoms. Other antidepressants have shown efficacy in the treatment of bulimia nervosa at the same dose as used for depression. They include the following:

- SSRIs sertraline (Zoloft), paroxetine (Paxil), and citalopram (Celexa)
- The tricyclic antidepressants imipramine (Tofranil), nortriptyline (Pamelor), and desipramine (Norpramin)
- The monoamine oxidase inhibitor tranylcypromine (Parnate)

Bupropion (Wellbutrin) is contraindicated in patients diagnosed with bulimia due to the increased risk of seizure with this medication. Serotonin-norepinephrine reuptake inhibitors (SNRIs) have not been evaluated through randomized controlled trials in patients with bulimia. Research is exploring the potential for second-generation antipsychotics, antiepileptics, and/or opioid antagonists for decreasing symptoms associated with bulimia.

Psychological Therapies

Advanced practice professionals are qualified to use the evidence-based CBT, which is considered a first-line treatment for bulimia. Additional modalities which have been explored and found to be helpful include dialectical behavioral therapy (DBT), interpersonal therapy (IPT), and acceptance and commitment therapy (ACT) (Mehler & Andersen, 2017). Chapter 29 provides a description of these models.

BINGE-EATING DISORDER

Individuals with binge-eating disorder engage in episodes of increased intake that occur beyond the point of satiety (fullness) and cause distress afterward. A key difference between this disorder and bulimia nervosa is that compensatory behaviors such as self-induced vomiting and laxatives are typically not used. Although individuals who start binge eating may be of normal weight, repeated binge eating inevitably results in obesity. Binge eating occurs once a week for 3 months.

Epidemiology

Binge eating is the most common eating disorder. The 12-month prevalence for adults is 1.6% in women and

0.8% in men. For women, the lifetime incidence of binge-eating disorder is 3.6% and the lifetime incidence for men is 2.1% (Rosenvinge & Petterson, 2015). This eating disorder is more prevalent in individuals who are overweight (3%) than in the general population (2%). All racial and ethnic groups seem to be represented fairly equally.

Risk Factors

Binge-eating disorder tends to run in families, which may be the result of additive genetic influences. As in the case of patients diagnosed with bulimia nervosa, individuals with binge eating have also exhibit altered processing in the orbitofrontal cortex (Donnelly et al., 2018). Body dissatisfaction, low self-esteem, and difficulty coping with feelings can also contribute to binge-eating disorder. Social pressures to be thin, which are typically influenced through media, can trigger emotional eating. Social weight stigma, which is stereotyping or discrimination based on a person's body, is common in the United States and perpetuates the cycle of binging. A history of trauma, particularly emotional neglect, increases the risk of binge eating.

Assessment

Signs and Symptoms
Psychological
- Feels out of control
- Distress
- Depression
- Grief
- Anxiety
- Shame
- Self-disgust

Behavioral
- Compulsive eating
- Eats rapidly
- Eats until feeling uncomfortably full
- Eats large amounts of food even when not hungry
- Eats alone
- Lack of control
- Isolation
- Stealing or hoarding food
- Creates a lifestyle or rituals to have time for binges

- Withdraws from others and activities
- Frequent diets

Physiological
- Normal weight, overweight, or obese
- Obesity may result in:
  - Type II diabetes
  - High blood pressure
  - High cholesterol
  - Gallbladder disease/gallstones
  - Cardiac disease
  - Joint pain
  - Sleep apnea
  - Cancer (e.g., gallbladder, esophagus)

Nursing Diagnoses

The nursing diagnosis *impaired high nutritional intake* is essential in structuring care for individuals with this disorder (International Council of Nurses, 2019). Because binge-eating disorder is similar to bulimia nervosa (without the purging behaviors), many of the same nursing diagnoses are applicable. These diagnoses include *compulsive eating behavior*, *powerlessness*, and *disturbed body image*.

Nursing Care for Binge-Eating Disorder

Impaired High Nutritional Intake
Related to
- Binge eating
- Lack of control overeating
- Eating rapidly
- Eating until uncomfortably full
- Eating when not hungry

Desired Outcome The patient will demonstrate decreased nutritional intake.

Assessment/Interventions and *Rationales*
1. Encourage the patient to keep a journal recording urges to binge eat, feelings or events immediately before, and responses to urges. *Understanding a pattern of binge eating will help to identify more adaptive responses to the urges.*

2. Identify ways to challenge irrational thoughts that may occur before binge eating. *Correcting faulty thinking is an evidence-based approach to managing this disorder.*
3. Encourage the exploration of alternative and healthy coping strategies. *Patients have been using food to regulate their mood and need new strategies.*
4. Help the patient to develop goals for adopting healthy eating patterns and exercise. *Self-care is promoted through the development of goals within the context of the nurse–patient relationship.*
5. Identify social support through friends and community (locally or online). *Social support makes one feel less alone and stronger and more likely to achieve goals.*
6. Identify support groups for eating disorders in general or binge-eating disorder specifically. Groups can be local in physical facilities or online forums. *Support groups are a powerful tool for reducing isolation, getting feedback, sharing, helping, and practicing relational skills.*

TREATMENT MODALITIES

Biological Treatments

Pharmacotherapy

Because of their efficacy with bulimia nervosa, researchers have studied the use of SSRIs at or near the high end of the dosage range to treat binge-eating disorder. Although these medications seem to help in the short term, patients regained significant weight after discontinuing them. Some evidence has been found to support SNRIs, including duloxetine (Cymbalta) or venlafaxine (Effexor XR) in the treatment of patients with comorbid binge-eating disorder and major depressive disorder (Brownell & Walsh, 2017). Other medications that are under investigation include the tricyclic antidepressants and antiepileptic agents.

Lisdexamfetamine (Vyvanse), a stimulant used to treat attention-deficit/hyperactivity disorder, also has FDA approval for the treatment of moderate to severe binge-eating disorder in adults. Lisdexamfetamine is correlated with a significantly lower risk of relapse in binge episodes compared with placebo at 6-month follow-up (Brownell & Walsh, 2017). In adults with binge-eating disorder, the most common side effects are dry mouth, insomnia, decreased appetite, increased heart rate, constipation, feeling jittery, and anxiety. The FDA includes a black box warning on the label of lisdexamfetamine due to the potential of misuse.

Surgical Interventions

Bariatric surgery is a controversial option for the treatment of obesity that is due to binge-eating disorder. Potential complications from this surgery require individuals to consider it carefully (Mitchell et al., 2015). Complications include impaired fasting glucose levels, high triglycerides, and urinary incontinence. Furthermore, surgery does not address psychiatric concerns associated with binge-eating disorder. It is quite common to require psychiatric counseling that addresses food-related thoughts and behaviors as a prerequisite to bariatric surgery.

Psychological Therapies

Advanced practice professionals provide CBT, DBT, and IPT to reduce binge frequency or eliminate them all together (Mehler & Andersen, 2017). See Chapter 29 for a description of these models.

 ## NURSE, PATIENT, AND FAMILY RESOURCES

Anorexia Nervosa and Related Eating Disorders
www.anred.com

Center for Discovery Eating Disorder Treatment Support Groups
https://centerfordiscovery.com/groups/

Families Empowered and Supporting Treatment of Eating Disorders
www.feast-ed.org

KidsHealth (Search for Eating Disorders)
www.kidshealth.org

Mirror Eating Disorder Help
www.mirror-mirror.org

National Association of Anorexia Nervosa and Associated Disorders (ANAD)
www.anad.org

National Eating Disorders Association
www.nationaleatingdisorders.org

CHAPTER 11

Sleep Disorders

For many people, sleep is an expendable commodity. In a fast-paced society, sleep is often forfeited, and people keep schedules that disrupt normal sleep physiology. The amounts of time spent working, engaging in academic activities, and traveling to and from work and school are the strongest determinants of total sleep time. The more time devoted to other activities, the less time spent sleeping.

Sleep requirements vary from individual to individual and are probably genetically mediated to some degree. While most adults require 7 to 8 hours of sleep for optimal functioning, a small percentage of individuals are considered to be long sleepers and require 10 or more hours per night or short sleepers and require less than 5 hours per night. The amount of sleep necessary to feel fully awake and able to sustain normal levels of performance is known as the basal sleep requirement.

Nurses routinely work with patients who are sleep deprived. Pain, noise, unfamiliar environments, and anxiety disrupt sleep patterns in hospitalized patients. Virtually all psychiatric disorders are associated with sleep disturbance. Sleep disruption itself may be a precipitating factor in psychiatric disorders and may increase the risk of relapse. Individuals with major depressive disorder accompanied by sleep disturbances demonstrate greater degrees of suicidal ideation. Long-standing insomnia is common in alcohol use disorder recovery. One of the strongest indications of recovery from any mental illness is a return to normal sleep patterns.

According to the American Psychiatric Association (APA; 2013), sleep disorders are classified into three specific categories:

1. **Sleep–wake disorders**: Insomnia (insufficient sleep), hypersomnolence (sleeping too much), and narcolepsy (attacks of falling asleep)

2. **Breathing-related sleep disorders:** Sleep apnea (breathing repeatedly stops and starts), sleep-related hypoventilation (restricted breathing), and circadian rhythm disorders (sleep–wake cycles out of sync with the environment)
3. **Parasomnias:** Nonrapid eye movement sleep arousal disorders (sleepwalking), sleep terrors nightmare disorder, rapid eye movement sleep behavior disorder (physically acting out dreams), and restless legs syndrome (irresistible urge to move legs)

This chapter first presents an overview of the most common sleep disorder, insomnia. Afterward, basic nursing care to address sleep disruptions is presented.

INSOMNIA DISORDER

Insomnia is characterized by dissatisfaction with the quantity or quality of sleep (APA, 2013). Individuals with insomnia may have difficulty initiating sleep, maintaining sleep, and trouble going back to sleep.

According to Spielman and Glovinsky (2004), three types of factors contribute to insomnia:

1. Predisposing factors: Internal attributes that lower the threshold for waking. They include a genetic predisposition to insomnia along with preexisting conditions such as major depressive disorder, chronic pain, and sleep-disordered breathing.
2. Precipitating factors: External events that trigger insomnia. Examples of precipitating factors are personal and occupational difficulties, changes in routine (e.g., hospitalization), loss and grieving, and changes in role or identity (e.g., retirement).
3. Perpetuating factors: Repeated behaviors that contribute to sleep inadequacy. These modifiable factors include excessive caffeine or alcohol use, spending too much time in bed or napping, and even worrying about insomnia.

EPIDEMIOLOGY

Insomnia is the most common sleep disorder and may affect up to 45% of adults (Sadock et al., 2015). Females are more commonly affected, as are older adults.

ASSESSMENT

Signs and Symptoms

- Fatigue
- Poor concentration
- Irritability, agitation
- Listlessness
- Complains of drowsiness
- Expresses dissatisfaction with sleep

ASSESSMENT GUIDELINES

The following questions are useful in determining the extent of the sleep problem:

A. When did you begin having trouble with sleep? Have you had trouble with sleep in the past?

B. Describe your sleep environment. What are the activities you usually engage in before sleep?

C. Describe your sleep environment. Are there things in your sleep environment that are hampering your sleep, such as noise, light, temperature, or overall comfort?

D. Do you use your bedroom for anything other than sleep or sexual activity (e.g., working, eating, or watching television)?

E. What time do you go to bed? How long does it take to fall asleep?

F. Once asleep, do you wake in the middle of the night? If so, what wakes you up? Are you able to return to sleep?

G. When you are unable to sleep, what do you do?

H. What time do you wake up? What time do you get out of bed?

I. How much time do you actually think you sleep? Are you tracking your sleep with smartwatch or tracker?

J. Do you sleep longer on weekends or days off?

K. Do you nap? If so, for how long? Do you feel refreshed after napping?

L. Can you identify any stress or problem that may have initially contributed to your sleep difficulties?

M. What are your daily habits, diet, exercise, and medications?

N. What changes, if any, have you made to improve your sleep? What were the results?

Nursing Diagnoses

There are several specific International Classification for Nursing Practice (ICNP) (International Council of Nurses, 2019) nursing diagnoses that address sleep disturbances.

The two that will be discussed in this chapter are *insomnia* and *impaired sleep*.

INTERVENTION GUIDELINES

Provide patients with education on the following topics:
A. Reserve the bedroom for sleep and as a place of intimacy (i.e., no electronics, reading, or other activities in the bedroom).
B. Avoid clock watching.
C. Avoid heavy meals before bedtime.
D. Use alcohol cautiously, and avoid use for several hours before bed.
E. Exercise daily, but not right before bed.
F. Get out of bed if unable to sleep and engage in a quiet acti-vity such as reading or crossword puzzles.
G. Avoid lighted activities, which stimulate the retina in the hour before bed (e.g., no television or computer).
H. Maintain a regular sleep–wake schedule, getting up at the same time each day being the most important factor.
I. Avoid daytime napping. If napping is necessary, limit to 20 to 30 minutes maximum, and set a timer.

Nursing Care for Insomnia

Insomnia

Related to
- Neurological dysfunction
- Anxiety
- Pain
- Grieving
- Daytime napping
- Inadequate physical activity
- Poor sleep hygiene
- Medication
- Caffeine
- Alcohol
- Unsuitable environment

Desired Outcome The patient will report and demonstrate improved sleep.

Assessment/Interventions and *Rationales*

1. Assess the patient's activity pattern and sleep pattern. *Baseline information sets the stage for successful interventions.*

2. Monitor the effects of hypnotic or other medications on the patient's sleep pattern. *If medication is effective, the patient may need to work with their healthcare provider to slowly withdrawal the sleeping medication as more permanent methods [e.g., antidepressants] take effect.*

3. Teach sleep hygiene measures such as limiting daytime naps, avoiding caffeine and nicotine near bedtime, increasing daytime exercise, establishing a relaxing bedtime routine, and avoiding light-producing electronics 1 hour before sleep. *These simple sleep hygene measures promote sleep.*

4. Provide a comfortable, cool, quiet, disturbance-free, and dark environment. *Heat, noise, people, and light impair an individual's ability to sleep.*

5. Encourage the use of blackout curtains, eyeshades, earplugs, white noise machines or cell phone apps, humidifiers, fans, and other devices. *Nonpharmacological sleep aids are often extremely successful in promoting sleep.*

6. Teach relaxation methods to promote sleep such as slow, deep breathing; guided imagery; and progressive muscle relaxation. *Relaxation methods reduce anxiety and muscle tension that interfere with sleep.*

7. Monitor the patient's sleep for physical problems such as sleep apnea, urinary frequency, or discomfort. *Many physical problems that interfere with sleep can be successfully treated.*

8. Encourage the patient to keep a sleep diary or use an sleep-tracking device. *Understanding and evaluating sleep practices promote self-care. Sometimes perceptions of sleep are inaccurate, and tracking sleep can improve self-perception.*

Impaired Sleep
Related to
- Neurological dysfunction
- Physical or psychological pain
- Age-related sleep pattern changes
- Circadian asynchrony
- Restless legs syndrome

- Sleep apnea
- Poor sleep hygiene
- Nightmares, sleepwalking, sleep terrors
- Caffeine
- Sleep interruption for treatments
- Unsuitable environment
- Life demands (e.g., caregiving responsibilities, parental duties, night shift work)

Desired Outcome The patient will report and demonstrate improved sleep.

Assessment/Interventions *(Rationales)*

1. Assess sleep patterns and document findings. *Accurate baseline data will inform interventions and provide a record for improvement or lack of improvement.*
2. Provide sedatives or hypnotics, antipsychotics, or other medications prescribed for sleep. *Medication can prevent sustained sleep loss, which could result in psychosis [i.e., disturbed thinking, delusions, hallucinations].*
3. Minimize sleep disruption in the hospital whenever possible by medicating before bed and in the morning, keeping lights dim and voices quiet if medications or treatments must be given at night. *Hospitals are notoriously noisy, and treatments can be intrusive at night. Minimizing sleep disturbances is essential to facilitate recovery.*
4. Promote a regular bedtime and wake time. *Reestablishing a normal period of sleep will improve functioning.*
5. As sleep normalizes, discourage sleep during the day. *Initially, patients may be so sleep deprived that short daytime naps are essential to restoring brain function and body homeostasis. After the crisis period, daytime naps will interfere with sleeping at night.*
6. Limit caffeine-containing drinks and food such as energy drinks, coffee, tea, colas, and chocolate. *Caffeine is a central nervous system stimulant and will interfere with sleep.*

TREATMENT FOR SLEEP DISORDERS

Biological Treatments

Pharmacotherapy

Generally, long-term sedative/hypnotic use is discouraged because nonpharmacological treatments have shown superior efficacy in reducing insomnia. Other classifications of drugs used for insomnia are antidepressants, anticonvulsants, and antihistamines, which are used off-label without specific approval from the US Food and Drug Administration (FDA). Second-generation antipsychotics improve sleep in people using them as indicated for other problems such as schizophrenia. Chapter 26 provides a list of FDA-approved drugs for the treatment of insomnia.

Over-the-counter sleeping aids have limited effectiveness. Melatonin, a naturally occurring hormone, is a popular over-the-counter product. To date, there are limited data to support its use in the management of insomnia disorder, but new research into prolonged-release forms of melatonin is demonstrating some promise.

Somatic Treatments

Functional magnetic resonance imaging studies indicate that the prefrontal cortex is overly active with insomnia. Racing thoughts interfere with the individual's ability to sleep. The Cerêve Sleep System has FDA approval and significantly reduced sleep latency from stage 1 to stage 2 in clinical trials. This product is a software-controlled bedside device that is placed on the forehead. A fluid-filled pad cools the forehead and reduces activity in the cerebral cortex.

Psychological Therapies

Successful treatment of insomnia involves the integration of basic principles of sleep hygiene, which are conditions and practices that promote continuous and effective sleep. Modifying poor sleep habits and establishing a regular sleep–wake schedule can be accomplished using sleep diaries (Fig. 11.1). A period of 2 weeks is helpful in establishing overall sleep patterns and determining overall sleep efficiency ([time in bed divided by total sleep time] × 100). After reviewing sleep diaries, patients are sometimes surprised to discover that their sleep problems are not as bad as previously believed.

Sleep restriction, or limiting the total sleep time, creates a temporary mild state of sleep deprivation and strengthens the sleep homeostatic drive. This helps decrease sleep latency and improves sleep continuity and quality. If, for example, if a sleep diary indicates that your patient is in bed for 8 hours but sleeping only 6 hours, sleep is restricted to 6 hours, and the bedtime and wake time are adjusted accordingly. Do not reduce the sleep time below 5 hours, regardless of sleep efficiency, and caution patients about the dangers of sleepiness

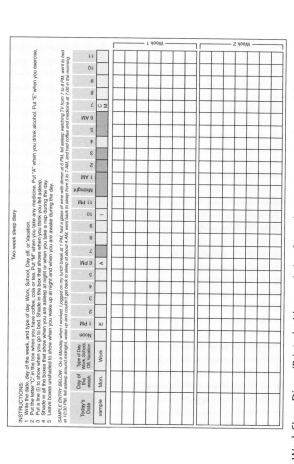

Fig. 11.1 Two-Week Sleep Diary. (Printed with permission from the American Academy of Sleep Medicine. Available from: http://sleepeducation.org/.)

with driving while undergoing a trial of sleep restriction. Once sleep efficiency is improved, total sleep time is gradually increased by 10- to 20-minute increments.

A specific type of cognitive–behavioral therapy (CBT) has been developed for insomnia (CBT-I). Patients are encouraged to identify misperceptions about sleep (e.g., I must have 9 hours of sleep). The focus is aimed at the quality of sleep rather than the number of hours slept. Other objectives of CBT-I are directed at identifying and correcting maladaptive attitudes and beliefs about sleep that perpetuate insomnia. For example, patients may rationalize behaviors such as excessive time in bed to "catch up" on lost sleep and may exhibit unrealistic expectations about sleep.

Nurse, Patient, and Family Resources

American Academy of Sleep Medicine
www.aasmnet.org

American Sleep Apnea Association
www.sleepapnea.org

American Sleep Medicine
www.americansleepmedicine.com

Centers for Disease Control and Prevention: Sleep and Sleep Disorders
www.cdc.gov/sleep/resources.html

Narcolepsy Network
www.narcolepsynetwork.org

National Sleep Foundation
www.sleepfoundation.org

Restless Legs Syndrome Foundation
www.rls.org

CHAPTER 12

Substance Use Disorders

Substance use disorders are not illnesses of choice. They are complex diseases of the brain characterized by craving, seeking, and using regardless of consequences. Continuous substance use results in changes in the brain structure and function. Substance use disorders are chronic and relapsing. Deficits in executive functioning that mediate self-control and decision making are both a risk factor for substance use and a consequence of substance use.

In 2019 about 7.7% (or about 19 million people) of the US population aged 18 or older had a substance use disorder (Substance Abuse and Mental Health Services Administration [SAMHSA], 2020). A substance use disorder is a pathological use of a substance that leads to a disorder of use. Symptoms include:

- Impaired ability to control use
- Social impairment
- Risky use
- Physical effects (i.e., addiction, intoxication, tolerance, withdrawal)

Substance use disorders encompass the use of a broad range of products that individuals take into their bodies through various means such as swallowing, inhaling, and injecting. These disorders range from fairly harmless and innocent-seeming substances such as caffeine to illegal mind-altering drugs such as lysergic acid diethylamide (LSD). No matter the substance, use disorders share many commonalities, intoxication characteristics, and withdrawal attributes.

The *Diagnostic and Statistical Manual of Mental Disorders*, 5th edition *(DSM-5)* (American Psychiatric Association [APA], 2013) provides diagnostic criteria for the following psychoactive substances:

- Alcohol
- Caffeine

- Cannabis
- Hallucinogen
- Inhalant
- Opioid
- Sedative, hypnotic, and antianxiety medication
- Stimulant
- Tobacco

In addition to substances, behaviors are also recognized as addictive. These behavioral addictions are also called process addictions. While the physical signs of drug addiction do not accompany behavioral addictions, compulsive actions activate the reward or pleasure pathways in the brain similarly to substances. The first process addiction, gambling, was established as a disorder in 2013. Excesses in internet gaming, social media use, shopping, and sexual activity are also process addictions that may be included in future *DSM* editions.

CONCEPTS CENTRAL TO SUBSTANCE USE DISORDERS

Addiction

Addiction is a chronic and progressive medical condition with roots in the environment, genetics, neurotransmission, and life experiences. Addiction is a physiological or psychological need for a habit-forming substance, activity, or behavior that results in negative consequences. Like other chronic diseases, there are cycles of relapse and remission. When the addiction is removed, there are typically well-defined withdrawal symptoms.

Intoxication

When a substance is used in excess, intoxication is experienced and a person's normal ability to act or reason is inhibited. Terminology used to describe intoxication may be different depending on the substance. For example, alcohol causes one to be drunk, while marijuana makes one high.

Tolerance

Tolerance occurs when a person experiences a diminished physical response to a substance due to repeated use. The person might never again achieve that initial high, leading them to constantly "chase the high" that was initially experienced.

Tolerance is not always synonymous with addiction. For example, individuals with chronic pain may develop tolerance to prescription medications without being addicted to them.

Withdrawal

Withdrawal is a set of symptoms that occur when a person stops using a substance. Withdrawal is specific to the substance being used, and each substance will have its own characteristic syndrome, which may be mild or life-threatening. The more intense symptoms a person has, the more likely the person is to start using the substance again to avoid the withdrawal symptoms.

This chapter focuses on substance use disorders. An overview of each major category is provided in the following sections. Nursing care for this population is then addressed.

SUBSTANCE USE DISORDERS

Caffeine

Caffeine is the most widely used psychoactive substance in the world. The typical side effects of caffeine include feeling more awake or alert; feeling restless, anxious, or irritable; increased body temperature; dehydration; headache; and increased respirations and pulse. Excessive caffeine use is not an official use disorder. However, caffeine can result in intoxication, withdrawal, and overdose.

Caffeine Intoxication

The stimulatory effects of caffeine may begin as early as 15 minutes after ingestion and last as long as 6 hours. Behavioral symptoms of caffeine intoxication include restlessness, nervousness, excitement, agitation, rambling speech, and inexhaustibility. Physical symptoms of intoxication are flushed face, diuresis, gastrointestinal disturbance, muscle twitching, tachycardia, and cardiac arrhythmia. These symptoms are distressing and result in impairment of normal areas of functioning. Individuals with tolerance are less sensitive to intoxication. Conversely, chronic use of high doses of caffeine can cause the body's stress system to produce hormones to counter the stimulation, causing a sedating response.

Caffeine Withdrawal

Removal of caffeine from daily use results in headache, drowsiness, irritability, and poor concentration. Some people experience flu-like symptoms such as nausea, vomiting, and muscle aches. Symptoms occur within 12 to 24 hours after the last dose, peak in 24 to 48 hours, and resolve within 1 week.

Caffeine Overdose

Although caffeine overdoses are rare, extremely high doses of caffeine may lead to death. With the advent of energy drinks, caffeine pills, and caffeinated alcoholic beverages more people are experiencing overdoses. Symptoms of a lethal concentration of caffeine include trouble breathing, vomiting, hallucinations, confusion, chest pain, irregular pulse, uncontrollable muscle movements, and seizures.

Overdose treatment is aimed at managing symptoms while eliminating the caffeine from the body. Activated charcoal, laxatives, or gastric lavage may be used.

Cannabis Use Disorder

Cannabis, or marijuana, comes from the dried leaves, flowers, stems, and seeds from the cannabis plant. A chemical, delta-9-tetrahydrocannabinol (THC), is responsible for its mind-altering effects.

The 12-month prevalence of cannabis use disorder in adolescents is about 3.5% and about 1.5% in adults (APA, 2013). Males are more likely to be affected.

Cannabis Intoxication

Cannabis intoxication heightens users' sensations. They experience brighter colors, see new details in common stimuli, and time seems slowl down. In higher doses, individuals may experience depersonalization and derealization. Motor skills are impacted for 8 to 12 hours, and driving and the use of machinery may be hazardous. Physical symptoms that support a diagnosis of cannabis intoxication are conjunctival injection (red eyes from vessel dilation), increased appetite, dry mouth, and tachycardia.

Cannabis Withdrawal

Withdrawal occurs within 1 week of cessation. Symptoms include irritability, anger, aggression, anxiety, restlessness, and depressed mood. Because people often use marijuana as a sleep aid, insomnia and disturbing dreams may develop without it. Decreased appetite may lead to weight loss. At least one of the following physical symptoms of withdrawal occurs: abdominal pain, shakiness, sweating, fever, chills, and headache.

Abstinence and support are the main principles of treatment for cannabis use disorder. Hospitalization or outpatient care may be required. Individual, family, and group therapies may provide support. Antianxiety medication is useful for short-term relief of withdrawal symptoms. Patients with underlying anxiety and major depressive disorder may respond to antidepressant therapy.

Hallucinogen Use Disorder

Hallucinogens cause a profound disturbance in reality. Hallucinogens are associated with flashbacks, panic attacks, psychosis, delirium, and mood and anxiety disorders. They are both natural and synthetic substances. Hallucinogens have no medical use. They are found in some plants and mushrooms, or they can be manufactured. Classic hallucinogens (e.g., LSD) and dissociative hallucinogens (e.g., phencyclidine [PCP] and ketamine) are used. A use disorder causes significant impairment or distress and results in craving, difficulty with role obligations, impairment, and tolerance.

Hallucinogen Intoxication

Intoxication is characterized by paranoia, impaired judgment, intensification of perceptions, depersonalization, and derealization. Illusions, hallucinations, and synesthesia (e.g., hearing colors or seeing sounds) are prominent. Physical symptoms include pupillary dilation, tachycardia, sweating, palpitations, blurred vision, tremors, and incoordination.

Treatment for hallucinogen intoxication includes reassurance that the symptoms are caused by the drug and that the symptoms will subside. In severe cases, an antipsychotic such as haloperidol (Haldol) or a benzodiazepine such as diazepam (Valium) can be used in the short term.

Phencyclidine Intoxication

PCP intoxication is a medical emergency. Behavioral symptoms include belligerence, assaultiveness, impulsiveness, and unpredictability. Physical symptoms include nystagmus (involuntary eye movements), hypertension, tachycardia, diminished response to pain, ataxia (loss of voluntary muscle control), dysarthria (unclear speech), muscle rigidity, seizures, coma, and hyperacusis (sensitivity to sound). Hyperthermia and seizure activity may also occur.

Patients who have ingested PCP cannot be talked down and may require restraint. Placing the patient in a quiet room with dim lights may be helpful. Mechanical cooling may be necessary for severe hyperthermia. Benzodiazepines such as lorazepam (Ativan) or diazepam (Valium) may be administered intramuscularly or intravenously to reduce hypertension, agitation, and control seizures.

Hallucinogen Withdrawal

There is no official withdrawal syndrome. However, hallucinogen-persisting perception disorder may be experienced by about 4% of users, particularly with LSD. The hallmark of this problem is the reexperiencing of perceptual symptoms that were experienced while intoxicated. These symptoms are distressing and impair the individual from normal functioning for weeks, months, or even years.

Inhalant Use Disorder

Inhalants are toxic gases inhaled through the nose or mouth and enter the bloodstream. Misused household products include:

- Solvents for glues and adhesives
- Aerosol propellant paint sprays, hair sprays, and shaving cream
- Thinners such as paint products and correction fluids
- Fuels such as gasoline and propane

Repeatedly inhaling substances results in increasing use, craving, and tolerance. Inhalant use impairs one's ability to fulfill life roles and causes problems in relationships. This disorder occurs primarily in youth, with 2.7% of adolescents between the ages of 12 and 17 being past-year users of inhalants (APA, 2013).

Inhalant Intoxication

Small doses of inhalants result in disinhibition and euphoria. High doses can cause fearfulness, illusions, auditory and visual hallucinations, and a distorted body image. Apathy, diminished social and occupational functioning, impaired judgment, impulsive behavior and aggression accompany intoxication. Physical responses include nausea, anorexia, nystagmus, depressed reflexes, and diplopia. High doses can lead to stupor, unconsciousness, and amnesia. Delirium, dementia, and psychosis are also possible outcomes of inhalant use.

Inhalant intoxication usually does not require treatment. However, serious and potentially fatal responses such as coma, cardiac arrhythmias, or bronchospasm do occur, and medical treatment is required. A psychotic response may be induced by inhalant intoxication.

Opioid Use Disorder

Opioid misuse, particularly with heroin and prescription drugs, is a chronic relapsing disorder. Cravings and tolerance are significant. The use of this substance results in significant impairment in life roles and interpersonal conflict and puts a person in physically hazardous situations.

In 2019 about 10 million people aged 12 or older misused opioids (SAMHSA, 2020). Specifically, 9.7 million people misused prescription pain relievers and 745,000 people used heroin.

Opioid use usually begins in the late teens or early 20s. Increasing age is associated with fewer affected individuals, probably due to early mortality and a cessation of use after age 40 years.

Opioid Intoxication

Opioid intoxication results in psychomotor retardation, drowsiness, slurred speech, altered mood (ranging from withdrawn to elated), and impaired memory and attention. Physical symptoms include pinpoint pupils (miosis), decreased bowel sounds, reduced respiratory rate, and normal to low heart rate. Skin disruptions in the form of track marks or fresh injection sites may confirm intravenous drug use.

Opioid Overdose

Death from an opioid overdose usually results from respiratory arrest due to respiratory depression. Symptoms include unresponsiveness, slow respiration, coma, hypothermia, hypotension, and bradycardia. Three symptoms—coma, pinpoint pupils, and respiratory depression—are strongly suggestive of overdose.

Overdose treatment begins with aspirating secretions, inserting an airway, and mechanical ventilation. Naloxone, a specific opioid antagonist, can be given intranasally, intramuscularly, or intravenously. Increased respirations and pupillary dilation happen quickly. Too much naloxone may produce withdrawal symptoms. Duration of action for naloxone is short compared with many opioids, so repeated administration may be required.

Opioid Withdrawal

Withdrawal symptoms occur after a reduction or cessation in heavy use or after an opioid antagonist has been administered. Symptoms include mood dysphoria, nausea, vomiting, diarrhea, muscle aches, fever, and insomnia. Other classic symptoms of withdrawal are lacrimation (watery eyes), rhinorrhea (runny nose), pupillary dilation, piloerection (bristling of hairs), and yawning. Males may experience sweating and spontaneous ejaculations.

Morphine, heroin, and methadone withdrawal begins at 6 to 8 hours. This withdrawal intensifies on the second or third day and then subsides during the next week. Meperidine (Demerol) withdrawal begins within 8 to 12 hours from abstinence and lasts about 5 days. See Chapter 27 for information regarding pharmacotherapy for opioid withdrawal and abstinence.

Sedative, Hypnotic, and Antianxiety Medication Use Disorder

Sedative, hypnotic, and antianxiety use disorder is applied to the misuse of all prescription sleeping medications and almost all prescription antianxiety drugs. These drugs include benzodiazepines, benzodiazepine-like drugs (e.g., zolpidem, zaleplon), carbamates, barbiturates (e.g., secobarbital), and barbiturate-like hypnotics (e.g., methaqualone). Misuse of these neural depressants negatively affects role performance and relationships. Craving, tolerance, and withdrawal can develop even when taken for their intended indication. However, a use disorder diagnosis is only given in the presence of clinically significant maladaptive behavior or psychological changes.

The 12-month prevalence of this problem is about 0.2% in adults (APA, 2013). It occurs in males slightly more often than in females. These disorders are highest among 18- to 29-year-olds (0.5%) and lowest among individuals 65 and older (0.04%).

Sedative, Hypnotic, and Antianxiety Medication Intoxication

Because they are depressants, intoxication from these drugs results in slurred speech, incoordination, unsteady gait, nystagmus, and impaired thinking. Inappropriate aggression and sexual behavior, mood fluctuation, and impaired judgment may also occur.

Sedative, Hypnotic, and Antianxiety Medication Overdose

Overdose treatment includes gastric lavage, activated charcoal, and vital sign monitoring. If conscious, patients are kept awake. If unconscious, an intravenous line is initiated. Endotracheal tubes may be required to provide a patent airway, and mechanical ventilation may be necessary.

Sedative, Hypnotic, and Antianxiety Medication Withdrawal

Repeated depression of the central nervous system, along with the body's attempts to return to homeostasis, results in rebound hyperactivity with the removal of the depressant. Hence autonomic hyperactivity, tremor, insomnia, psychomotor agitation, anxiety, and grand mal seizures may occur. The drug's half-life is an important predictor of withdrawal time.

Gradual reduction of benzodiazepines will prevent seizures and other withdrawal symptoms. Barbiturate withdrawal can be aided by using a long-acting barbiturate such as phenobarbital.

Stimulant Use Disorder

Amphetamine-type, cocaine, or other stimulant drugs are second only to cannabis as the most widely used illicit substances in the United States (SAMHSA, 2020). They typically produce a euphoric feeling and high energy. Long-distance truckers, students studying for examinations, soldiers in wartime, and athletes in competition may use these drugs. As with all use disorders, increased use, craving, and tolerance are accompanied by a reduced ability to function in major roles. Stimulants represent a significant problem, as a use disorder pattern can occur in as little as 1 week.

The estimated 12-month prevalence for amphetamine-type stimulants is about 0.2% in adults (APA, 2013). Females and males are affected equally. Intravenous stimulant use is greater in males, around 4:1. Cocaine use disorder is higher, 0.3%, with more male users.

Stimulant Intoxication

Stimulants make people feel elated, euphoric, and sociable. They also make people hypervigilant, sensitive, anxious, tense, and angry. Physical symptoms include chest pain, cardiac arrhythmias, high or low blood pressure, tachycardia or bradycardia, and respiratory depression. Other physical symptoms are evident with dilated pupils, perspiration, chills, nausea or vomiting, weight loss, psychomotor agitation or retardation, weakness, confusion, seizures, and coma.

Stimulant Withdrawal

Withdrawal symptoms begin within a few hours to several days. Symptoms include fatigue, vivid nightmares, increased appetite, insomnia or hypersomnia, and psychomotor retardation or agitation. Functionality is impaired during this period. Depression and suicidal thoughts are the most serious side effects of stimulant withdrawal.

Depending on the amphetamine used, specific drugs may be helpful in the short term during withdrawal. Antipsychotics may be prescribed for a few days. If there is no psychosis, diazepam (Valium) is useful in treating agitation and hyperactivity. Once the patient has been withdrawn from the amphetamine, major depressive symptoms can be treated with antidepressants.

For cocaine, the 1- to 2-week withdrawal period has no physiological disturbances that require inpatient care. However, hospitalization may be helpful to remove the affected individual from the usual social settings and drug sources. Some patients experience fatigue, mood changes, disturbed sleep, craving, and depression. There are no drugs that reliably reduce the intensity of these symptoms.

Tobacco Use Disorder

Craving, persistent use, and tolerance are all symptoms of tobacco use disorder. Dependence happens quickly. The 12-month prevalence of tobacco use disorder is about 13% in adults (APA, 2013). Rates are slightly higher in males compared with females. Most people who use tobacco begin before the age of 18 years.

Tobacco Withdrawal

Tobacco withdrawal is distressing and results in irritability, anxiety, depression, difficulty concentrating, restlessness, and insomnia. Within days of smoking cessation, heart rates decrease by 5 to 12 beats/minute. Within the first year of smoking cessation, people gain an average of 4 to 7 pounds.

Behavioral therapy helps patients recognize cravings and respond to them. Hypnosis is used to treat tobacco withdrawal. Nicotine replacement therapies in the form of gum, lozenges, nasal sprays, and patches are successful treatments. The antidepressant bupropion (Zyban) reduces cravings for nicotine. Varenicline (Chantix) is a nicotinic receptor partial agonist that provides mild nicotine-like effects. It also blocks the effects of nicotine from cigarettes if smoking is resumed.

Gambling Disorder

Gambling may become a compulsive activity that causes severe financial problems and significant disturbances in personal, social, or occupational functioning. Affected individuals are preoccupied with gambling, experience an increasing desire to gamble, and lie to conceal the extent of the problem. They may try to control the behavior, cut back, or stop gambling. Otherwise honest people may commit illegal acts to finance this addiction. They may rely on others to help pay off debts and gamble in an attempt to recoup losses.

The 1-year prevalence rate of gambling disorder in females is about 0.2% and in males is about 0.6% (APA, 2013). Early expression of gambling disorder is more common in males, although the progression is more rapid for females. Gambling may be regular or episodic. Heavy gambling may be interspersed with abstinence. Stress and depression may increase this behavior.

Legal problems, pressure from family, and other psychiatric illnesses may bring the person who gambles excessively into treatment. Gamblers Anonymous (GA) is a 12-step program modeled on Alcoholics Anonymous (AA). GA involves public confession, peer pressure, and peer counselors who are reformed gamblers. Hospitalization may help by removing patients from gambling environments. Individual, group, and family therapy are useful in supporting the patient.

Medications are used to decrease either the urge to gamble or the thrill involved in doing so. Antidepressants such as selective serotonin reuptake inhibitors and bupropion (Wellbutrin), mood stabilizers (lithium), and anticonvulsants such as topiramate (Topamax) may be helpful. Second-generation antipsychotics are also used. Naltrexone, an opioid antagonist, may be given to individuals with the most severe symptoms of gambling disorder.

ALCOHOL USE DISORDER

Although alcohol is a sedative, it creates an initial feeling of euphoria. This is probably related to decreased inhibitions. A cluster of behavioral and physical symptoms characterizes alcohol use disorder.

Types of Problematic Drinking

Amounts of alcohol that are considered safe vary depending on individual factors. Table 12.1 identifies the numbers of drinks that are considered acceptable depending on the gender, age, and pregnancy status.

Excessive drinking is described with two different terms: binge drinking and heavy drinking. Binge drinking

Table 12.1 **Maximum Safe Number of Drinks**

	Men	Women	Pregnant	Adolescent	Older Adults
Day	4	3	0	0	3
Week	14	7	0	0	7

National Institute on Alcohol Abuse and Alcoholism (n.d.). *What is a standard drink?* https://www.niaaa.nih.gov/alcohols-effects-health/overview-alcohol-consumption/what-standard-drink#:~:text=In%20the%20United%20States%2   C%20one,which%20is%20about%20 40%25%20alcohol refers to drinking too much alcohol quickly. This amount is four or more drinks for women and five or more drinks for men in about 2 hours. Heavy drinking is characterized by drinking too much, too often. Consuming eight or more drinks in a week constitutes heavy drinking in women. Men who drink more than 14 drinks in a week are considered heavy drinkers.

Alcohol Intoxication

In the United States, a standard drink contains about 14 g of pure alcohol (National Institute on Alcohol Abuse and Alcoholism, n.d.). This amount is found in 12 ounces of beer with 5% alcohol content, 5 ounces of wine with 12% alcohol content, and 1.5 ounces of distilled spirits with 40% alcohol content.

The legal definition of intoxication in most states requires a blood concentration of 0.08 to 0.10 g/dL. Blood alcohol levels, numbers of drinks, and symptoms of alcohol intoxication are listed in Table 12.2.

Table 12.2 **Blood Alcohol, Drinks, and Symptoms**

Blood Alcohol	Drinks	Symptoms
0.02 g/dL	2	Slower motor performance, decreased thinking ability, altered mood, and reduced ability to multitask
0.05 g/dL	3	Impaired judgment, exaggerated behavior, euphoria, and lower alertness
0.08 g/dL	4	Poor muscle coordination, altered speech and hearing, difficulty detecting danger, impaired judgment, poor self-control, and decreased reasoning
0.10 g/dL	5	Slurred speech, poor coordination, and slowed thinking
0.15 g/dL	6	Vomiting (unless high tolerance) and major loss of balance
0.20 g/dL	8–10	Memory blackouts, nausea, and vomiting
0.30 g/dL	10+	Reduction of body temperature, blood pressure, and respiratory rate; sleepiness; and amnesia
0.40 mg/dL	—	Impaired vital signs and possible death

Excessive amounts of alcohol may result in blackouts in which new memories cannot be consolidated. During blackouts, a person actively engages in behaviors, can perform complicated tasks, and may appear normal.

Alcohol Withdrawal

Alcohol withdrawal occurs after reducing or quitting alcohol after heavy and prolonged use. A summary of symptoms is provided here. See Chapter 27 for a more thorough discussion of alcohol withdrawal and treatment.

- The classic sign of alcohol withdrawal is tremulousness, commonly called the shakes or the jitters, which begins 6 to 8 hours after alcohol cessation.
- Mild-to-moderate alcohol withdrawal includes agitation, lack of appetite, nausea, vomiting, insomnia, impaired cognition, and mild perceptual changes. Both systolic and diastolic blood pressure increase, as do pulse and body temperature.
- Psychotic and perceptual symptoms may begin in 8 to 10 hours. Patients undergoing withdrawal to the point of psychosis should be treated promptly because of the risks of unconsciousness, seizures, and delirium.
- Withdrawal seizures may occur within 12 to 24 hours after alcohol cessation. These seizures are generalized and tonic-clonic.
- Alcohol withdrawal delirium or delirium tremens (DTs) may happen anytime in the first 72 hours. This is a medical emergency that may be fatal in untreated patients, usually as a result of pneumonia, renal disease, hepatic insufficiency, or heart failure. Autonomic hyperactivity is accompanied by delusions and visual and tactile hallucinations.

Cognitive Disturbances

Wernicke–Korsakoff Syndrome. Heavy alcohol use may result in a memory-reducing problem called Wernicke's (alcoholic) encephalopathy, an acute and reversible condition. It is characterized by altered gait, vestibular dysfunction, confusion, and several ocular motility abnormalities. Sluggish reaction to light and anisocoria (unequal pupil size) are also symptoms. Wernicke's encephalopathy responds rapidly to large doses of intravenous thiamine two to three times daily for 1 to 2 weeks.

Untreated Wernicke's encephalopathy may progress into Korsakoff's syndrome, the more severe and chronic version of this problem. Treatment for Korsakoff's syndrome is thiamine for 3 to 12 months. Most patients with Korsakoff's syndrome never fully recover, although cognitive improvement may occur with thiamine and nutritional support.

Fetal Alcohol Syndrome

Alcohol use during pregnancy is the most common cause of intellectual disability in the United States. The condition in the infant is known as fetal alcohol syndrome. Alcohol during pregnancy inhibits intrauterine growth and postnatal development resulting in microcephaly, craniofacial malformations, and limb and heart defects. As adults, affected individuals tend to have a short stature. Pregnant women with alcohol-related disorders have a significant risk of having a child with defects.

Systemic Effects

Alcohol overuse results in damage to just about every system in the body. Conditions associated with alcohol use disorder include the following:
- Peripheral neuropathy
- Alcoholic myopathy
- Alcoholic cardiomyopathy
- Esophagitis
- Gastritis
- Cirrhosis of the liver
- Leukopenia
- Thrombocytopenia
- Cancer
- Pancreatitis
- Alcoholic hepatitis

ASSESSMENT

A substance use assessment is part of a more comprehensive assessment that evaluates the individual holistically. Ideally, this assessment involves an addiction professional with specialized knowledge and skills to make a diagnosis. The Screening, Brief Intervention, and Referral to Treatment (SBIRT) is a comprehensive, integrated, public health approach to the delivery of early intervention and treatment services for persons with substance use disorders, as well as those who are at risk of developing these disorders. SBIRT identifies at-risk substance users for early intervention (SAMHSA, 2021) and consists of three major components:

- Screening: A nurse or other health care professional in any health care setting assesses the severity of substance use and identifies the appropriate level of treatment.
- Brief Intervention: A nurse or other health care professional focuses on increasing insight and awareness regarding substance use and motivation toward behavioral change.
- Referral to Treatment: A nurse or other health care professional provides those identified as needing more extensive treatment with access to specialty care.

Assessment Tool

A variety of other screening tools are available to assist health care practitioners in gaining important information on which to base plans of care. A simple, crosscutting measure for most misused substances is provided in Table 12.3.

Table 12.3 **CAGE* Questions Adapted to Include Drug Use (CAGE-AID)**

Item	0 = No 1 = Yes
1. Have you ever felt you ought to cut down on your drinking or drug use?	
2. Have people annoyed you by criticizing your drinking or drug use?	
3. Have you felt bad or guilty about your drinking or drug use?	
4. Have you ever had a drink or used drugs first thing in the morning to steady your nerves or to get rid of a hangover (eye-opener)?	
Total	

Scoring: Item responses on the CAGE questions are scored 0 for "no" and 1 for "yes" answers, with a higher score being an indication of alcohol problems. A total score of two or greater is considered clinically significant.

*Cut down, annoyed, guilty, and eye opener.

ASSESSMENT GUIDELINES

A. Is immediate medical attention necessary for a severe or major withdrawal syndrome? For example, alcohol and sedative use can be life-threatening during a major withdrawal.
B. Is the patient experiencing an overdose of a substance that requires immediate medical attention? For example, opioids or depressants can cause respiratory depression, coma, and death.
C. Does the patient have physical complications related to substance use (e.g., acquired immunodeficiency syndrome [AIDS], abscess, tachycardia, hepatitis)?
D. Does the patient have suicidal thoughts or indicate, through verbal or nonverbal cues, a potential for self-destructive behaviors?
E. Does the patient seem interested in doing something about the substance use problem?

Nursing Diagnoses

Nurses care for patients with substance use disorders in a variety of settings and situations. Some conditions call for medical interventions and skilled nursing care, whereas others call for effective use of communication and counseling skills. Use of substances can cause intoxication, overdose, and withdrawal, making *risk for injury* a priority nursing diagnosis.

Patients often have difficulty taking care of their health in areas such as finances, nutrition, sleep, and coping skills. The nursing diagnoses *impaired health maintenance* and *impaired coping* are important. Also, given that individuals have difficulty viewing their use as a problem, the nursing diagnosis *denial* is essential.

INTERVENTION GUIDELINES

A. Support the patient during detoxification.
B. Assess for feelings of hopelessness, helplessness, and suicidal thinking.
C. Determine whether the patient is being treated for a comorbid physical condition (e.g., liver disease or infections) or psychiatric condition (e.g., depression or panic attacks).
D. Intervene with the patient's use of denial, rationalization, projection, and other defenses that interfere with motivation for change.

E. Involve family members and support them. Be aware that they may minimize the problem or enable the patient.

F. Emphasize abstinence.

G. Provide referrals to self-help groups (e.g., AA, Narcotics Anonymous [NA], Cocaine Anonymous [CA]) or a recovery program early in treatment.

H. Teach the patient to avoid medications that may be habit forming such as antianxiety agents or pain medications.

I. Emphasize personal responsibility, placing control within the patient's grasp.

J. Support residential treatment when appropriate, particularly for patients with multiple relapses.

K. Provide support if the patient relapses.

L. Provide education on the physical and psychological consequences of substance use.

M. Provide verbal and written education regarding pharmacotherapy for addictions (e.g., naltrexone or methadone to help prevent relapse in alcoh use disorder and narcotic addiction).

Nursing Care for Substance Use Disorders

Risk for Injury

Related to

- Neurological dysfunction
- Perceptual alteration, loss, or disorientation
- Chemical toxicity (e.g., poisons, drugs, alcohol, nicotine, pharmacological agents)
- Impaired judgment (disease, drugs, reality testing, risk-taking behaviors)
- Substance withdrawal
- Severe and panic levels of anxiety and agitation
- Potential for electrolyte imbalance or seizures
- Hallucinations (bugs, animals, snakes)
- Elevated temperature, pulse, and respirations
- Agitation, trying to escape, or climb out of bed
- Combative behaviors
- Misinterpretation of reality (illusions)

Desired Outcome The patient will remain free from injury.

Assessment/Interventions and *Rationales*

1. Take vital signs frequently, at least every 15 minutes until stable, and then every hour for 4 to 8 hours

according to hospital protocol or care provider's order. *Withdrawal from depressants, particularly alcohol, can result in significant and dangerous autonomic hyperactivity. Pulse is a strong indicator of impending DTs, signaling the need for more rigorous sedation.*

2. Provide the patient with a quiet room with limited environmental stimulation, such as a single room near the nurses' station if possible. *Low stimulation reduces irritability and confusion.*

3. Approach the patient in a calm and reassuring manner. *Patients need to feel that others are in control and that they are safe.*

4. Use simple, concrete language and directions. *The patient is able to follow simple commands but unable to process complex or abstract ideas.*

5. Orient the patient to time, place, and person during periods of confusion. Point out the patient's progress during periods of lucidity. *Fluctuating levels of consciousness occur during intoxication, withdrawal, and overdose of some drugs. Orientation can help reduce anxiety.*

6. Institute seizure precautions according to hospital protocol as needed. *Seizures might occur during intoxication, overdose, and withdrawal, and precautions for patient safety are a priority.*

7. Carefully monitor intake and output. Check for dehydration or overhydration. *Dehydration can aggravate electrolyte imbalance. Overhydration can lead to congestive heart failure.*

8. If hallucinations are present, let the patient know that although they seem real, that you cannot hear/see them. Offer to stay with the patient to provide support (e.g., "I don't see rats on the wall. You sound frightened right now. I will stay with you for a few minutes."). *Instilling reasonable doubt as to the reality of the hallucinations is supportive when carefully presented. Staying nearby a frightened patient provides reassurance.*

9. If the patient is experiencing illusions, correct the patient's misinterpretation in a calm and matter-of-fact manner (e.g., "This is not a snake around my neck ready to bite you, it is my stethoscope…let me show you."). *Illusions can be explained to a patient who is misinterpreting environmental cues. When the patient recognizes normal objects for what they are, anxiety is reduced.*

10. Administer medications ordered to treat use disorders, intoxication, overdose, and withdrawal. *Medication can reverse uncomfortable responses and prevent mortality when treating responses to use disorders.*

11. Use the least restrictive environment to maintain safety. Restraints and seclusion are used with caution if the patient is combative. Always follow unit protocol. *Myocardial infarction, cardiac collapse, and death have occurred when patients have fought against restraints.*

12. Maintain frequent, accurate documentation of the patient's vital signs, behaviors, medications, interventions, and effects of interventions. *Documentation provides a record of progress, identifies what works best, and alerts for potential complications.*

Impaired Health Maintenance
Related to
- Neurological dysfunction
- Inability to make appropriate judgments
- Ineffective coping skills
- Perceptual or cognitive impairment
- Focus on obtaining and using the drug
- Finances depleted because of substance use leaving little or none left for health care, nourishing food, or safe shelter
- Poor nutrition related to prolonged drug binges, taking drug instead of eating nourishing food, or diminished appetite related to choice of drug (e.g., cocaine)
- Malabsorption of nutrients caused by chronic alcohol use
- Sleep deprivation related to decreased rapid eye movement (REM) sleep as a result of use of stimulants, alcohol, or central nervous system depressants
- Lack of regular health care (e.g., mammograms, dentist, yearly physicals) because of either being intoxicated, being hung-over, or withdrawing from an illicit substance

Desired Outcome The patient will demonstrate improved health maintenance.

Assessment/Interventions and *Rationales*
1. Encourage small feedings if appropriate. Check nutritional status (e.g., conjunctiva, body weight, eating history). *Pale conjunctiva can signal anemia. If the patient*

has a loss of appetite, small feedings are better tolerated. Bland foods are often more appealing.

2. Monitor fluid intake and output. Check skin turgor and ankle edema. As ordered, perform a urine-specific gravity if skin turgor is poor. *Patients can have potentially serious electrolyte imbalances. Deficient fluid intake can cause or signal renal problems. If the patient is retaining too much fluid, congestive heart failure may result.*

3. When skin turgor is poor, encourage fluids that contain protein and vitamins (e.g., milk, milkshakes/smoothies, juices). *Proteins and vitamins help build nutritional status.*

4. Promote rest and sleep by providing a quiet environment. *Restorative rest and sleep are disrupted during substance use. Sleep hygiene measures are emphasized during recovery.*

5. Explore the patient's understanding of the detrimental impact of alcohol or substances use (e.g., fetal alcohol syndrome, hepatitis or AIDS, fertility issues). *Before teaching, the nurse must identify what the patient knows about the drugs and evaluate readiness to learn. Patient education allows for personal control over health care.*

6. Review the patient's blood work and physical examination results and discuss these findings with the patient. *Assessment informations helps the nurse identify potential causes of symptoms [e.g., infection] and initiate counseling. Sharing this information allows the patient to take an active role in health care.*

7. Set up an appointment for medical follow-up and encourage the patient to record the event on a calendar, cell phone, or appointment book. If possible, follow up reminders through calls, e-mails, and texts. *Follow-up is essential in monitoring physical status. Concrete reminders increase the likelihood of appointments being kept.*

Denial
Related to
- Substance use or process addiction and a need to maintain the status quo
- Fear of acknowledging the destructiveness of the substance or process
- Feelings of hopelessness and helplessness without the substance
- Ineffective coping strategies

Desired Outcome The patient will acknowledge and demonstrate responsibility for behavior.

Assessment/Interventions and *Rationales*

1. Maintain an interested, nonjudgmental, and supportive approach. *A professional and caring approach based on a therapeutic relationship is most effective.*

2. Initially, focus on reducing or eliminating high levels of anxiety due to current crisis situations. *Patients are unable to address higher-level needs while experiencing situational anxiety [e.g., practical living problems, family crisis].*

3. Avoid criticizing the patient's behaviors. *Disapproval is a nontherapeutic approach to communication with a patient. These reactions will only make the patient more defensive.*

4. Suggest the role of denial in continuing addictive behaviors. *Denial is a primary obstacle to seeking treatment for addictive behaviors.*

5. Explore goals and what the patient wants to change. *Initially, the patient's goal might not be abstinence. Identifying areas the patient wants to change gives the patient a motivation to change.*

6. Use of miracle questions can help identify what patients want to change. For example, "What if your worst problem were miraculously solved overnight. What would be different about your life the next day?" *Miracle questions help patients perceive their future without some of their problems and give direction to moving forward and identifying long- and short-term goals.*

7. Encourage the patient to explore the pros and cons of substance use. *Analyzing the pros and cons helps the patient look at what substances will and will not do for them in a clear light. This analysis may help strengthen personal motives for change.*

8. Encourage the patient to explore the relationship between external problems (e.g., relationships, job-related, legal) and substance use. *Denial of the destructive nature of addiction is a major component of addiction. Patients may gradually view external problems as the result of addictive behaviors and not the cause.*

9. Assist the patient to identify behaviors that have contributed to problems (e.g., family dysfunction, social difficulties, job-related problems, legal difficulties). *When individuals take responsibility for maladaptive*

behaviors, they are more prepared to take responsibility for learning effective and satisfying behaviors.

10. Encourage the patient to stay in the here and now (e.g., "Let's focus on how you want to respond when you feel criticized by your boss"). *Focusing on past disappointments is not useful to developing new and more adaptive coping methods.*

11. Encourage the patient to find a sponsor within a 12-step program or another therapeutic mode. *Having a sponsor and being a sponsor support success.*

12. Assist the patient to identify times of vulnerability to substance use and strategies to use at those times. *Considering alternative strategies to drinking or taking drugs in vulnerable situations gives the patient a ready choice.*

13. Encourage family and friends to seek support, education, and ways to recognize and refrain from enabling the patient's substance use. *Enabling behavior supports the patient's use of drugs by taking away incentive for change.*

14. Educate the patient and family regarding the physical and neurological effects of the substance or process, potential treatment, and aftercare. *Education allows the patient to take responsibility for personal care. Educating the family provides clarity for them and, ideally, support for the patient.*

15. Recognize that treatment is a long process. *Patience and external support help the patient make a commitment to treatment.*

16. Refer and encourage the patient to attend a 12-step support group, recovery program, or residential program. *External supports are effective tools in overcoming addiction.*

17. Attend several open meetings in your local community. *Attending the meeting helps the nurse understand how the 12-step fellowship process works.*

Impaired Coping
Related to
- Neurological dysfunction
- Inadequate resources
- Disturbance in pattern of stress management
- Inadequate level of or perception of control
- Knowledge deficit

- Coping styles no longer adaptive in present situations
- Insufficient social support

Desired Outcome The patient will report and demonstrate improved coping.

Assessment/Interventions and *Rationales*
1. Set small, easy to reach goals in the beginning of treatment. *Patients with substance use problems have mild-to-moderate cognitive deficits while using substances, deficits which may continue months after sobriety.*
2. Encourage the patient to write notes and self-memos (e.g., enter them into a smartphone or computer calendar) to help keep appointments and follow the treatment plan. *Cognition usually gets better with long-term abstinence, but initially memory aids prove helpful.*
3. Encourage the patient to join relapse prevention groups. *Attending these groups helps the patient anticipate and rehearse healthy responses to stressful situations.*
4. Encourage the patient to identify or find role models (e.g., peers in recovery). *Role models increase motivation and hope for recovery by abstaining from substance use.*
5. Help the patient to identify triggers for substance use (e.g., people, feelings, situations) that help drive the patient's addiction. *Identifying triggers to substance use supports change and targets areas for acquiring new skills.*
6. Practice and role-play alternative responses to triggers for substance use. *Increases patient confidence of handling drug triggers effectively.*
7. Give positive feedback when the patient applies new and effective responses to difficult trigger situations. *Validates the patient's positive steps toward growth and change.*
8. Address denial throughout recovery. *Denial can interfere with sobriety during all stages of recovery.*
9. Explore coping in these areas: (1) personal issues (e.g., relationships), (2) social issues (e.g., family violence, unemployment), and (3) feelings of self-worth. *In the absence of substance use, healing and growth in other areas of life can be accomplished.*
10. Recommend family therapy. *Enhanced strategies for dealing with family conflict are essential to recovery. Family therapy also improves the family's sense of empowerment and increase's familial support.*
11. Stress that substance use is a disease of the entire family. *Family members also need encouragement and support.*

12. Discuss the potential for relapse and reaffirm the patient's ability to attain sobriety. *Reaffirmation helps minimize shame and guilt and rebuild self-esteem.*

TREATMENT MODALITIES FOR SUBSTANCE USE DISORDERS

Biological Treatment

Pharmacotherapy

Pharmacotherapy for substance use withdrawal and abstinence varies depending on the substance. Pharmacological treatments for substance use disorders are provided in Chapter 27.

Psychological Therapies

Cognitive–behavioral therapy (CBT) and motivational interviewing are commonly used evidence-based therapies for substance use disorders. CBT helps patients explore destructive and negative thinking patterns so that the core belief system and any irrational core beliefs can be identified. Positive and negative consequences of substance use are explored. Patients learn to self-monitor their cravings and challenge these cravings realistically. Chapter 27 provides more information about CBT.

Motivational interviewing is an approach based on the transtheoretical or stages of change theory. It has gained popularity in its use as a brief, long-term, and supplementary intervention, particularly in the treatment of substance use disorders. It uses a person-centered approach to strengthen motivation for change.

Twelve-Step Programs

Twelve-step programs are peer aid groups for the purpose of recovery from substance addictions, behavioral addictions, and compulsions. AA, founded in 1930, is the oldest and most well-known of the 12-step programs. Anyone with the desire to quit drinking or using substances is welcome to attend meetings. Individuals learn how to be sober through the support of other members and the 12 steps. In most suburban and urban areas, meetings can be found every day around the clock. Virtual meetings are also available online.

All groups are structured for confidentiality and anonymity. Family members and other support are often welcome.

There are also meetings to address the special needs of family and significant others, such as Al-Anon for friends and family members and Alateen for teenage relatives. Other substance-based support groups include Narcotics Anonymous (NA), Pills Anonymous (PA), Cocaine Anonymous (CA), and others.

Nurse, Patient, and Family Resources

Addictions.com
www.addictions.com

Alcoholics Anonymous
www.aa.org

Al-Anon
www.al-anon.org

Cocaine Anonymous
www.ca.org

Center for Substance Abuse Treatment (CSAT) National Drug Helpline (bilingual)
1-800-662-HELP (4357)

Marijuana Anonymous
www.marijuana-anonymous.org

Nar-Anon Family Groups
www.nar-anon.org

Narcotics Anonymous
www.na.org

National Association for Children of Alcoholics
www.nacoa.org

National Institute on Drug Abuse (NIDA)
www.drugabuse.gov/

National Mental Health Consumers' Self-Help Clearinghouse
www.mhselfhelp.org/

CHAPTER 13

Neurocognitive Disorders

The clarity and purpose of an individual's journey in life depend in large part on the ability to reflect on its meaning. Disturbances in cognitive processing cloud or cut short the meaning of the journey. Cognition represents a fundamental human feature that distinguishes living from existing.

Cognitive processes function on two hierarchical domains. Lower-level cognitive domains include the attention and orientation to the environment as well as the recognition of previously acquired information. Higher-level cognitive domains are more complex and include the following:

- Sustained attention and information processing
- Planning, decision making, problem solving, and abstract thinking (i.e., executive function)
- Learning and memory, including retention, recall, and immediate and long-term memory
- Using of language, both expressive and receptive
- Perceiving and navigating the environment through motor and visual senses (e.g., using a fork/spoon)
- Processing, storing, and applying information about other people and social situations (i.e., social cognition)

Psychiatric disorders have a profound impact on cognitive functioning. The three main neurocognitive classifications in the *Diagnostic and Statistical Manual of Mental Disorders*, 5th edition (*DSM-5*) are delirium, mild neurocognitive disorders, and major neurocognitive disorders (American Psychiatric Association [APA], 2013).

In this chapter, delirium, which is an acute and reversible condition affecting lower-level functioning, is discussed and nursing care is addressed. Mild and major neurocognitive disorders, where there is a decline in higher-level cognitive functioning, are then discussed. Mild neurocognitive disorders may or may not progress to the major type. Major neurocognitive disorders, commonly referred to as dementia, are progressive and irreversible.

DELIRIUM

Delirium is an acute cognitive disturbance that is usually reversible. It is common in patients who are hospitalized, especially older patients. Delirium is characterized as a syndrome, that is, a constellation of symptoms rather than a disorder. The chief symptoms of delirium are an inability to direct, focus, sustain, and shift attention; an abrupt onset with clinical features that fluctuate with periods of lucidity; and disorganized thinking. Other characteristics include disorientation (often to time and place, but rarely to person), anxiety, agitation, poor memory, and delusional thinking. When hallucinations are present, they are usually visual. These visual hallucinations can be formed (e.g., people, animals) or unformed (e.g., spots, flashes of light).

Epidemiology

About 10% to 30% of all general hospital patients develop delirium. In older frail individuals, the prevalence of delirium can be as high as 60% (Siddiqi et al., 2016). In critically ill patients, the prevalence varies from 20% to 84% (Herling et al., 2018).

Risk Factors

Delirium is always related to underlying physiological causes. These underlying causes put a patient at risk for developing delirium, and there are immediate factors that precipitate the syndrome. The interaction of the two results in delirium. The risk factors that are modifiable through nursing care are listed in Box 13.1.

ASSESSMENT GUIDELINES

A. Do not assume that acute confusion in an older person is due to dementia.
B. Assess for acute onset and fluctuating levels of awareness.
C. Assess the person's ability to attend to the immediate environment, including responses to nursing care.

Box 13.1 **Risk Factors for Delirium**

- Pain
- Infection
- Dehydration
- Hypoxia
- Immobilization
- Poor or inadequate nutrition
- Environmental noise, lack of orienting material (e.g., calendars, clocks, whiteboards), movement to new area
- Sleep deprivation
- Lack of eyeglasses or hearing aids
- Restraint use

D. Establish the person's usual level of cognition by talking with family or other caregivers.
E. Assess for past cognitive impairment—especially an existing dementia diagnosis—and other risk factors.
F. Identify disturbances in physiological status, especially infection, hypoxia, and pain.
G. Identify physiological abnormalities documented in the patient's record.
H. Assess vital signs, level of consciousness, and neurological signs.
I. Assess potential for injury, especially in relation to potential for falls and wandering.
J. Maintain comfort measures, especially in relation to pain, cold, or positioning.
K. Monitor situational factors that worsen or improve symptoms.

INTERVENTION GUIDELINES

A. Delirium is transitory when treated and if delirium does not last a prolonged period of time. Immediate intervention for the underlying cause of the delirium is needed to prevent irreversible damage to the brain. Medical interventions are the first priority.
B. Safety becomes a priority since confusion and fear may make patients more prone to accidents.
C. Since delirium is a terrifying experience, preventive counseling and education after recovery from acute delirium are helpful.

D. Avoid the use of restraints, which are themselves risk factors for developing delirium.

Nursing Care for Delirium

Delirium

Related to
- Neurological dysfunction
- Medical condition (e.g., urinary tract infection, pneumonia)
- Fluid and electrolyte imbalance
- Substance use or intoxication
- Substance withdrawal
- Toxin exposure

Desired Outcomes The patient will be free from symptoms of delirium.

Assessment/Interventions and *Rationales*

1. Introduce yourself and call patient by name at the beginning of each contact. *With short-term memory impairment the patient is often confused and needs reintroductions and orienting.*

2. Maintain face-to-face contact. *If the patient is easily distracted, this helps focus on one stimulus at a time.*

3. Use short, simple, concrete phrases. *The patient is not able to process complex information.*

4. Briefly explain everything you are going to do before doing it. *Even if you are not sure that the patient is comprehending your explanation, this explanation reduces misinterpretation of actions and provides a reassuring reminder of your presence.*

5. Encourage the patient's family and friends to provide a non-stimulating and supportive presence one at a time. *A familiar presence lowers anxiety and increases orientation. Many visitors at one time can be a distraction and anxiety provoking.*

6. Keep the room well lit, preferably with windows, during the day and darken the room at night if possible. *Lighting that mirrors the 24-hour cycle of light and darkness will help preserve circadian rhythms and promote a normal sleep cycle and increase orientation.*

7. Keep environmental noise to a minimum (e.g., television, visitors). *Noise interferes with rest and can be misconstrued as something frightening or threatening.*

8. Keep the head of the bed elevated. *This position can help provide important visual cues and minimize illusions.*

9. Provide clocks, calendars, and whiteboards with information about caregivers and activities.. *These cues help orient the patient to time.*

10. Encourage and help the patient to wear prescribed eyeglasses or hearing aids. *This intervention is often overlooked because the patient does not seem to miss these sensory aids. However, wearing glasses or hearing aids supports accurate perceptions of visual and auditory stimuli.*

11. When possible, assign the same personnel on each shift to care for patient. *Familiar faces minimize confusion and enhance nurse–patient relationships.*

12. When hallucinations are present, assure patients that they are safe (e.g., "I know you are frightened. I'll sit with you a while and make sure you are safe."). *The patient feels reassured, and fear and anxiety often decrease.*

13. When illusions are present, clarify reality (e.g., "This is a coat rack, not a man with a knife…see?"). *With illusions, misinterpreted objects or sounds can be clarified when pointed out.*

14. Update and reorient the patient of progress during lucid intervals. *Consciousness and lucidity may fluctuate during delirium. When oriented, the patient feels less anxious.*

15. Ignore insults and name-calling, and acknowledge how upset the person might be feeling. For example:
    Patient: "You are an incompetent idiot! Get me a real nurse, someone who knows what they are doing."
    Nurse: "What you are going through is very difficult. I'll stay with you." *Feelings of fear are often projected onto the environment. Arguing or becoming defensive only increases the patient's anger and aggressive behaviors. Support and reassurance will decrease anxiety.*

16. If the patient's behavior becomes physically assaultive:
    a. First, set limits on behavior (e.g., "Mr. Jones, you may not hit me or anyone else. Tell me how you feel." "Mr. Jones, if you have difficulty controlling your actions, we will help you gain control.").
    b. Second, check orders for medication to reduce agitation.
    c. Finally, if the patient's behavior becomes extreme and dangerous to the patient or others, you may need to consider obtaining an order for physical restraints.

Clear limits need to be set to protect the patient, staff, and others. Sometiems the patient cannot respond to verbal requests. Chemical and physical restraints are used as a last resort.

17. After the patient returns to a premorbid cognitive state, educate and offer counseling for frightening memories and images. *Patients will have varied recollections of the events that occurred during states of delirium. The patient may believe that illusions or hallucinations were real. Developing a realistic narrative is an important part of healing.*

MILD AND MAJOR NEUROCOGNITIVE DISORDERS

Dementia is a broad term used to describe deterioration and global impairment of cognitive functioning. It is a term that does not refer to specific disease but rather to a collection of symptoms. The *DSM-5* incorporates forms of dementia into the diagnostic categories of mild and major neurocognitive disorders. When mild, impairments do not interfere with essential activities of daily living, although the person may need to make extra efforts. These impairments may or may not progress to a major neurocognitive disorder.

While the remainder of this chapter focuses on Alzheimer's disease (AD), nursing care is essentially the same with other dementia disorders. A brief description of the various forms of dementia is listed in Table 13.1.

ALZHEIMER'S DISEASE

AD, the most common cause of dementia, is a devastating disease. It not only impacts the person experiencing it, but also results in a tremendous emotional toll and burden for the families and caregivers. AD is classified according to the stage of the degenerative process: mild, moderate, and severe. The first stage roughly corresponds to the *DSM-5* criteria for mild neurocognitive disorders. Stages two and three correspond to the *DSM-5* criteria for major neurocognitive disorder. Table 13.2 describes the stages of AD.

Epidemiology

Although Alzheimer's disease can occur at a younger age (early onset), most of those affected are 65 years of age or

Table 13.1 **Common Types of Dementia**

Type of Dementia	Symptoms
Alzheimer's disease (60%–80% of dementias)	Early: difficulty remembering recent conversations, names, or events; apathy; and depression Middle: Impaired communication, disorientation, confusion, poor judgment, and behavioral changes Late: Difficulty speaking, swallowing, and walking
Cerebrovascular disease (5%–10% of dementias)	One or more documented cerebrovascular events; impaired judgment; poor decision making, planning' and organizing; slow gait; and poor balance
Frontotemporal lobar degeneration (<10% of dementias)	Onset is usually between 45 and 64 years old; marked changes in personality, disinhibition, and difficulty with communication
Lewy body disease (5%–10% of dementias)	Same as Alzheimer's disease but includes sleep disturbance, visual hallucinations, movement, and visuospatial impairment
Parkinson's disease dementia	Change in memory, cognition, and judgment; visual hallucinations; paranoid delusions; depression; irritability; and rapid eye movement sleep disorder
Mixed pathologies	Brain changes of more than one cause of dementia are apparent; over 50% of patients with dementia have more than one cause.

older (late onset). An estimated 6.2 million in the United States age 65 and older were living with Alzheimer's dementia in 2021 (Alzheimer's Association, 2021). Seventy-two percent are age 75 or older. Two-thirds of individuals with dementia are women.

Risk Factors

There is an increased risk for individuals with an affected immediate family member. There are also some rare genetic mutations that guarantee that a person will develop AD. Cardiovascular disease and head injury/traumatic brain injury also contribute to the development of AD and other

Table 13.2 **Stages of Alzheimer's Disease**

Mild Alzheimer's Disease (Early Stage)

Noticeable memory lapses. May still function independently but will experience:

- Difficulty remembering correct words or names
- Trouble remembering names when introduced to new people
- Challenges in performing tasks in social or work settings
- Forgetting what they have just read
- Losing or misplacing valuable objects
- Difficulty with planning or organizing

Moderate Alzheimer's Disease (Middle Stage)

Confuses words, gets frustrated or angry, or acts in unexpected ways such as refusing to bathe. Symptoms become noticeable to others, and these. Individuals may:

- Forget events or their personal history
- Become moody or withdrawn, especially in socially or mentally challenging situations
- Be unable to recall their address, phone number, or the school from which they graduated
- Become confused about where they are or what day it is
- Need help choosing appropriate clothing for the season or the occasion
- Change sleep patterns, such as sleeping during the day and becoming restless at night
- Be at risk of wandering and becoming lost
- Become suspicious, delusional, or compulsive

Severe Alzheimer's Disease (Late Stage)

Loses the ability to respond to the environment, to carry on a conversation, and, eventually, to control movement. May still say words or phrases. Personality changes occur. The person may:

- Require full-time, around-the-clock assistance with daily activities and personal care
- Lose awareness of recent experiences and surroundings
- Experience changes in physical abilities, including the ability to walk, sit, and, eventually, swallow
- Have increasing difficulty communicating
- Become vulnerable to infections, especially pneumonia

Adapted from Alzheimer's Association. (2019). *Stages of Alzheimer's.* https://www.alz.org/alzheimers-dementia/stages

dementias. Modifiable factors that reduce risk include engaging in mentally stimulating activities, physical exercise, social engagement, healthy diet, and sufficient sleep.

Assessment

Signs and Symptoms

- Memory impairment, usually short-term memory first
- Loss of executive functioning (i.e., the ability organize, plan, and carry out a tasks efficiently)
- The A's of Alzheimer's:
  Amnesia: Memory loss
  Aphasia: Word loss with impaired communication, language disturbance, difficulty finding words, using words incorrectly
  Apraxia: Motor loss with the inability to carry out activities despite motor functions being intact (e.g., putting on clothes)
  Agnosia: Sensory loss with an inability to recognize or identify familiar objects (e.g., a toothbrush) or sounds (e.g., telephone ringing)
  Agraphia: Loss of the ability to write
  Alexia: Loss of the ability to read
  Anomia: inability to find the right word
- Gradual decline in previous level of functioning
- Poor judgment
- Mood disturbances, anxiety, hallucinations, delusions
- Impaired sleep

Assessment Tools

A variety of tools are available to measure mental status in individuals with dementia. The Montreal Cognitive Assessment (MOCA) is an evidence-based tool to detect cognitive changes in the early stages of dementia. The tool is provided in Fig. 13.1.

ASSESSMENT GUIDELINES

Because the symptoms of other problems may look like neurocognitive disorders, determine whether the patient has symptoms or a history of such problems as major depressive disorder, substance use, or delirium (e.g., urinary tract infections). Box 13.2 lists potential diagnostic tests to rule out other problems.

A. Evaluate the current level of cognitive and daily functioning.
B. Evaluate the safety of the home environment if possible (e.g., with regard to wandering, eating inedible objects, falling, hostile behaviors toward others).

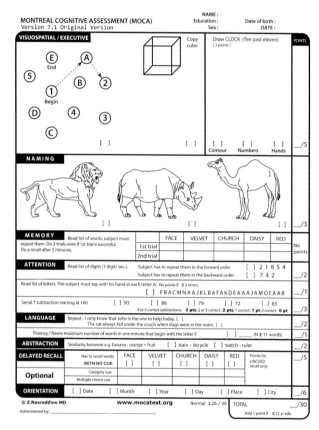

Fig. 13.1 Montreal Cognitive Assessment (MOCA). From Nasreddine, Z. S., Phillips, N. A., Bedirian, V., Charbonneau, S., Whitehead, V., Collin, I. et al. (2005). The Montreal Cognitive Assessment, MoCA: A brief screening tool for mild cognitive impairment. *Journal of the American Geriatric Society, 53*(4), 695–699.

C. Review medications, including herbs and complementary therapy and distress.
D. Ask the family to describe the patient background and personality.
E. Identify the needs of the family for teaching and guidance.
F. Assess the level of family coping.
G. Review the resources available to the family.

Box 13.2 **Diagnostic Tests to Rule Out Other Problems**

- Chest x-ray
- Electrocardiograph (ECG)
- Urinalysis
- Basic metabolic panel
- Complete blood count (CBC)
- Sequential multiple analyzers: 13-test serum profile
- Liver panel
- B12 and folate levels
- Thyroid function studies
- Venereal disease research laboratories (VDRL)
- Human immunodeficiency (HIV) tests
- Serum creatinine assay
- Electrolyte assessment
- Vision and hearing evaluation
- Neuroimaging (computed tomography [CT], magnetic resonance imaging [MRI] and positron emission tomography [PET])

INTERVENTION GUIDELINES

A. Educate the patient's family on safety measures for the impaired family member living at home (see Box 13.3):
   1. Precautions for wandering (e.g., identification bracelet, complex locks on top of doors)
   2. Home safety (e.g., eliminating slippery rugs, labeling of rooms and drawers, grab bars in showers and bathtubs)
   3. Guidelines on maintaining optimal nutrition, bowel and bladder habits, optimal sleep patterns, and optimizing activities of daily living
B. Support the family's use of effective communication strategies:
   1. Alternate methods of communication when a patient is aphasic (e.g., give the person time to speak; use drawings, gestures, writing, and facial expressions in addition to speech; use yes and no questions)
   2. Basic communication techniques for patients who are confused (e.g., re-introduce yourself; use simple, short sentences; maintain eye contact; focus on one topic at a time; talk about familiar and simple topics)

Box 13.3 **Home Safety for Individuals With Cognitive Impairment**

Avoid Injury During Daily Activities
Install walk-in showers.
Add grab bars to the shower or bathtub and next to the toilet to allow for independent, safe movement.
Add textured stickers to slippery surfaces.
Apply adhesives to keep throw rugs, or remove rugs completely.
Monitor the hot water temperature in the shower or bath. Consider installing an automatic thermometer.
Install locks out of sight. Place a latch or deadbolt either above or below eye level on all doors. Remove locks on interior doors to prevent the person from locking themselves in. Keep an extra set of keys hidden near the door.

Adapt to Vision Limitations
Encourage use of prescription glasses changes in levels of lights can be disorienting. Create an even level by adding extra lights in entries, outside landings, and in areas between rooms, stairways, and bathrooms.
Use nightlights in hallways, bedrooms, and bathrooms.

Beware of Dangerous Objects and Substances
Use appliances that have an automatic shut-off feature.
Disconnect the garbage disposal.
Install a hidden gas valve or circuit breaker on the stove so a person with dementia cannot turn it on. Consider removing the knobs.
Store grills, lawn mowers, power tools, knives, and cleaning products in secure places.
Discard toxic plants and decorative fruits that may be mistaken for real food.
Remove vitamins, prescription drugs, sugar substitutes, and seasonings from the kitchen table and counters. Medications should be kept in a locked area.
Remove guns and firearms from the home or lock them up—can have disastrous results. Firearm accessibility combined with impaired judgment and forgetting who people are could be disastrous.

From Alzheimer's Association.Alz.org. (n.d.). *Home safety and Alzheimer's.* www.alz.org/care/alzheimers-dementia-home-safety.asp

C. Family and caregiver support is a priority. Provide information regarding support groups, respite care, day care, protective services, recreational services, Meals on Wheels, and hospice services
D. Provide the family with information on medications the patient is taking, including purpose, side effects, and potential adverse effects.

Nursing Diagnoses

Because the symptoms of delirium and major neurocognitive disorders are similar, the following nursing diagnoses can be individualized and applied to patients with either diagnosis. One of the most important areas of concern is the patient's safety due to wandering, falls, burns, and accidental ingestion of poisons/medications. Therefore, *risk for injury* is always a priority diagnosis.

Patients often have difficulty with their activities of daily living, making *self-care deficit* an important nursing diagnosis. As the person's ability to process information and speak declines, *impaired verbal communication* becomes a problem.

An important aspect of the patient's care is the support, education, and referrals for the family. *Caregiver stress* is always present, and planning with the family and offering community support are integral parts of appropriate care.

Other nursing diagnoses that may be useful in caring for patients with delirium and dementia include *impaired cognition, acute/chronic confusion, impaired sleep, anxiety, family grief,* and *hopelessness*.

Nursing Care for Major Neurocognitive Disorders

Risk for Injury
Related to
- Neurological dysfunction
- Sensory dysfunction
- Cognitive or emotional impairment
- Confusion, disorientation
- Loss of executive functioning
- Initial loss of short-term memor; eventual loss of long-term memory

Desired Outcomes Patient will remain free of injury.

Assessment/Interventions and *Rationales*

1. Restrict driving. *Cognitive impairment may lead to accidents or result in the individual becoming lost lead to accidents.*

2. Remove area rugs and other objects that could lead to falls. *Removing these hazards minimizes tripping, falling, and serious injury.*

3. Minimize sensory stimulation; provide meaningful stimulation. *Minimizing unhelpful and unnecessary sensory stimulation decreases sensory overload, which can increase anxiety and confusion.* Providing meaningful verbal stimulation and welcome background music or other media supports cognitive functioning.

4. If patients become upset, listen, give support, and then change the topic. *When attention span is short, patients can be distracted to more productive topics and activities.*

5. Label objects used for activities of daily living with words and pictures. In residential care, label the patients' rooms with their names and photographs. *Labeling objects (e.g., hairbrushes and toothbrushes) supports the patient's functioning. Labeling rooms helps prevent wandering into other patients' rooms and increases autonomy.*

6. Recommend safety bars reduces near the toilet and in the shower and bathtub. *Use of safety bars can prevent falls.*

7. If the patient wanders during the night, consider putting their mattress on the floor. *Putting the mattress on the floor reduces falls when the patient is confused.*

8. Provide an identification bracelet that cannot be removed (with a name, address, and phone number). *The patient can be easily identified by police, neighbors, or hospital personnel.*

9. Place locks at the top of the door. *In moderate and late neurocognitive disorders, the ability to look up and reach upward is lost.*

10. Place large black doormats in front of external doors. *Individuals with dementia often think that dark areas of the floor are holes and will not walk over them.*

11. Encourage physical activity during the day. *Physical activity during the day helps to decrease wandering at night.*

12. Explore the possibility of installing sensor devices. *Sensor devices can provide a warning if the patient wanders.*
13. Enroll the patient in the Alzheimer's Association's MedicAlert Safe Return program (www.alz.org). *This program helps track individuals who wander and are at risk for getting lost or injured.*

Self-Care Deficit
Related to
- Neurological dysfunction
- Perceptual or cognitive impairment
- Neuromuscular impairment
- Decreased strength and endurance
- Confusion
- Apraxia (inability to perform tasks that were once routine)
- Agnosia (inability to recognize familiar items)
- Memory impairment

Desired Outcome The patient will demonstrate improved self-care.

Assessment/Interventions and *Rationales*
Dressing and Bathing.
1. Encourage patients to perform tasks of which they are capable. *Maintains self-esteem, uses muscle groups, and minimizes further regression.*
2. Encourage patients to wear their own clothes, even if in the hospital or residential care. *Helps maintain the patient's identity and dignity.*
3. Use clothing with elastic, and substitute Velcro for buttons and zippers. *Minimizes frustration and increases independence of functioning.*
4. Label clothing items with the patient's name and the name of the item. *Helps identify patients if they wander, and gives patients additional clues when agnosia occurs.*
5. Give step-by-step instructions if necessary (e.g., "Take this blouse…put in one arm…now the other arm… pull it together in the front…now…"). *Patients can focus on small pieces of information more easily, allowing the patient to perform at an optimal level.*

Eating and Drinking.

6. Monitor food and fluid intake. *The patient might have limited appetite or be too confused to eat.*
7. Offer finger foods. *The patient might eat only small amounts while sitting at meals.* Offering on-the-go finger foods increases intake throughout the day.
8. If hyperorality is a problem, ensure that the patient does not eat nonfood items (e.g., ceramic fruit or food-shaped soaps). *Hyperorality results in the patients putting inedible objects into their mouths and may result in choking or poisoning.*

Elimination.

9. Begin a bowel and bladder program early using a regular schedule for toileting. For example, direct the patient to the toilet early in the morning, after meals and snacks, and before bedtime. *A toileting routine will reduce episodes of incontinence and help to maintain dignity.*
10. Evaluate the need for adult disposable undergarments. *If disposable undergarments prevents embarrassment and soiling of their surroundings if incontinent.*
11. Label the bathroom door, as well as doors to other rooms, with a picture. *Additional environmental clues can maximize independent toileting. Pictures may be more easily interpreted than words.*

Sleep Hygiene.

12. Provide dim lighting at night. *Dim lighting reinforces orientation while supporting sleep hygiene through normal light/dark rhythms.*
13. Monitor for side effects if using sleep-promoting medications. *Because of metabolic changes, older adults experience more severe side effects including the potential for dangerous falls.*

Impaired Verbal Communication
Related to
- Neurological dysfunction
- Deterioration or damage to neurological centers that regulate speech and language
- Decreased circulation to the brain
- Severe memory impairment
- Escalating anxiety

Desired Outcome The patient will demonstrate optimal communication.

Assessment/Interventions and *Rationales*
In addition to the interventions for delirium in the first half of this chapter, communication techniques specific to neurocognitive disorders follow.

1. Use a variety of nonverbal techniques to enhance communication:
   a. Point, touch, or demonstrate an action while talking about it.
   b. Ask patients to point to parts of their body or things they want to communicate about.
   c. When the patient is searching for a particular word, guess at what is being said and ask whether you are correct (e.g., "You are pointing to your mouth, saying pain. Is it your dentures? No. Is your mouth sore? Yes. Okay, let me take a look to see if I can tell what is hurting you."). Always ask the patient to confirm whether your guess is correct.
   d. The use of cue cards, flash cards, alphabet letters, signs, and pictures on doors to various rooms is often helpful for many patients and their families (e.g., bathroom, "Charles's bedroom"). Use of pictures is helpful when ability to read decreases. *Both delirium and dementia can cause huge communication problems, and often alternative nonverbal or verbal methods are helpful.*
2. Encourage reminiscing about life's highlights. *Remembering accomplishments and shared joys reinforces language use and gives meaning to existence.*
3. If a patient gets into an argument with another patient, stop the argument and separate them. After a short time (5 minutes), explain to each patient matter-of-factly why you had to intervene. *Separation prevents escalation to physical acting out and shows respect for the patient's right to know. Explaining in an adult manner helps maintain self-esteem.*
4. Reinforce the patient's speech through pictures, nonverbal gestures, Xs on calendars, and other methods used to anchor the patient in reality. *When aphasia starts to hinder communication, alternate methods of communication must be instituted.*

Caregiver Stress

Related to

- Complexity of activities and severity of the illness
- 24-hour care responsibility
- Lengthy (e.g., years) periods of caregiving
- Lack of support
- Caregiver isolation
- Inadequate use of community support
- Inadequate physical environment (transportation, housing) for providing care

Desired Outcomes Caregivers will demonstrate and verbalize reduced stress.

Assessment/Interventions and *Rationales*

1. Assess what caregivers know about the patient's disorder and provide education. *Empowering caregivers with knowledge of the disorder promotes patience, reduces the tendency to view the patient's actions as bad behavior, and helps them to anticipate further deterioration and plan accordingly.*

2. Provide community agencies and support groups where the family and primary caregiver can receive support, education, and information regarding respite care. *This support helps diminish a sense of hopelessness, increase a sense of empowerment, and provide a much-needed break from 24-hour care.*

3. Assist the caregiver and family to identify areas that need intervention. *Health care providers are knowledgeable and have experience in the care of individuals with dementia. This makes them able to anticipate specific areas that need assistance and those that may need assistance in the future.*

4. Teach the caregiver and family specific interventions to use in response to behavioral or social problems that results in dementia. *Caregivers are supported by learning new ways to intervene in situations that are common in patients with dementia, such as agitation, sleep–wake disturbances, and wandering.*

5. Safety is a major concern. Box 13.3 identifies some steps the caregiver and family can take to make the home a safer place. *These steps can help make the home safe for individuals with dementia.*

6. Encourage the family to engage in activities with the patient based on the current level of functioning

(e.g., watching a favorite movie together; reading a simple book with pictures together; performing simple tasks like setting the table, washing dishes, or washing the car). *This encourages the patient to participate as much as possible in family life and helps reduce feelings of isolation and alienation. Engagement and generativity help to reduce self-absorption and improve self-image.*

7. Encourage the caregiver or family to follow family traditions such as church activities, holidays, and vacations as much as possible and reasonable. *Continuing customary activities helps the family transition to and make peace with the eventual loss of a loved one. These experiences also increase the patient's sense of belonging.*

8. Encourage the caregiver or family to use respite care at regular intervals such as every 2 weeks and during vacations. *Regular periods of respite can help prevent burnout, allow caregivers to continue participating in their life, and help minimize feelings of resentment.*

9. Identify financial burdens. Refer to community, national associations, or other resources that can help. *Any long-term illness may place devastating financial burdens on the family.*

10. Suggest legal and financial planning and preparation for care as the patient's condition worsens. *Advanced planning for eventual deterioration and death will make these transitions less difficult.*

TREATMENT MODALITIES

Biological Treatment

Pharmacotherapy

Medications with US Food and Drug Administration approval for the treatment of cognitive symptoms of AD fall into two categories. The first is the cholinesterase inhibitors, which includes donepezil (Aricept), rivastigmine (Exelon), and galantamine (Razadyne). These drugs are used for mild, moderate, and severe AD symptoms. The other category is an N-methyl-D-aspartate inhibitor, memantine (Namenda), which is used for moderate-to-severe symptoms.

Although these medications are used widely and have shown statistically significant effects compared with placebos, they produce only a marginal clinical improvement in cognition and functioning. The benefits of these medications diminish after 1 to 2 years. Patients and families should weigh the potential side effects against the potential benefits. See Chapter 28 for more information about neurocognitive medications.

Integrative Therapies

Nutrition may play a role in both the prevention and treatment of dementia. One nutritional substance, omega-3 fatty acids, has been promoted as modulating these diseases. Although some studies have found an association between omega-3 fatty acids and a lower incidence of dementia, their use in the treatment of dementia is controversial. See Appendix B for more information on integrative therapies.

Community Resources

The Alzheimer's Association is a national agency that provides assistance to individuals with the disease and their families. The Alzheimer's Association has a Community Resource Finder that is useful in locating local resources.

Some families manage the care of their loved one until death. Other families eventually find that they can no longer deal with the labile and aggressive behavior, incontinence, wandering, unsafe habits, or disruptive nighttime activity. Families need information, support, and legal and financial guidance at this time. Include information regarding advance directives, durable power of attorney, guardianship, and conservatorship in the communication with the family.

 # NURSE, PATIENT, AND FAMILY RESOURCES

AlzConnected
www.alzconnected.org

Alzheimer's Association
www.alz.org

Alzheimer Society of Canada
www.alzheimer.ca

Association for Frontotemporal Degeneration
www.theaftd.org

Lewy Body Dementia Association
www.lbda.org

National Institute on Aging
www.nia.nih.gov

National Parkinson's Foundation
www.parkinson.org

CHAPTER 14

Personality Disorders

Personality disorders are among the most challenging and complex group of disorders to treat. Individuals who meet criteria for these disorders display significant challenges in self-identity or self-direction, and they have problems with empathy or intimacy within their relationships.

Personality can be described operationally in terms of functioning. Personality is an individual's characteristic, relatively permanent, pattern of thoughts, feelings, and behaviors that define the quality of experiences and relationships. A personality is considered unhealthy when interpersonal relationships and functioning are consistently maladaptive or complicated. Personality can be protective for a person in times of difficulty, but it may also be a liability if it results in ongoing relationship problems or leads to constant emotional distress.

People with these disorders have difficulty recognizing or owning personality problems. Some individuals believe the problems originate outside of themselves. Still others may be unaware that their behavior is unusual, and they may not experience any distress. It is rare for people to seek help for a personality disorder, although they may seek treatment for comorbid conditions such as major depressive disorder or generalized anxiety disorder.

TYPES OF PERSONALITY DISORDERS

According to the American Psychiatric Association (APA, 2013), there are 10 personality disorders. They are grouped into clusters of similar behavior patterns and personality traits, as follows:

Cluster A: Behaviors described as odd or eccentric
　　Paranoid personality disorder
　　Schizoid personality disorder
　　Schizotypal personality disorder

Cluster B: Behaviors described as dramatic, emotional, or erratic
   Borderline personality disorder
   Narcissistic personality disorder
   Histrionic personality disorder
   Antisocial personality disorder
Cluster C: Behaviors described as anxious or fearful
   Avoidant
   Dependent
   Obsessive–compulsive

This chapter begins with a discussion of eight personality disorders, including their prevalence, characteristics, nursing care guidelines, and treatment modalities. Afterward, two of the most common and challenging personality disorders—antisocial and borderline—are described in more detail. An application of the nursing process is provided for both of these personality disorders. A short and useful personality disorder questionnaire is provided in Figure 14.1

CLUSTER A PERSONALITY DISORDERS

Paranoid Personality Disorder

Paranoid personality disorder is characterized by a distrust and suspiciousness of others based on the belief, unsupported by evidence, that others want to exploit, harm, or deceive the person. Relationships are difficult because of jealousy, controlling behaviors, and grudge-holding.

The prevalence of paranoid personality disorder is about 2% to 4% (APA, 2013). Slightly more men than women are diagnosed with this disorder. Relatives of patients with schizophrenia are more commonly affected. Symptoms may be apparent in childhood or adolescence.

Nursing Guidelines

- Due to mistrust, all prearranged promises, appointments, and schedules should be strictly adhered to.
- Being too friendly may be met with suspicion. Give clear and straightforward explanations of tests and procedures beforehand.
- Use simple language and project a neutral, but kind approach.
- Provide limits for threatening behaviors.

Treatment

Individuals with paranoid personality disorder tend to reject treatment. If they somehow end up in treatment, they may be suspicious about why this is happening. Paranoia makes communication difficult. The establishment of a professional and trusting relationship is essential. Although it may be threatening, group therapy is often useful in improving social skills. Role-playing and group feedback can help reduce suspiciousness.

Antianxiety agents such as diazepam (Valium) may be used short-term to reduce anxiety and agitation Also, short-term use of antipsychotic medication such as haloperidol (Haldol) in small doses may reduce delusional thinking or severe agitation. Another first-generation antipsychotic medication, pimozide (Orap), may also be useful in reducing paranoid thoughts.

Schizoid Personality Disorder

People with schizoid personality disorder exhibit a lifelong pattern of social withdrawal. They have a restricted range of emotional expression. Others tend to view them as odd or eccentric. People with this disorder do not seek out or enjoy close relationships. Neither approval nor rejection from others seems to have much effect.

Individuals with schizoid personality disorder may be able to function well in a solitary occupation such as being a security guard on the night shift. They often express feelings of being an observer rather than a participant in life. They may describe feelings of depersonalization or detachment from both themselves and the world.

The prevalence rate for schizoid personality disorder may be as high as 5% (APA, 2013). Males are more commonly affected. Symptoms of schizoid personality disorder appear before adulthood. There is an increased prevalence of the disorder in families with a history of schizophrenia or schizotypal personality disorder. Abnormalities in the dopaminergic systems may underlie this disorder.

Nursing Guidelines

- Avoid being overly friendly and use a neutral approach.
- Avoid efforts to increase socialization.
- Patients may be open to discussing topics such as coping and anxiety.

- Perform a thorough assessment to identify symptoms or problems the patient is reluctant to discuss.
- Monitor for rejection by group members due to the patient's unusual interests, ideas, and interaction.

Treatment

Because individuals with schizoid personality disorder tend to be introspective, they may be good, but distant, candidates for psychotherapy. As trust develops, they may describe a fantasy life and fears, particularly of dependence. Group therapy may also be helpful, even though the patient may be frequently silent. Group members can actually become important to the person with schizoid personality disorder, and the group may be their dominant form of socialization.

Antidepressants such as bupropion (Wellbutrin) may increase pleasure in life. Second-generation antipsychotics, such as risperidone (Risperdal) or olanzapine (Zyprexa), are used to improve emotional expressiveness.

Schizotypal Personality Disorder

Schizotypal (ski·zuh·**tai**·pl) personality disorder is classified as both a personality disorder and the first of the schizophrenia spectrum disorders (APA, 2013). Characteristics of this disorder include magical thinking, odd beliefs, strange speech patterns, and inappropriate affect.

These individuals have severe social and interpersonal deficits. They tend to ramble with lengthy, unclear, and overly detailed and abstract content. As a result of suspiciousness, they tend to misinterpret the motives of others as being out to get them. Odd beliefs (e.g., being overly superstitious) or magical thinking (e.g., "He tripped because I wanted him to") are also common.

Psychotic symptoms such as hallucinations and delusions may be present in schizotypal personality disorder, but to a lesser degree with schizophrenia, and only briefly. As opposed to schizophrenia, people with this disorder can be more easily made aware of their suspiciousness, magical thinking, and odd beliefs.

The prevalence of schizotypal personality disorder ranges from 0.6% to 4.6% (APA, 2013). It is more common in men. Symptoms are evident in young people. Having a first-degree relative with schizophrenia increases the risk. Abnormalities in brain structure, physiology, chemistry, and functioning are similar to those found in schizophrenia.

Nursing Guidelines
- Respect the patient's need for privacy.
- Monitor for increasing suspiciousness.
- Assess for other medical or psychological symptoms that may need intervention (e.g., chest pain, suicidal thoughts).
- Monitor for and modify personal responses to the patient's strange beliefs and activities.

Treatment

Because it is difficult to develop a therapeutic relationship or alliance, the goal should be to provide supportive care. Helping the patient to identify cognitive distortions may be useful. It is helpful to know that individuals with schizotypal personality disorder may actually be involved in groups such as unusual religious sects or occult-type societies that can complicate the clinical picture.

People with schizotypal personality disorder may benefit from low-dose antipsychotic agents such as risperidone (Risperdal) or olanzapine (Zyprexa) to improve functioning and to reduce psychotic-like symptoms, and improve day-to-day functioning. These agents help with such symptoms as ideas of reference or illusions. Antidepressants are used to treat comorbid major depressive disorder and anxiety disorders.

CLUSTER B PERSONALITY DISORDERS

Histrionic Personality Disorder

People with histrionic personality disorder are often high functioning. Characteristics of this disorder include being overly dramatic, extroverted, flamboyant, and colorful. Despite this bold exterior, they tend to have a limited ability to develop meaningful relationships.

Histrionic personality disorder occurs at a rate of nearly 2% (APA, 2013). It tends to be diagnosed more frequently in women than in men. Symptoms begin by early adulthood. Inborn character traits such as emotional expressiveness and egocentricity have been identified as predisposing an individual to this disorder.

Nursing Guidelines

- Encourage and model the use of concrete and descriptive rather than vague and dramatic language.
- Help patients clarify inner feelings, as they often have difficulty identifying them.
- Teach and role model assertiveness.

Treatment

Individuals with histrionic personality disorder have difficulty regulating their feelings and the expression of those feelings. Psychotherapy may promote clarification of these feelings and appropriate expression. Both individual and group therapy are useful in this population.

There are no specific pharmacological treatments for people with histrionic personality disorder. Antidepressants can be used for depressive, anxiety, or somatic symptoms. Antipsychotics may be used if the patient exhibits derealization or illusions.

Narcissistic Personality Disorder

Narcissistic personality disorder is characterized by feelings of entitlement, an exaggerated belief in one's own importance, and a lack of empathy. In reality, people with this disorder suffer from weak self-esteem and hypersensitivity to criticism. Narcissistic personality disorder is associated with less impairment in individual functioning and quality of life than the other personality-based disorders.

The prevalence of narcissistic personality disorder ranges from 0% to about 6% (APA, 2013). It tends to be more common in males than in females. Age of onset is difficult to determine because of the narcissistic traits that are commonly found in adolescents. Genetics is a risk factor for the development of this personality disorder (Luo & Cai, 2018). This risk, may be increased by parents with narcissm who may attribute an unrealistic sense of talent, importance, and beauty to their children, thus putting the children at higher risk.

Nursing Guidelines

- Maintain a neutral tone.
- Avoid engaging in power struggles or becoming defensive in response to the patient's controversial remarks.
- Do not directly challenge grandiose statements.
- Role model empathy.

Treatment

If a person with narcissistic personality disorder seeks treatment, individual cognitive–behavioral therapy (CBT) helps to deconstruct faulty thinking and promote realistic thoughts. Group therapy can also assist the person in sharing with others, seeing their own qualities in others, and learning empathy.

Lithium (Eskalith, Lithobid) has been used in patients with narcissism who demonstrate mood swings. Antidepressants can also be used if the person has depressive symptoms.

CLUSTER C PERSONALITY DISORDERS

Avoidant Personality Disorder

People with avoidant personality disorder avoid interpersonal contact due to extreme fears of rejection, criticism, or failure. These individuals are overly sensitive to rejection, feel inadequate, and are socially inhibited.

Avoidant personality disorder occurs in 2.4% of the population (APA, 2013) and is found equally in men and women. Early symptoms include shyness and avoidance in childhood that increase during adolescence and early adulthood.

Nursing Guidelines

- Use a friendly, accepting, and reassuring approach.
- Remember that social situations can cause severe anxiety.
- Convey an attitude of acceptance toward patient fears.
- Provide exercises to enhance new social skills with caution, since failure can increase feelings of poor self-worth.
- Role play assertive responses to help the person to learn to express needs.

Treatment

Individual and group therapy are useful in processing anxiety-provoking symptoms and in planning methods to approach and handle anxiety-provoking situations. Psychotherapy focuses on trust and assertiveness training.

Antianxiety agents can help. Beta-adrenergic receptor antagonists (e.g., atenolol) reduce autonomic nervous system hyperactivity. Antidepressants such as selective serotonin reuptake inhibitors (SSRIs) like citalopram (Celexa) and serotonin–norepinephrine reuptake inhibitors (SNRIs) such as venlafaxine (Effexor) may reduce social anxiety. Serotonergic agents may help individuals with avoidant personalities feel less sensitive to rejection.

Dependent Personality Disorder

Dependent personality disorder is characterized by a pattern of submissive and clinging behavior related to an overwhelming need to be cared for. This results in intense fears of separation. These individuals may experience intense anxiety when left alone for even brief periods of time (APA, 2013).

The prevalence is estimated at about 0.5% (APA, 2013). Dependent personality disorder may be the result of chronic physical illness or punishment for independent behavior in childhood. The inherited trait of submissiveness may be a factor in the development of this disorder.

Nursing Guidelines
- Encourage the patient to identify and address current stressors.
- Monitor for strong countertransference that may develop because of the patient's demands of extra time and crisis states.
- Use the therapeutic relationship as a testing ground for increased assertiveness through role modeling and teaching of assertive skills.

Treatment
Psychotherapy is the treatment of choice for dependent personality disorder. CBT can help in the development of new perspectives and attitudes about other people.

There are no specific medications indicated for this disorder, but symptoms of depression and anxiety may be treated with appropriate antidepressant and antianxiety agents. Panic attacks can be helped with the tricyclic antidepressant imipramine (Tofranil).

Obsessive–Compulsive Personality Disorder

Obsessive–compulsive personality disorder is characterized by limited emotional expression, stubbornness, perseverance, and indecisiveness. Preoccupation with orderliness, perfectionism, and control are the hallmarks of this disorder. Rigidity and inflexible standards of self and others persist even if they are self-defeating or relationship defeating. Preoccupation with the activity often results in losing the major point of the activity. Projects are often incomplete because of overly strict standards.

A distinction should be made: Obsessive–compulsive *disorder* is characterized by repetition or adherence to rituals. Obsessive–compulsive *personality disorder* is characterized more by an unhealthy focus on perfectionism.

Obsessive–compulsive personality disorder is one of the most prevalent personality disorders. Prevalence rates range from about 2% to 8% (APA, 2013). It is more common in men than in women. Risk factors for this disorder include a background of harsh discipline and having a first-degree relative with the disorder.

Nursing Guidelines

- Avoid power struggles with patients whose need for control is high.
- Provide structure since patients with this disorder have difficulty dealing with unexpected changes.
- Provide patients extra time to complete rituals.
- Help patients identify ineffective coping and explore alternative coping methods.

Treatment

Typically, individuals seek help for obsessive–compulsive personality disorder, because they are uncomfortable with the symptoms. Treatments are often long and complicated. Both group and behavioral therapy can help the person learn new coping skills, manage anxiety, and receive feedback from the group.

Clomipramine (Anafranil) may help reduce the obsessions, anxiety, and depression associated with this disorder. Other serotonergic agents such as the SSRI fluoxetine (Prozac) may also be helpful.

ANTISOCIAL PERSONALITY DISORDER

In this section, we focus on one cluster B personality disorder, antisocial personality disorder. This disorder is characterized by a pattern of disregard for the rights of others and their frequent violation. The main pathological traits that characterize antisocial personality disorder are antagonistic behaviors such as being deceitful and manipulative for personal gain or being hostile if needs are blocked. People with this disorder also exhibit disinhibited behaviors such as risk-taking, disregard for responsibility, and impulsivity. Criminal misconduct and substance use are common.

One of the most disturbing qualities associated with antisocial personality disorder is a lack of empathy, also known as callousness and unemotional traits. This results in a lack of concern about the feelings of others; the absence of remorse or guilt except in the face of punishment; and a disregard for meeting school, family, and other obligations. They may seem concerned and caring if these attributes help them manipulate and exploit others. Wittiness, charm, and flattery may accompany manipulation and exploitation.

Epidemiology

The prevalence of antisocial personality disorder is between 0.2% and 3.3% (APA, 2013). The highest prevalence is among males with substance use disorders and in incarcerated individuals.

Risk Factors

Antisocial personality disorder is genetically linked, and twin studies indicate a predisposition to this disorder. An alteration in serotonin transmission, childhood mistreatment, and cultural bias have also been implicated.

ASSESSMENT

Signs and Symptoms

- History of violence
- Violates rights of others
- Anger and aggression
- Impulsivity
- Substance use
- Illegal and reckless behaviors
- Unstable relationships
- Lacks empathy, callous, unemotional

ASSESSMENT GUIDELINES

A. Assess current life stressors
B. Assess for criminal history
C. Assess for suicidal, violent, and/or homicidal thoughts
D. Assess anxiety, aggression, and anger levels
E. Assess motivation for maintaining control
F. Assess for substance use (past and present)

Nursing Diagnoses

The International Classification for Nursing Practice (International Council for Nurses [ICN], 2019) provides useful nursing diagnoses for individuals with antisocial personality disorder. Because the main characteristics of antisocial personality disorder are callous disregard for others and antagonistic behaviors, *risk for violence* is a top priority. Individuals with antisocial personality disorder demonstrate irresponsibility and fail to maintain work and financial obligations. Therefore *impaired coping* is a useful nursing diagnosis to address those behaviors.

INTERVENTION GUIDELINES

A. Recognize attempts to manipulate (e.g., flattery, seductiveness, and instilling guilt).
B. Set clear and realistic limits for specific behaviors.
C. Inform all staff of the treatment plan and discuss importance of adherence to the treatment plan.
D. Assist patients to recognize feelings of anger and their source. Identify options for handling anger.
E. Document behaviors objectively (i.e., provide times, dates, circumstances).
F. Establish and communicate clear boundaries and consequences.

Nursing Care for Antisocial Personality Disorder

Risk for Violence

Related to
• Neurological dysfunction
• Impulsivity
• Inability to control temper
• Emotional dysregulation (e.g., anger, hostility)
• Lack of empathy (callousness)
• Antagonistic behaviors (e.g., deceitfulness, manipulation, hostility)

Desired Outcome The patient will refrain from violence.

Assessment/Interventions and *Rationales*
1. Use one-to-one or appropriate level of observation to determine emotional and situational triggers. *Monitoring patients who may exhibit hostility provides external support and helps to prevent acts of aggression and violence.*
2. Intervene early to calm the patient and defuse a potential incident. *Learning can take place before the patient loses control. New ways to cope can be discussed and role modeled.*
3. Set clear, consistent limits in a calm, nonjudgmental manner. *This provides structure, safety, and control.*
4. Avoid power struggles and repeated negotiations about rules and limits. *When limits are realistic and enforceable, manipulation is minimized.*
5. Redirect agitation with physical outlets in areas of low stimulation (e.g., punching bag, exercise bike). *Learning how to use anger constructively is essential for self-control.*
6. Encourage feelings of concern for others and remorse for wrongdoings and verbal disrespect. *Development of empathy is a therapeutic goal.*
7. Alert staff if the potential for restraint or seclusion appears imminent. The usual priority of interventions is (1) setting limits, (2) encouraging time out, (3) offering as-needed medication, and (4) restraint or seclusion. *A team approach to aggression is essential. Always use the least restrictive intervention when managing potentially violent behavior.*
8. Document the patient behaviors, interventions, what seemed to escalate agitation, what helped to calm agitation, if and when as-needed medications were given and their effect, and what proved most helpful. *Documentation provides staff with guidelines for future interventions and legal evidence if necessary.*

Impaired Coping
Related to
- Neurological dysfunction
- Genetic predisposition
- Chaotic environment in childhood
- Inadequate coping strategies
- Impulsivity and failure to plan ahead
- Irritability and aggressiveness
- Reckless in regards to safety
- Consistent irresponsibility
- Lack of remorse

Desired Outcome Patient will demonstrate improved coping.

Assessment/Interventions and *Rationales*
1. Provide the patient with a clear overview of expectations for behavior in regard to unit rules, routine, and engagement with other individuals. *Since the patient has a history of coping ineffectively and inappropriately, a clear understanding of expectations is essential.*
2. Consequences for breaking the behavior code should be established by the treatment team and communicated with the patient. *Undesirable consequences may help to decrease repetition of undesirable behaviors.*
3. Discuss the patient's goals for the hospitalization or treatment period. *Although most people with this disorder do not seek treatment for it, they may seek help for other problems such as major depressive disorder, anxiety, or anger management. Engaging the patient in care by identifying goals is a strong first step.*
4. Encourage the patient to identify usual coping methods such as deceit or aggression. *Identifying coping methods helps to clarify nonproductive responses to stress.*
5. Explore alternate potential coping methods and link these coping methods to their goals. *Understanding that there are choices in the way the patient responds opens the door to change.*
6. Provide positive feedback for the use of new coping methods. *Positive feedback reinforces new learning and the use of prosocial behaviors.*

TREATMENT MODALITIES FOR ANTISOCIAL PERSONALITY DISORDER

Biological Therapies

Pharmacotherapy

There are no medications specifically approved by the Food and Drug Administration (FDA) for antisocial personality disorder. However, mood-stabilizing medications such as lithium or valproic acid (Depakote) may help with aggression, depression, and impulsivity. SSRIs such as fluoxetine (Prozac) and sertraline (Zoloft) may be used to decrease irritability and help with anxiety and depression. Benzodiazepines may reduce anxiety but are used with caution because they are addictive. Methylphenidate (Ritalin) may help if there is a comorbidity of attention-deficit/hyperactivity disorder.

Psychological Therapies

Behavioral therapy is a basic approach that uses a system of rewards and punishment to promote positive behavior. CBT, specifically mentalization behavioral therapy (MBT) and dialectical behavior therapy (DBT), goes deeper and is useful in helping individuals to recognize sociopathic ways of thinking and then altering such behaviors. Group therapy has the additional benefits of learning from others, supporting others, and experiencing the camaraderie of working together.

BORDERLINE PERSONALITY DISORDER

As previously identified, borderline personality disorder is a nother cluster B diagnosis. People with borderline personality disorder exhibit patterns of marked instability in emotional regulation (dysregulation), impulsivity, identity, unstable mood, and unstable interpersonal relationships. Emotional lability is exhibited in moving from one emotional extreme to another, usually in response to a pathological fear of separation and intense sensitivity rejection.

Another disruptive trait is impulsivity. Impulsivity is manifested in acting quickly in response to emotions without considering the consequences. This impulsivity results in damaged relationships and even in suicide attempts. Self-destructive behaviors such as cutting, promiscuous sexual behavior, and numbing with substances are common. Chronic suicidal ideation is common and increases the likelihood of accidental deaths. Co-occurring mood, anxiety, or substance disorders complicate the treatment and prognosis. Antagonism is manifested in hostility, anger, and irritability in relationships. Violence may occur in relationships and against property.

Splitting, a primitive defense mechanism, refers to the inability to view both positive and negative aspects of others as part of a whole. This results in seeing someone as either a wonderful person or a horrible person. Initially, the individual may idealize another person such as a nurse. At the first disappointment or frustration, the nurse's status quickly shifts to one of devaluation, and the nurse is then despised.

Epidemiology

Borderline personality disorder occurs at a rate of about 1.6% in the general population, and up to 20% of the inpatient psychiatric population (Skodol et al., 2019). It is more commonly diagnosed in women. It is likely that the rates are about the same in men and women, and that men are underdiagnosed or misdiagnosed. Symptoms seem to decrease with age.

Risk Factors

Borderline personality disorder seems to have a genetic component. It is about five times more common in first-degree biological relatives with the same disorder compared with the general population (APA, 2013). Serotonergic dysfunction may accompany the borderline trait of impulsivity. Mahler and colleagues (1975) suggest that such psychological problems are due to disruption of the normal separation–individuation between the child and the mother.

Assessment

Signs and Symptoms
- Feelings of emptiness
- May engage in risky behaviors such as reckless driving, unsafe sex, substance use, binge eating, gambling, and overspending
- Intense feelings of abandonment that result in paranoia or feeling spaced out
- Idealization of others with quick attachment
- A tendency toward anger, sarcasm, and bitterness
- Nonsuicidal self-injury
- Suicidal ideation, behaviors, gestures, or threats
- Sudden shifts in self-evaluation that result in changing goals, values, and career focus
- Extreme mood shifts in a matter of hours or days
- Intense, unstable romantic relationships

Nursing Diagnoses

People with borderline personality disorder are usually admitted to psychiatric treatment programs because of symptoms of comorbid disorders or dangerous behavior. Emotions such as anxiety, rage, depression, and behaviors such as withdrawal, paranoia, and manipulation are among the most frequent problems that health care workers must address.

The International Classification for Nursing Practice (ICN, 2019) provides the nursing diagnosis *risk for self-mutilation*. This diagnosis is most often associated with borderline personality disorder. Self-mutilation involves deliberate non-suicidal self-injurious behavior that causes tissue damage. The intent of this behavior is to attain relief of tension and perhaps to enlist the aid and support of others. Other nursing diagnoses directly relevant to borderline personality disorder are *chronic low self-esteem*, *impaired socialization*, and *impaired coping*.

INTERVENTION GUIDELINES

A. Set realistic goals, using clear action words.
B. Assess for manipulative behaviors (e.g., flattery, seductiveness, guilt instilling).
C. Provide clear and consistent boundaries and limits.
D. Use clear and straightforward communication.
E. When behavioral problems emerge, calmly review the therapeutic goals and boundaries of treatment.
F. Avoid rejecting or rescuing.
G. Assess for suicidal ideation and non-suicidal self-injury, especially during times of stress.

Nursing Care for Borderline Personality Disorder

Risk for Self-Mutilation
Related to
- Neurological dysfunction
- Borderline personality disorder
- History of self-mutilation
- Impulsivity
- Poor self-esteem
- Unstable self-image
- Feelings of emptiness
- Impaired problem-solving abilities

- Culture of self-mutilation
- Efforts to avoid abandonment
- Intense anger

Desired Outcome Patient will refrain from self-injurious behaviors.

Assessment/Interventions and *Rationales*

1. Assess the patient's history of self-mutilation including:
   a. Types of mutilation
   b. Frequency of self-mutilation
   c. Stressors preceding self-mutiliation
   Identifying patterns and circumstances surrounding self-injury helps the nurse plan patient-centered interventions and teach strategies.
2. Identify feelings experienced by the patient around the time of self-mutilation. *Feelings are a guideline for future intervention (e.g., rage at feeling left out or abandoned).*
3. Explore what these feelings might mean. *Self-mutilation might be a way to relieve anxiety, feel alive through pain, express guilt, or self-hate, or manipulation.*
4. Identify specific steps (e.g., persons to call upon) when feeling the urge to self-mutilate. *Talking to others can reduce the frequency and severity self-injury until the behavior ceases.*
5. Use a matter-of-fact approach when self-mutilation occurs. Avoid criticizing or giving sympathy. *A neutral approach prevents blaming that increases anxiety, or giving special attention that encourages acting out.*
6. After treatment of the wound, discuss what happened right before and the thoughts and feelings the patient had immediately before self-mutilating. *Identifying warning signs and triggers for self-mutilation helps the patient know when to self-manage behavior or when to seek help from others.*
7. Develop alternatives to self-mutilating behaviors.
   a. Anticipate certain situations that might lead to increased stress (e.g., anger or frustration).
   b. Identify actions that might modify the intensity of such situations.
   c. Identify two or three people whom the patient can contact to discuss and examine intense feelings (e.g., rage, self-hate) when they arise.

Planning for stressful situations provides the patient with increasing self-agency rather than relying on external controls.

8. Set and maintain limits on acceptable behavior and make clear the patient's responsibilities. If the patient is hospitalized, be clear regarding unit rules. *Clear and nonpunitive limit setting is essential for decreasing negative behaviors.*

Chronic Low Self-Esteem
Related to
- Neurological dysfunction
- Borderline personality disorder
- Repeated failures
- Childhood abuse and/or neglect
- Avoidant and dependent patterns
- Lack of integrated self-view
- Shame and guilt
- Inconsistent affection and discipline in family of origin

Desired Outcome The patient will report and demonstrate improved self-esteem.

Assessment/Interventions and *Rationales*
1. Maintain a respectful and empathetic approach to the patient. *This helps Feeling respected as a person, even when behavior might not be appropriate, promotes trust and builds on the therapeutic relationship.*
2. Assess for blaming, projection, anger, passivity, and demanding behaviors. *Many behaviors seen in patients with personality disorders cover a fragile sense of self. Often these behaviors are the crux of the patient's interpersonal difficulties in all relationships.*
3. Assess the patient's self-perception. Target a variety of aspects in the patient's life:
   a. Strengths and weaknesses in performance at work, school, and daily life tasks
   b. Strengths and weaknesses in relation to physical appearance, sexuality, and personality
   After identifying realistic areas of strengths and weaknesses, the patient and nurse can work on the realities of the self-appraisal and target the areas that seem inaccurate.
4. Review the types of cognitive distortions that affect self-esteem (e.g., self-blame, mind reading, overgeneralization, selective inattention, all-or-none thinking). *These are*

the most common cognitive distortions. Identifying them is the first step to correcting false thoughts.

5. Help the patient to recognize cognitive distortions, their impact on emotion, and influence on behavior. Encourage the patient to keep a log. *Cognitive distortions are automatic. Keeping a log helps make automatic, unconscious thinking clear.*

6. Teach the patient to reframe and dispute cognitive distortions. Disputes need to be strong, specific, and nonjudgmental. *Practice and belief in the disputes over time help patients gain a more realistic appraisal of events, the world, and themselves.*

7. Discourage the patient from dwelling on and reliving past mistakes. *The past cannot be changed. Dwelling on past mistakes prevents the patient from appraising the present and planning for the future.*

8. Discourage the patient from making self-blaming and negative remarks. *Words become feelings, thoughts, and beliefs that result in a negative cycle of more negative verbalizations. Stopping negative is a step in breaking the cycle.*

9. Focus questions in a positive and active way to help the patient refocus on the present and look to the future. For example: "What could you do differently now?" or "What have you learned from that experience?" *Focusing questions in an active light allows the patient to look at past behaviors differently with have a sense of control over the future.*

10. Provide honest and genuine feedback regarding your observations as to strengths and areas that could use additional skills. *Feedback helps give the patient a more accurate view of self, strengths, and areas to work on, as well as a sense that someone understands.*

11. Set goals realistically, and revise goals as needed in small steps. *The patient's negative self-view and distrust of the world took years to develop. Unrealistic goals can set up hopelessness in patients and frustration in staff.*

12. Help the patient to set realistic short-term goals for the future. Identify skills the patient will need to reach these goals. *Looking toward the future minimizes dwelling on the past and negative self-rumination. When realistic short-term goals are met, the patient gains a sense of accomplishment, direction, and purpose in life. Accomplishing goals can bolster a sense of control and enhance self-perception.*

Impaired Socialization
Related to
- Neurological dysfunction
- Inability to engage in mature interactions
- Manipulative behavior
- Self-concept disturbance
- Unacceptable social behavior or values
- Disruptive or abusive early family background

Desired Outcome The patient will demonstrate improved socialization.

Assessment/Interventions and *Rationales*
1. Assist the patient to recognize maladaptive patterns of social interaction. *The patient does not recognize patterns of maladaptive behaviors. Change cannot happen until this recognition occurs.*
2. Identify alternative social interaction methods. *Once maladaptive behavior is eliminated, new methods of social interaction must be identified and adopted.*
3. Role-play and practice successful social interaction. *The nurse–patient relationship is an ideal testing ground for developing relationship skills.*
4. Encourage attendance at group therapy and group work. *Group member influence, confrontation, altruistic learning, and recognition of own behaviors in others are often more valuable than one-to-one encounters.*

Impaired Coping
Related to
- Neurological dysfunction
- Disturbance in patterns of tension relief
- Intense emotional state
- Failure to intend to change behavior
- Lack of motivation to change behaviors
- Negative attitudes toward health behavior

Desired Outcome The patient will report and demonstrate improved coping.

Assessment/Interventions and *Rationales*
1. Assess for suicidal ideation and non-suicidal self-injury. *Maintaining safety by monitoring for urges or acts of self-mutilation and suicidal thoughts is a priority.*

The Personality Inventory for DSM-5—Brief Form (PID-5-BF)—Adult

Name: _____ Age: ____ Sex: ☐ Male ☐ Female Date:_____

Instructions: This is a list of things different people might say about themselves. We are interested in how you would describe yourself. There are no right or wrong answers. So you can describe yourself as honestly as possible, we will keep your responses confidential. We'd like you to take your time and read each statement carefully, selecting the response that best describes you.

		Very False or Often False	Sometimes or Somewhat False	Sometimes or Somewhat True	Very True or Often True	Clinician Use Item score
1	People would describe me as reckless.	0	1	2	3	
2	I feel like I act totally on impulse.	0	1	2	3	
3	Even though I know better, I can't stop making rash decisions.	0	1	2	3	
4	I often feel like nothing I do really matters.	0	1	2	3	
5	Others see me as irresponsible.	0	1	2	3	
6	I'm not good at planning ahead.	0	1	2	3	
7	My thoughts often don't make sense to others.	0	1	2	3	
8	I worry about almost everything.	0	1	2	3	
9	I get emotional easily, often for very little reason.	0	1	2	3	
10	I fear being alone in life more than anything else.	0	1	2	3	
11	I get stuck on one way of doing things, even when it's clear it won't work.	0	1	2	3	
12	I have seen things that weren't really there.	0	1	2	3	
13	I steer clear of romantic relationships.	0	1	2	3	
14	I'm not interested in making friends.	0	1	2	3	
15	I get irritated easily by all sorts of things.	0	1	2	3	
16	I don't like to get too close to people.	0	1	2	3	
17	It's no big deal if I hurt other peoples' feelings.	0	1	2	3	
18	I rarely get enthusiastic about anything.	0	1	2	3	
19	I crave attention.	0	1	2	3	
20	I often have to deal with people who are less important than me.	0	1	2	3	
21	I often have thoughts that make sense to me but that other people say are strange.	0	1	2	3	
22	I use people to get what I want.	0	1	2	3	
23	I often "zone out" and then suddenly come to and realize that a lot of time has passed.	0	1	2	3	
24	Things around me often feel unreal, or more real than usual.	0	1	2	3	
25	It is easy for me to take advantage of others.	0	1	2	3	
					Total/Partial Raw Score:	
				Prorated Total Score: (if 1-6 items left unanswered)		
					Average Total Score:	

Fig. 14.1 Reprinted with permission from The Personality Inventory for DSM-5, (Copyright ©2013). American Psychiatric Association. All Rights Reserved.

2. Intervene in times of intense and labile mood swings, anxiety, depression, and irritability. *Many dysfunctional behaviors of patients (e.g., parasuicidal, anger, manipulation, substance use) are used as behavioral solutions to intense pain.*

   a. Anxiety: Teach stress-reduction techniques such as deep breathing, relaxation, meditation, and exercise. *Patients experience intense anxiety and fear of abandonment. Stress-reduction techniques help the patient focus more clearly.*

   b. Depression: The patient might need medications to improve mood. Assess for side effects. *Medication combined with talk therapy and exercise is effective in decreasing depression. Side effects should be managed or medication changed to promote adherence.*

    c. Irritability, anger: Use interventions early before anxiety and anger escalate. *Intervening early can help reduce or eliminate escalation.*

3. Reduce manipulation through consistency, limit setting, and unit or community rules. *External structure will decrease negative behaviors, while patients develop internal control.*

4. Be assertive when setting limits on the patient's demands for time and attention. *Firm, clear, nonjudgmental limits give the patient structure.*

5. Be nonjudgmental and respectful when listening to the patient's thoughts, feelings, or complaints. *Developing a trusting relationship with the nurse lays the groundwork for future relationships.*

6. Encourage the patient to explore feelings and concerns (e.g., identify fears, loneliness, self-hate). *The patient is used to acting out feelings rather than expressing them verbally. Appropriate self-expression is an essential new skill.*

7. When the patient is ready and interested, teach coping skills to help diffuse tension and troubling feelings (e.g., anxiety reduction, assertiveness skills). *Increasing skills helps the patient to use healthier ways to diffuse tensions and get needs met.*

8. Patients with personality disorders often benefit from additional training (e.g., dialectical behavioral therapy, interpersonal skills, anger management skills, emotional regulation skills). Provide referrals or involve professional experts. *Training teaches the patient to refine skills in changing behaviors, emotions, and thinking patterns associated with problems in living that are causing misery and distress.*

9. Treatment of substance use is best handled by well-organized treatment professionals. *Keeping detailed records and having a team involved with each patient can minimize manipulation.*

10. Provide and encourage the patient to use professionals in other disciplines such as social services, vocational rehabilitation, social work, or the law. *Patients with borderline personality disorder often have multiple social problems and do not know how to obtain these services.*

TREATMENT FOR BORDERLINE PERSONALITY DISORDER

Biological Treatments

Pharmacotherapy

There are no medications specifically approved by the FDA for treating borderline personality disorder. This means that prescribers use medications off-label until evidence-based pharmacotherapies are proven to be safe and effective.

Psychotropic medications geared toward maintaining cognitive function, symptom relief, and improved quality of life are available. People with borderline personality disorder often respond to antidepressants such as SSRIs, anticonvulsants, and lithium for mood and emotional dysregulation. Naltrexone (Revia, Vivitrol), an opioid receptor antagonist, reduces self-injurious behaviors. Second-generation antipsychotics may control anger and brief episodes of psychosis. Chapters 22–24 and 27 discuss the medications mentioned in this paragraph.

Psychological Therapies

There are two three essential therapies for borderline personality disorder, CBT, DBT and schema-focused therapy. CBT helps individuals to identify and change inaccurate core perceptions of themselves and others and problems interacting with others. DBT combines cognitive and behavioral techniques with mindfulness, which emphasizes being aware of thoughts and actively shaping them. Schema-focused therapy combines parts of CBT with other forms of therapy that focus on the ways that individuals view themselves. These therapies are discussed in Chapter 29.

 ## NURSE, PATIENT, AND FAMILY RESOURCES

Borderline Personality Disorder Central
www.bpdcentral.com

Internet Mental Health
www.mentalhealth.com

MedlinePlus
www.medlineplus.gov/personalitydisorders.html

National Alliance on Mentally Illness (NAMI)
www.nami.org

Self-Injury Outreach and Support
sioutreach.org

CHAPTER 15

Suicide

Suicide can have long-lasting and devastating effects on family, friends, and communities. Yet, suicide is largely a preventable problem. In fact, a 2018 (Stone et al.) study found that in the year before their deaths by suicide, 83% used health care services and 54% of those who died by suicide did not have a mental health diagnosis. These findings highlight the need for mental health screening in all settings, not just psychiatric settings.

This chapter focuses on self-harm and interventions to keep people safe. Terms associated with self-harm include:

- *Suicidal ideation* is thinking about wanting to be dead or active thoughts about killing oneself, not accompanied by preparatory behavior.
- A *suicide attempt* is self-injurious behavior with the intention of death, also referred to a nonfatal suicide attempt or suicidal act.
- *Suicide* is death caused by self-directed injurious behavior with the intent to die as a result of the behavior.
- *Suicidality* is a broad term that encompasses suicidal ideation, plans, suicide attempts, and suicide.
- *Suicide survivors* are family members, significant others, or acquaintances who have experienced a loss due to suicide. This term may also refer to suicide attempt survivors.

Some words used to describe suicide concepts are problematic and are avoided. One familiar term is to commit suicide. However, using the word "commit" is discouraged due to its association with a criminal activity. This term is linked to the past when it was actually illegal to kill oneself. Other troublesome terms connote a positive tone when a suicide is carried through, and a negative tone when a suicide is attempted but does not result in death. These terms are "completed suicide," "successful suicide," or "failed suicide attempt."

EPIDEMIOLOGY

According to the Centers for Disease Control and Prevention ([CDC]; 2018), nearly 47,000 people died by suicide in 2017, making it the 10th leading cause of death in the United States. In 2020, COVID-19 was the third leading underlying cause of death, replacing suicide as one of the top 10 leading causes of death (CDC, 2021).

This entirely preventable cause of death is especially prominent in younger people. In 2017, suicide was the second leading cause of death for 10- to 34-year-olds, the fourth leading cause of death in 35- to 54-year-olds, and the eighth leading cause of death for 55- to 64-year-olds.

Men died by suicide about 3.5 times more often than women, while over a lifetime, women attempted suicide almost 1.5 times more often than men. White males accounted for almost 70% of all suicide deaths. Non-Hispanic American Indian or Alaska Natives had the highest suicide rates for both males and females in age groups from 15 to 44 years old in 2017.

RISK FACTORS

Twin and adoption studies suggest genetic factors in suicide since concordance rates are higher in monozygotic (identical) twins than in dizygotic (fraternal) twins. Low serotonin levels are related to depressed mood. Postmortem examinations of individuals who have died by suicide reveal low levels of serotonin in the brainstem and/or the frontal cortex.

The central emotional factor underlying suicide intent is hopelessness. Cognitive styles that contribute to higher risk are rigid all-or-nothing thinking, inability to see different options, and perfectionism. Adolescents are at especially high risk due to their immature prefrontal cortex, the portion of the brain that controls the executive functions involving judgment, frustration tolerance, and impulse control.

Assessment

- History of suicide attempts or self-mutilation
- Family history of suicide attempts or death by suicide
- History of bullying and/or victimization
- History of a mood disorder, schizophrenia, or drug or alcohol use
- History of chronic pain, recent surgery, or chronic physical illness
- History of personality disorder (e.g., borderline, paranoid, antisocial)
- Bereavement or another significant loss (e.g., divorce, job, home)
- Legal or disciplinary problems

Signs and Symptoms

- Talking or writing about death, dying, or suicide
- Making comments about being hopeless, helpless, or worthless
- Expressions of having no reason to live; no sense of purpose in life; saying things like "It would be better if I wasn't here"
- Increased alcohol and/or substance use
- Withdrawal from friends, family, and community
- Reckless behavior or more risky, impulsive activities
- Dramatic mood changes
- Talking about being a burden to others

Assessment Tools

There are a variety of assessment tools to measure suicide risk. The Columbia-Suicide Severity Rating Scale (C-SSRS) assesses patients through a series of simple questions. Answers to these questions can assist in identifying suicide risk, determine the severity and immediacy of that risk, and determine the level of support that the person needs. The C-SSRS is in Box 15.1.

Assessment Guidelines
Suicide

1. Assess risk factors (Box 15.2).
2. Assess protective factors (see Box 15.2).

Box 15.1 **Columbia-Suicide Severity Rating Scale (C-SSRS)**

Suicide Ideation Definitions and Prompts	Past Month	
Ask Questions That Are Bolded and <u>Underlined</u>	Yes	No

Ask Questions 1 and 2

1) Wish to be Dead:

Have you wished you were dead or wished you could go to sleep and not wake up?

2) Suicidal Thoughts:

Have you actually had any thoughts of killing yourself?

If YES to 2, Ask Questions 3, 4, 5, and 6. If NO to 2, go Directly to Question 6

3) Suicidal Thoughts with Method (Without Specific Plan or Intent to Act):

E.g. "I thought about taking an overdose, but I never made a specific plan as to when, where, or how I would actually do it….and I would never go through with it."

Have you been thinking about how you might do this?

4) Suicidal Intent (Without Specific Plan):As opposed to *"I have the thoughts, but I definitely will not do anything about them."*

Have you had these thoughts and had some intention of acting on them?

5) Suicide Intent With Specific Plan:

Have you started to work out or worked out the details of how to kill yourself? Do you intend to carry out this plan?

6) Suicide Behavior Question:

Have you ever done anything, started to do anything, or prepared to do anything to end your life?

Examples: Collected pills, obtained a gun, gave away valuables, wrote a will or suicide note, took out pills but didn't swallow any, held a gun but changed your mind or it was grabbed from your hand, went to the roof but didn't jump; or actually took pills, tried to shoot yourself, cut yourself, tried to hang yourself, etc.

If YES, ask: **Was this within the past 3 months?**

Continued

Box 15.1 **Columbia-Suicide Severity Rating Scale (C-SSRS)—cont'd**

Suicide Ideation Definitions and Prompts	Past Month	
Ask Questions That Are Bolded and <u>Underlined</u>	Yes	No

Response Protocol to C-SSRS Screening (linked to last item marked Yes)

Item 1: Behavioral health referral

Item 2: Behavioral health referral

Item 3: Behavioral health consult and consider patient safety precautions

Item 4: Immediate notification of physician and/or behavioral health and safety precautions

Item 5: Immediate notification of physician and/or behavioral health and safety precautions

Item 6 (over 3 months ago): Behavior health consult and consider patient safety precautions

Item 6 (3 months ago or less): Immediate notification of physician and/or behavioral health and safety precautions

---

From Posner, K., Brent, D., Lucas, C., Gould, M., Stanley, B., Brown, G. et al. (2009). Columbia-Suicide Severity Rating Scale. Retrieved from http://www.integration.samhsa.gov/clinical-practice/Columbia_Suicide_Severity_Rating_Scale.pdf

3. Determine the level of suicide precautions for the patient based on the following questions:
   a. Are you thinking of killing/hurting yourself?
   b. How long have you been thinking about suicide (i.e., frequency, intensity, duration)?
   c. Do you have a plan? Obtain specific information if there is a plan.
   d. Do you have the means to carry out the plan (e.g., accessibility of a weapon, medications, drugs)?
   e. Have you attempted suicide in the past? If yes, how?
   f. Has someone in your family died by suicide? If yes, how?
   g. Is there anything or anyone to stop you such as religious beliefs, children left behind, or pets?
4. Assess for a sudden mood improvement. Often a decision to die by suicide provides a way out of severe emotional pain.
5. Assess social supports and helpfulness of significant other(s).

Box 15.2 **Risk and Protective Factors for Suicide**

Risk Factors:
- Previous suicide attempt
- A history of suicide in the family
- Substance use
- Mood disorders (depression, bipolar disorder)
- Access to lethal means (e.g., keeping firearms in the home)
- Losses and other events (e.g., breakup of a relationship or a death, academic failure, legal difficulty, financial problems, bullying)
- History of trauma or abuse
- Chronic physical illness including chronic pain
- Exposure to the suicidal behavior of others

Protective Factors:
- Effective and accesible mental health care clinical interventions
- Strong connections to individuals, family, community, and social institutions
- Significant other
- Having children
- Problem-solving skills

Nursing Diagnoses

A thorough assessment provides the framework for determining the level of protection the patient requires. Therefore, *risk for suicide* is the first area of concern (International Council of Nurses, 2019). Believing that one's situation or problem is intolerable, inescapable, and interminable leads to feelings of hopelessness. *Hopelessness* is often associated with suicide and is a priority nursing diagnosis.

Reinforcing the patient's own problem-solving skills and helping to reframe life difficulties as events that can be controlled are strategic parts of the counseling process. Therefore, *impaired coping* is the third point of intervention. Other potential nursing diagnoses include *low self-esteem, impaired socialization, spiritual distress, and impaired family process.*

Nursing Care for Patients With Suicidality

Risk for Suicide

Related to

- History of prior suicide attempt
- Family history of suicide
- Suicidal ideation
- Suicide plan
- Alcohol and substance use
- Adverse childhood experiences
- At-risk demographics (e.g., older adult, young adult male, adolescent, widowed, white, American Indian)
- Physical illness, chronic pain, terminal illness
- Grief, bereavement, loss of important relationship, job, home
- Psychiatric disorder (e.g., major depressive disorder, schizophrenia, bipolar disorder)
- Poor support system, loneliness
- Legal or disciplinary problems
- Hopelessness or helplessness

Desired Outcome The patient will be free from suicidal risk.

Assessment/Interventions and *Rationales*
Hospitalized

1. Follow agency protocol for suicide regarding providing a safe environment (e.g., removing potential weapons such as belts and sharp objects, checking what visitors bring into the patient's room). *While having suidcidal ideation, the availability of means of harming oneself could result in death.*

2. Suicide precautions range from one-on-one with a staff member at arm's length at all times to less frequent checks. *Close contact with healthcare workers not only provides safety for a patient with suicidal ideation but also improves socialization and self-esteem.*

3. If there is fear of imminent harm to self, seclusion or restraint may be required. *For patients with the most severe suicidal ideation, temporary seclusion or restraint may be the safest option.*

4. Follow unit protocol and document the patient's behavior and statements along with nursing interventions. *Documentation provides for continuity of care with*

other health care workers, tracks progress, and provides a legal record of nursing care.

5. Encourage the patient to talk about stressors, responses to stressors, and alternative responses to stressors. *Talking about feelings, responses to stressors, and looking at alternatives can reduce suicidal thinking.*

Outside the Hospital

1. If an individual is managed outside the hospital, notify the family, significant other, or friends to the risk and treatment plan. Provide education about signs of worsening depression such as hopelessness. *Family and friends can support the individual and also facilitate access to healthcare if suicidal ideation continues or increases.*

2. Provide education or referral for medication, counseling (i.e., a general nursing intervention), and/or psychotherapy (i.e., advanced practice interventions). *Antidepressants are initiated quickly due to the significant lag time before they take effect. Counseling and psychotherapy will provide immediate support.*

3. Provide the patient, family, and friends with the number for the emergency department, crisis care facilities, or an emergency hotline (i.e., 988 for the US mental health hotline). *Patients, family, and friends need access to 24/7 support.*

4. Schedule a follow-up visit as early as the next day if decisions concerning hospitalization need to be reconsidered. *During a crisis period, individuals are monitored carefully for increasing suicidal ideation.*

5. Educate friends and family regarding signs of increased suicidal ideation. These signs include withdrawal, preoccupation, silence, remorse, and sudden mood change from sad to happy and carefree. *Friends and family can intervene and facilitate the patient receiving more acute care.*

6. Identify social supports and encourage the patient to initiate contact. *Social connections reduce self-absorption and hopelessness. Talking with other people is one of the best activities for improving mood and reducing suicidal thoughts.*

7. List support people and agencies to use as outpatient and crisis hotline numbers. Significant others. *Suicide attempts are often impulsive. Immediate access to another person can be lifesaving.*

Hopelessness

Related to
- Deteriorating physical or psychiatric condition
- Social isolation
- Long-term stress
- Spiritual distress
- Severe loss (financial hardship, termination of a relationship, loss of job)
- Chronic pain
- Negative perception of the future

Desired Outcome The patient will demonstrate and verbalize hopefulness for the future.

Assessment/Interventions and *Rationales*

1. Encourage the patient to reframe negative thinking into neutral objective thinking. *Cognitive reframing helps a person look at situations in more productive and positive ways.*
2. Point out unrealistic and perfectionistic thinking. *Constructive interpretations of events and behavior open up more realistic and satisfying options for the future.*
3. Work with the patient to identify strengths. *When people are feeling overwhelmed, they no longer view their lives or behavior objectively and dismiss strengths.*
4. Spend time discussing the patient's dreams and wishes for the future. Identify short-term goals for the future. *Renewing realistic dreams and hopes can give promise to the future and meaning to life.*
5. Identify aspects of life that have given meaning and joy in the past. Discuss how these aspects of life can be reincorporated into the present lifestyle (e.g., religious or spiritual beliefs, group activities, creative endeavors). *Reawakens the patient abilities and experiences that tapped areas of strength and creativity. Creative activities give people intrinsic pleasure, joy, and life satisfaction.*
6. Encourage contact with religious or spiritual individuals or groups that have supplied comfort and support in the patient's past. *During times of hopelessness, people might feel abandoned and too paralyzed to reach out to caring people or groups.*

Impaired Coping
Related to
- Situational or maturational crises
- Disturbance in pattern of tension release
- Inadequate social support
- Inadequate coping skills
- Impulsive use of extreme solutions
- Inadequate resources

Desired Outcome The patient will demonstrate improved coping.

Assessment/Interventions and *Rationales*
1. Identify situations that trigger suicidal thoughts. *Identifying triggers for suicidal thoughts helps to identify targets for learning more adaptive coping skills.*
2. Assess the patient's strengths and positive coping skills (e.g., talking to others, creative outlets, social activities, problem-solving abilities). *Use these strengths and skills when planning alternatives to self-defeating behaviors.*
3. Assess the patient's ineffective coping behaviors (e.g., drinking, angry outbursts, withdrawal, denial, procrastination) that result in negative emotions. *This helps to identify areas to target for teaching and planning strategies for more effective and self-enhancing behaviors.*
4. Role-play adaptive coping strategies that can be used when suicidal thinking begins to emerge. *Practice helps the patient use skills when/if suicidal thoughts occur.*
5. Assess the need for assertiveness training. *Assertiveness skills can help the patient develop a sense of control and balance.*
6. Clarify aspects of life that are not under the patient's control such as other's actions, likes, choices, or health status. *Recognizing one's limitations in controlling others is, paradoxically, a beginning to finding one's own strength.*
7. Assess the patient's social supports. *Social supports reduce isolation, thereby reducing the possibility of suicide attempts.*
8. Encourage the patient to identify two potential social activities with others who share mutual interests such as walking, books, or dining. These groups are easy to find online. *Involvement in outside activities with others reduces introspection and self-absorption.*

NURSE, PATIENT, AND FAMILY RESOURCES

Alliance of Hope for Suicide Survivors
www.allianceofhope.org

American Association of Suicidology
www.suicidology.org

American Foundation for Suicide Prevention
www.afsp.org

Crisis Text Line
www.crisistextline.org

Friends for Survival, Inc.
www.friendsforsurvival.org

(If You Are Thinking About) Suicide... Read This First
www.metanoia.org/suicide

National Suicide Prevention Lifeline
1-800-273-8255

Samaritans
www.samaritans.org

Suicide Awareness Voices of Education
www.save.org

CHAPTER 16

Crisis Intervention

This edition of the *Manual of Psychiatric Nursing Care* was revised in the midst of a global pandemic. Any nursing student reading this chapter experienced this crisis/disaster situation firsthand. Most of us were afraid, if not for ourselves, for loved ones who were older or had preexisting conditions. Anxiety levels ran high as the country and states wrestled with the accompanying economic disaster. People were isolated and cut off from their usual supports and social outlets. For some vulnerable individuals, the stress of the coronavirus pandemic caused an emergence or exacerbation (i.e., worsening) of psychiatric symptoms.

Despite stress, the human organism's internal environment maintains a relatively stable state while interacting with external forces. This stable state is referred to as *homeostasis* or *equilibrium*. A crisis, which is a major disturbance caused by a stressful event or threat, disrupts this homeostasis. In a crisis, normal coping mechanisms fail, resulting in an inability to function as usual. Equilibrium is replaced by disequilibrium. Crisis intervention efforts are aimed at promoting (1) a realistic perception of the event, (2) adequate situational supports, and (3) adequate coping skills.

PERCEPTION OF THE EVENT

Perception of a crisis may range from realistic to distorted. People vary in the way they absorb, process, and use information from the environment. Some people may respond to a minor event as if it were life-threatening, whereas others may calmly assess a life-threatening event.

SITUATIONAL SUPPORT

Situational support includes all the people who are available and who can be depended upon to help during the time of a crisis. Nurses and other health care professionals who use crisis intervention are providing situational support. Family members and friends may also provide individuals with support.

COPING SKILLS

The quality and quantity of a person's usual coping skills affect a person's ability to cope with a crisis situation. Other factors may compromise a person's ability to cope with a crisis event. These factors include the number of other stressful life events with which the person is coping, other unresolved losses, the presence of psychiatric disorders or other medical problems, and excessive fatigue or pain.

Crisis by definition is self-limiting and is resolved within 4 to 6 weeks. The overall goal of crisis intervention is to regain the pre-crisis level of functioning. However, an individual can emerge from the crisis at a lower or higher level of functioning. This variation in functional outcome is why crisis intervention and community services are so vitally important.

TYPES OF CRISES

Crises are organized in a variety of nomenclatures. One categorization is to use three basic types of situations: (1) maturational (or developmental) crises, (2) situational crises, and (3) adventitious crises. Identifying which type of crisis the individual is experiencing or has experienced helps in the development of a patient-centered plan of care in childhood, adolescence, and adulthood.

Maturational

Erikson (1963) identified eight stages of growth and development. Each stage is defined by two opposing psychological tendencies – one positive and one negative - with specific tasks that must be mastered to progress through the growth process. Former coping styles may no longer be age appropriate, and new coping mechanisms have yet to be developed.

A maturational crisis occurs when former coping mechanisms are inadequate in dealing with a stress common to a particular stage in the life cycle. Temporary disequilibrium might affect interpersonal relationships, body image, and social and work roles. Examples of precipitants to a maturational crisis include leaving home for the first time, marriage, the birth of a child, retirement, and the death of a parent.

Situational

A situational crisis arises from events that are unusually distressing and often unanticipated. Examples of precipitants to a situational crisis include a job loss or change, the death of a loved one, a change in financial status, divorce, and psychiatric or physical illness. These situations are often referred to as life events or crucial life problems, because most people encounter some of these problems during the course of their lives.

Adventitious

An adventitious crisis is a traumatic and external event that happens unexpectedly. This type of rare crisis may be natural, human, or accidental. Natural disasters may be the result of pandemics, epidemics, floods, fires, and earthquakes. Humans may be the source of adventitious crises through one-on-one violence—such as rape and murder—acts of terrorism, wars, riots, shootings, and bombings. Accidents are another source of adventitious crises and include airline crashes, structural collapses, and nuclear power plant failures. In addition to injury and loss of life, adventitious crises may result in long-term psychological trauma.

PHASES OF CRISIS

Through extensive study of individuals experiencing crisis, Caplan (1964) identified behaviors that followed a fairly distinct path. Caplan categorized these behaviors as four distinct phases of a crisis.

Phase 1

When a person is exposed to a serious stressor or problem, increased anxiety is experienced. The increase in anxiety stimulates the use of coping methods in an effort to solve the problem and decrease anxiety.

Phase 2

If the usual coping methods fail and the threat persists, anxiety will continue to rise and produce increased discomfort. Individual functioning becomes disorganized. Trial-and-error attempts at solving the problem and restoring balance begin.

Phase 3

If the trial-and-error attempts fail, anxiety may escalate to severe and panic levels. At this point, the person mobilizes automatic relief behaviors, such as withdrawal and flight. Resolution (e.g., compromising needs or redefining the situation to reach an acceptable solution) may occur at this stage.

Phase 4

If the problem is not solved and new coping skills are ineffective, anxiety may overwhelm the person. These powerful feelings may lead to serious personality disorganization, depression, confusion, violence against others, or suicidal behavior.

ASSESSMENT

Assessing History

A history for potential crises might include the following:
- Overwhelming life event (i.e., maturational, situational, or adventitious)
- Previous violent behavior
- Previous suicidal behavior
- A psychiatric disorder (e.g., major depressive disorder, personality disorder, bipolar disorder, schizophrenia, anxiety disorder)
- A physical condition (e.g., cancer, cardiac problems, uncontrolled diabetes, lupus, multiple sclerosis)

Signs and Symptoms

People in crisis exhibit a variety of behaviors, such as the following:
- Confusion, disorganized thinking
- Immobilization, social withdrawal
- Violence against others, suicidal thoughts or attempts

- Agitation, increased psychomotor activity
- Crying, sadness
- Flashbacks, intrusive thoughts, nightmares
- Forgetfulness, poor concentration

Sample Questions

Three main areas are assessed during a crisis: (1) perception of the event, (2) support system, and (3) coping skills. Nurses use a variety of therapeutic techniques to obtain the answers to the following questions.

1. **Perception of the Event**
   "What happened in your life before you started to feel this way?"
   "What does this event/problem mean to you?"
   "How does this event/problem affect your life?"
   "How do you see this event/problem affecting your future?"

2. **Support System**
   "Is there anyone—family or friends—you would like to have involved in your care?"
   "Are these people available now?"
   "Do you have a religious affiliation?"
   "Where do you go to school? Are you involved in any community-based activities?"

3. **Coping Skills**
   "What do you usually do when you feel stressed or overwhelmed?"
   "What has helped you get through difficult times in the past?"
   "What have you done so far to cope with this situation?"
   "Do you have any thoughts of killing yourself?"
   "Do you have any thoughts of killing or hurting someone else?"

ASSESSMENT GUIDELINES

- Determine whether the patient is able to identify the precipitating event.
- Assess the patient's situational supports.
- Identify the patient's usual coping styles, and determine what coping mechanisms may help the present situation.
- Determine whether there are religious or cultural beliefs that need to be considered in assessing and intervening with a patient in crisis.

- Assess whether this situation is one in which the patient needs health promotion (e.g., education, environmental manipulation, or new coping skills), crisis intervention, or rehabilitation.

Nursing Diagnoses

When anxiety levels escalate to moderate, severe, or panic levels, the ability to problem solve is impaired. In an acute crisis, an individual's usual coping skills are not effective in meeting the challenges of the crisis situation. For individuals with already compromised coping skills, this situation is compounded. The International Council Nurses (2019) provides useful and logical nursing diagnoses. The first is impaired coping, which is evidenced by... the inability to meet basic needs, use of inappropriate defense mechanisms, or alteration in social participation. In this chapter, *impaired coping* is addressed both in the context of acute crisis intervention and separately with the rehabilitation phase.

Other nursing diagnoses that are essential targets of intervention are anxiety and family coping. *Anxiety (moderate, severe, panic)* is always present in various levels in crisis situations. Reducing anxiety so that individuals can begin problem solving on their own is key in crisis management.

Because a crisis in a family member results in stress to the whole family, *impaired family processes* is an important area to address. Family members might have difficulty responding helpfully to each other. Communication becomes disorganized and the ability to express feelings appropriately may be problematic. Interventions support the individual and family to engage in healthy interactions.

INTERVENTION GUIDELINES

LEVELS OF CRISIS INTERVENTION

Crisis interventions levels correlate with the public health levels of prevention model. The levels are health promotion (primary prevention), acute crisis intervention (secondary prevention), and stabilization and rehabilitation (tertiary prevention).

Health Promotion

The goal of health promotion is to prevent crisis responses from occurring. Nurses help to promote mental health with the following interventions:

- Evaluating the patients experience of stressful life events.
- Provide education regarding specific coping skills, such as decision making, problem solving, assertiveness, meditation, and relaxation techniques.
- Encourage the patient to reduce or eliminate stress by postponing major changes in life events such as moving to a new residence or changing jobs.

Acute Crisis Intervention

Acute crisis intervention measures are taken to identify and reduce prolonged crisis responses once they occur. This care is provided in hospital units, emergency departments, clinics, or mental health centers.

Essential nursing interventions for acute crisis intervention are to:

- Conduct regular screening to detect psychiatric symptoms that may lead to crisis responses. Important symptoms include depressive, anxious, obsessive-compulsive, psychosis, and suicidality.
- An initial focus on safety from harmful thoughts and impulses.
- Assess problems, support systems, and coping styles.
- Promote a realistic perception of events, increasing social support, and exploring alternate coping methods.
- Provide an active and directive approach to care.

Crisis Stabilization and Rehabilitation (Tertiary Prevention)

Crisis stabilization and rehabilitation programs and services provide long-term support for individuals who have experienced a crisis. The goals are to facilitate optimal levels of functioning and prevent further emotional disruptions. This care occurs in rehabilitation clinics and centers, day hospitals, sheltered workshops, and outpatient clinics. Individuals with serious mental illness are more susceptible to crisis, and community facilities provide a supportive structured environment that reduces stress and provides support. Nurses promote stabilization and rehabilitation with the following interventions.

- Assess and provide for the patient's and family's educational needs.
- Assess and provide for social skills training as needed.

Table 16.1 **Responses to Stress in Mental Health and Mental Illness**

Mental Health	Mental Illness
Able to adapt to day-to-day disappointments and changes	May respond to a mild disruption as a crisis situation (e.g., a cancelation of a health care provider appointment)
Has a healthy sense of self, place, and purpose in life; good problem-solving abilities	Inadequate sense of self and purpose or abilities. Inadequate problem-solving abilities
Usually has adequate situational supports and is able to activate them during stressful times	May have no family or friends, might be living in isolation, and may be homeless
Usually has adequate coping skills with a number of techniques that can be used to lower anxiety and adapt to the situation	Coping ability tends to be compromised, and more support is required

- Assess and refer to vocational rehabilitation program when appropriate.
- Evaluate and refer to supportive group therapy.
- Teach cognitive techniques and/or refer patients to cognitive-behavioral therapy programs.

Table 16.1 describes the impact of stress based on mental health and mental illness.

ACUTE CRISIS

- Assess for suicidal or homicidal thoughts or plans.
- Focus on promoting safety and decreasing anxiety.
- Take an active and directive approach (e.g., make telephone calls, set up and mobilize social supports).
- Monitor the patient's progress.

Crisis Stabilization and Rehabilitation

- Individuals with serious mental illness are more susceptible to crises.
- Adapting the crisis model to this group includes focusing on the patient's strengths, modifying and setting realistic goals, and taking a more active role.

After Crisis Stabilization

- Assess and provide for the patient's and family's educational needs.
- Assess and provide for social skills training as needed.
- Assess and refer to a vocational rehabilitation program when appropriate.
- Evaluate and refer to supportive group therapy.
- Teach cognitive techniques and/or refer patients to cognitive–behavioral therapy programs.

Acute Crisis Intervention

Impaired Coping
Related to

- Maturational crisis
- Situational crisis
- Adventitious crisis
- Inadequate social support
- Inadequate level of perceived control
- Inadequate resources available
- High degree of threat
- Lack of opportunity to prepare for stressors
- Disturbance in pattern of appraisal of threat
- Disturbance in pattern of tension release

Desired Outcome The patient will demonstrate improved coping.

Assessment/Interventions and *Rationales*
 1. Provide a liaison such as a social worker who has expertise in community resources to link the patient to emergency support. *The patient's physical needs (e.g., shelter, food, protection from abuser) are the initial priority.*
 2. Facilitate making appointments for medical or other health care providers. *During an acute crisis, patients' attention may be limited. Making sure that healthcare appointments are made reduces the potential for missing other health problems.*
 3. Document the date and time of appointments, their purpose, and location. *A written reminder for follow-up is essential because anxiety reduces the capacity for attention and memory formation.*
 4. Assess for patient safety. Examples of questions to ask include: Do you have suicidal thoughts? Is there child

or spouse abuse? Are you living in unsafe living conditions? *The patient's physical safety is the priority.*

5. Identify the patient's perception of the event. Help the patient to reframe this perception of the event if memories of the event seem to be unrealistic or distorted. *The patient's distorted perception increases anxiety.*

6. Identify whether helplessness or hopelessness has interfered with the patient's usual coping skills. *Help the patient to view the event as a problem that can be solved.*

7. Assess stressors and the precipitating cause of the crisis. *Assessing for these stressors helps identify areas for change and intervention.*

8. Identify the patient's current skills, resources, and knowledge to deal with problems. *This reminder supports the patient's self-esteem while encouraging the patient to use strengths and usual coping skills.*

9. Identify other skills that may be helpful (e.g., decision-making skills, problem-solving skills, communication skills, relaxation techniques) and support the patient's use of these skills through patient education. *Teaching the patient additional skills helps to regain more control over the present situation and helps minimize crisis situations in the future.*

10. Assess the patient's support systems. Encourage the patient to contact these supports or, with the patient's consent, make the contact yourself if the patient is overwhelmed. *Engaging a support system often reduces anxiety. Helping the patient to make contact if the patient is initially immobilized is a useful intervention.*

11. Identify and arrange for external support such as self-help groups. These groups are especially important if the patient's current support system is unavailable or insufficient. *The patient might have lost important supports because of death, divorce, or distance, for example, or the patient may simply not have sufficient supports in place.*

12. Take an active role in crisis intervention (e.g., make telephone calls; arrange temporary child care; arrange for shelters, emergency food, or first aid). *Patients in crisis are often incapacitated by anxiety and unable to problem solve. The nurse can provide much-needed organization so the patient views the situation as solvable and controllable.*

13. Provide small amounts of information at a time. *Only small pieces of information can be understood when a person's anxiety level is high.*

14. Encourage the patient to stay in the present to deal with the immediate situation. *Crisis intervention deals with the immediate problem disrupting the patient's present situation.*

15. Listen to the patient's story. Avoid interrupting. *Telling the story can be healing in itself. Allowing the patient to set the pace is important in processing facts and feelings.*

16. Help the patient set achievable goals. *Working in small, achievable steps helps the patient gain a sense of control and mastery.*

17. Work with the patient on devising a plan to meet goals. *A realistic and specific plan helps decrease anxiety and promote hopefulness.*

18. Identify and contact other members of the health care team who can support the patient in addressing specific concerns after a crisis event. *Other members of the health care team with specific expertise broaden the base of support and increase the patient's network for future problems.*

19. Provide debriefing for patients and family members after a crisis and for staff after a serious unit event such as a suicide attempt. *Survivors, family members, and staff all need to discuss the effects of a crisis, and debriefing provides the structure in which to do so.*

Crisis Stablization and Rehabilitation

Crisis stabilization and rehabilitation addresses long-term needs of individuals with limited resources or support. This care may address deficits that result in a lower level of functioning after the crisis than prior to the crisis. This may happen to veterans who return from war after prolonged exposure to traumatic events. At other times, individuals with limited coping skills are faced with overwhelming situations, which for many people would not result in a crisis. For example, individuals with serious mental illness such as schizophrenia may experience a situational crisis based on seemingly trivial events such as a canceled therapist appointment.

The nursing diagnosis *impaired coping* applies to people with serious mental illness. These disorders usually impact multiple areas of functioning including activities of daily living (e.g., cooking, hygiene), health maintenance, relationships, leisure activities, safe movement within the community, finances, vocational and academic activities, and coping with stressors.

Impaired Coping
Related to
- Situational crisis
- Maturational crisis
- Adventitious crisis
- Serious mental illness
- Inadequate social supports
- Impaired ability to reduce anxiety
- Impaired ability to accurately appraise threat
- Poor coping skills
- Inability to problem solve
- Inadequate level of personal resources

Desired Outcome The patient will demonstrate improved coping.

Assessment/Interventions and *Rationales*
1. Nurses and trained mental health care workers meet with the patient and family to assess the patient's various needs. *Patients with psychiatric disabilities have a wide range of needs that are best addressed in the context of the health care team.*
2. Identify the patient's highest level of functioning in terms of:
   a. Living skills
   b. Learning skills
   c. Working skills
   Identifying the highest level of functioning provides a baseline evaluation of whether interventions help maintain or improve the patient's level of functioning.
3. Identify the social supports available to the family:
   a. Community support to help the patient function optimally
   b. Community supports that offer family support groups and education
   Family members need a variety of supports to prevent family deterioration.
4. Identify community support that can promote continuity of care, such as:
   a. Residential services
   b. Transportation services
   c. Outpatient services
   d. Case management
   e. Peer support and peer-led services

    f. 24/7 emergency and crisis stabilization services
    g. Crisis lines and text services
    h. Homeless and crisis hotlines
    Comprehensive community support services are available to help individuals function at optimal levels and slow their rate of relapse.

5. Obtain a referral for social skills training, especially if the patient is living with family. *Social skills training is an evidence-based practice that helps individuals understand and improve social behavior. This training is associated with decreased relapses and improved interactions with others, including families.*

6. Work with the patient and family to identify the patient's prodromal (early) signs of impending relapse. *The patient and family can access professional services before a full exacerbation of the illness occurs.*

7. Assist patient and family to identify a vocational rehabilitation service for the patient. *Vocational rehabilitation prepares individuals with serious mental illness for work. Employment makes a significant contribution to relapse prevention, improved clinical outcomes, and enhanced self-image.*

8. Teach the patient and family about medications for psychiatric disorders:
    a. Purpose
    b. Benefits
    c. Side effects
    d. Adverse effects
    e. Who to contact with questions or concerns
    Medication teaching empowers the patient to provide self-care, reduces relapse rates, and eliminates or prolongs the time between relapses.

Nurse, Patient, and Family Resources

Crisis Text Line
www.crisistextline.org

Emotions Anonymous
www.emotionsanonymous.org

Lifeline Chat
https://suicidepreventionlifeline.org/chat/

Mental Help Net
www.mentalhelp.net

NAMI (National Alliance on Mental Illness)
www.nami.org

Red Cross Disaster Mental Health Services (DMHS)
www.redcross.org
(Contact local Red Cross for information)

Teenline Online
www.teenlineonline.org/talk-now

CHAPTER 17

Anger, Aggression, and Violence

Anger, aggression, and violence are emotional and behavioral responses that challenge the skills and resources of health care providers and society as a whole. Understanding the differences between these terms provides a starting point for intervening and preventing potentially damaging outcomes.

- Anger is a primal and normal human emotion. Anger can motivate and energize individuals to act productively. Unfortunately, anger can become overwhelming or uncontrollable and lead to aggressive and violent behavior.
- Aggression is the behavioral manifestation of anger. It is characterized by directing angry or violent feelings toward others.
- Violence is an extreme subtype of aggression. Violence is the intentional physical manifestation of anger and aggression, threatened or actual, that may result in psychological harm, physical injury, or death.

Some people are more prone toward angry feelings and aggressive and violent behaviors than others. Individuals who may be at higher risk include those who use substances or have poor coping skills; are psychotic or have antisocial, borderline, or narcissistic traits; or suffer from cognitive disorders, paranoia, or mania.

The management of anger, aggression, and violence in the health care setting is a priority because safety is always a priority. Fortunately, most patients demonstrate signs of increasing anxiety before escalating to destructive levels. The most useful nursing interventions are implemented during the initial phases, before a patient's anger escalates out of control. However, there are times when anger has already escalated, aggression is evident, and the threat of violence is imminent. At this time, different intervention strategies are necessary.

RISK FACTORS

Anger, aggression, and even violence were once necessary for survival. As a result, some individuals may be more biologically predisposed to respond to life events with irritability, easy frustration, and anger. Neurobiological conditions such as brain tumors, Alzheimer's disease, temporal lobe epilepsy, and traumatic brain injuries can result in disinhibition that may result in increased violence. Abnormalities in the amygdala, hippocampus, hypothalamus, and prefrontal cortex are associated with anger and aggression. Altered neurotransmitters, especially serotonin, dopamine, and gamma-aminobutyric acid (GABA), may play a role in anger and aggression.

Nursing Care for Anger, Aggression, and Violence

The following sections offer nursing guidelines for (1) assessing anger and potential aggression when a patient's behavior is escalating and (2) interventions, sometimes in the form of restraints or seclusion when a patient's anger has escalated to physical violence. Hospital protocols that follow legal and ethical guidelines are always followed when restraining or secluding patients.

Assessment

- History of violence (the best predictor of future behavior is past behavior)
- Paranoia
- Alcohol or drug use
- Mania or agitated depression
- Personality disorders (e.g., antisocial, borderline, or narcissistic)
- Oppositional defiant disorder or conduct disorder
- Psychosis (i.e., hallucinations, delusions, and disorganized thought)
- Command hallucinations
- Neurocognitive disorder
- Intermittent explosive disorder
- Physical conditions (e.g., chronic illness, pain, or loss of body function)

Important questions:
- Have you thought of harming someone else?
- Have you ever seriously injured another person?
- What is the most violent thing you have ever done?

ASSESSMENT GUIDELINES: VIOLENCE AND AGGRESSION

- History of violence is the single best predictor of violence.
- Does the patient have a violent wish or intention to harm another?
- Does the patient have a plan?
- Does the patient have the availability or means to carry out a plan?
- Demographics: sex (male), age (14–24 years), socioeconomic status (low), and support systems (few)

Self-Assessment

Assess yourself for defensive response or taking the patient's anger personally, which may accelerate the anger cycle. For example, are you:

- Responding aggressively toward the patient?
- Avoiding the patient?
- Suppressing or denying either your own or the patient's anger?

Assess your level of comfort in the situation and the need for support of other staff to work with you to deal with a potentially explosive situation.

Interventions for Anger, Aggression, and Violent Behavior

Guidelines for working with angry and aggressive patients who are potentially violent follow the least restrictive means of helping them gain control. Least restrictive usually starts with verbal and nonverbal interventions, then pharmacological interventions, and finally moves to physical seclusion and restraints as a last resort.

Verbal and Nonverbal Interventions

Begin by telling the patient that you are concerned and want to listen. It is important to clearly state your expectations for the patient's behavior: "I expect that you will stay in control."

Approach the patient in a controlled, nonthreatening, and caring manner. Allow enough personal space so that you are not perceived as threatening. Stay about 1 foot farther than the patient can reach with arms or legs. Make sure that the patient is not between you and the door. Choose a quiet place to talk to the patient but one that is visible to other staff. Inform the staff about the situation so they can be prepared to intervene if the situation escalates.

When anger is escalating, a patient's ability to mentally process information decreases. It is important to speak to the patient slowly and in short sentences, using a low and calm voice. Use open-ended statements and questions such as "You think people are treating you unfairly?" Ask what is behind the angry feelings and behaviors. You may want to give two options such as, "Do you want to go to your room or to the quiet room for a while?" This approach decreases the sense of powerlessness that often precipitates violence while also providing external boundaries.

Pharmacological Interventions

When a patient is showing increased signs (e.g., pacing, hitting the wall, or yelling) or symptoms (e.g., "I'm so angry!") of anxiety or agitation, it is appropriate to offer the patient an as-needed medication, as ordered, to relieve symptoms. When used in conjunction with psychosocial interventions and deescalation techniques, medication can prevent an aggressive or violent incident.

Inhaled loxapine (Adasuve), a first-generation antipsychotic, has US Food and Drug Administration approval for the acute treatment of agitation associated with schizophrenia or bipolar I disorder in adults. Loxapine's use is limited due to the potential for a fatal bronchospasm.

Second-generation injectable antipsychotics, such as olanzapine (Zyprexa) and ziprasidone (Geodon), are useful in reducing agitation. An orally disintegrating tablet version of olanzapine (Zyprexa Zydis) is an alternative to injectable medication. The tablets disintegrate in saliva almost immediately, and the effects occur rapidly.

A combination of an antipsychotic and a benzodiazepine can be administered intramuscularly. Diphenhydramine or benztropine added to the injection reduces extrapyramidal side effects. Table 17.1 lists medications that have been found useful in managing aggression.

Seclusion or Restraints

Occasionally, aggression and the potential for violence require seclusion or restraint for the safety of the patient and others. Seclusion is confinement in a room that is

Table 17.1 **Drugs Used for Acute Management of Violent Behavior**

Generic (Trade)	Forms	Considerations
Antianxiety Agents (Benzodiazepines)		
Lorazepam (Ativan)	PO, SL, IM, IV	Drug of choice in this class. Short half-life and less hepatic metabolism relative to most other agents in class.
Alprazolam (Xanax)	PO	Paradoxical (opposite response) with personality disorders and the older adults.
Diazepam (Valium)	PO, IM, IV	FDA approved for alcohol withdrawal agitation. Rapid onset of calming and sedating. Long half-life; use with caution in the older adults.
First-Generation Antipsychotics		
Haloperidol (Haldol)	PO, IM, IV	Favorable side effect profile. IV administration requires ECG monitoring. Due to risk of neuroleptic malignant syndrome, keep hydrated, check vital signs, and test for muscle rigidity.
Loxapine (Adasuve)	Inhalation	Rapid systemic delivery. Available only through a restricted program. Risk for fatal bronchospasm—contraindicated for individuals with breathing disorders.
Perphenazine	PO	Risk of neuroleptic malignant syndrome increases; keep hydrated. Frequent vital sign checks and testing for muscular rigidity are recommended.
Chlorpromazine (Thorazine)	PO, PR, IM	Very sedating. Injections can cause pain; watch for hypotension.

Second-Generation Antipsychotics

Risperidone (Risperdal)	PO, disintegrating tablet	Calms while treating the underlying condition. Watch for hypotension with reflex tachycardia. Increased risk of stroke in older adults.
Olanzapine (Zyprexa, Zyprexa Zydis)	PO, IM, disintegrating tablet	IM is FDA approved for agitation with schizophrenia or bipolar I in adults. Useful in patients unresponsive to haloperidol. Calms while treating underlying condition. Avoid IM combination with lorazepam. Increased risk of stroke in older adults.
Ziprasidone (Geodon)	PO, IM	IM is FDA approved for agitation with schizophrenia in adults. Use cautiously with QT prolongation. Less sedating.
Combinations		
Haloperidol (Haldol), lorazepam (Ativan), and diphenhydramine (Benadryl) or benztropine (Cogentin)	IM	Commonly used in the acute setting. Men who are young and athletic are at increased risk of dystonia. Consider akathisia if agitation increases.

FDA, Food and Drug Administration; *IM,* intramuscularly; *IV,* intravenously; *PO,* orally; *PR,* per rectum (rectally); *SL,* sublingually. From US Food and Drug Administration (2021). *Online label repository.* https://labels.fda.gov/.

not within the control of the person to leave. Restraint is any method that immobilizes or reduces the movement of arms, legs, body, or head freely. These interventions require an order from a licensed provider, although the order may have to be secured subsequent to the emergency event. Licensing and accreditation agencies mandate how frequently patients in seclusion and restraint are observed and assessed.

Each team member is trained in the correct use of seclusion and physical restraint. A clear leader communicates with the patient and directs the activity of the team. The leader informs the patient of the team's intent to either seclude or restrain and the reason for the actions. Once the patient is secluded or restrained, the nurse may get an order for medication and administer it. Box 17.1 provides guidelines for the use of seclusion and restraints.

Signs and Symptoms

Violence is usually preceded by the following:
- Hyperactivity is the most important predictor of imminent violence (e.g., pacing, restlessness)
- Increasing anxiety and tension: clenched jaw or fist, rigid posture, fixed or tense facial expression, mumbling to self, shortness of breath, sweating, rapid pulse
- Verbal aggression (e.g., uses profanity, is argumentative, makes intrusive demands)
- Loud voice; change of pitch; or very soft voice, forcing others to strain to hear
- Changes in level of consciousness (e.g., confusion, disorientation, memory impairment)
- Intense eye contact or avoidance of eye contact
- Recent acts of violence, including property violence
- Verbal silence
- Alcohol or substance intoxication
- Possession of a weapon or object that might be used as a weapon (e.g., fork, knife, meal tray)
- Conditions conducive to violence:
  - Overcrowding
  - Inexperienced staff
  - Confrontational/controlling staff
  - Poor limit setting
  - Arbitrary revocation of privileges

Box 17.1 Guidelines for the Use of Seclusion and Restraint

Indications for Use
- To protect the patient from self-harm
- To prevent the patient from assaulting others

Legal Requirements
- Multidisciplinary involvement
- Appropriate health care provider's signature according to state law
- Patient advocate or relative notification
- Restraint or seclusion discontinued as soon as possible

Documentation
- Behaviors leading to restraint or seclusion
- Least restrictive interventions used before restraint
- Response to interventions
- Plan of care for seclusion or restraint use implemented
- Ongoing evaluations by appropriate health care providers

Clinical Assessments
- Patient's mental status at time of restraint
- Physical examination for medical problems that may contribute to behaviors
- Need for restraints

Observation
- 1:1 observation by staff
- Document every 15 minutes
- Range of movement
- Monitor vital signs
- If restrained, observe blood flow in the hands and feet and chafing
- Provide for nutrition, hydration, and elimination

Release Procedure
- Patient is able to follow instructions and stay in control
- Terminate seclusion or restraints
- Debrief with the patient

Other Tips
- Physically holding patients is a restraint
- Four side rails up is a restraint except in seizure precautions
- Tucking sheets in so tightly that a patient cannot move is a restraint
- Orders for seclusion or restraint are never written on an as-needed basis

Nursing Diagnoses

Impaired coping is an appropriate nursing diagnosis for patients who have angry and aggressive responses to stressful, frustrating, or threatening situations (International Council of Nurses, 2019). When a patient's anxiety and anger escalate to levels at which there is a potential for harm to self and others, *risk for violence* is the priority. During this time, talking-down skills are used first. Offering as-needed medication is the next step. If pharmacotherapy is ineffective, restraint or seclusion of an aggressive patient may be necessary.

Patients Who Are Angry and Hostile

Impaired Coping

Related to
- Neurological dysfunction
- Inadequate perception of control
- Perception of being threatened
- Impaired tension management
- Misperception of others' motives
- Knowledge deficit
- Overwhelming crisis situations
- Impaired reality testing
- Severe anxiety
- Substance use, intoxication, or withdrawal
- Ineffective problem-solving strategies or skills
- Personal vulnerability

Desired Outcome The patient will demonstrate improved coping.

Assessment/Interventions and *Rationales*

1. Assess your own feelings in the situation. Do not take the patient's abusive statements personally or becoming defensive. *Although patients are often skillful at making personal and pointed statements, they do not know nurses personally and have no basis on which to make accurate judgments.*
2. Avoid angry responses, no matter how threatened or angry you feel. *Confrontational responses by an authority figure will increase hostility.*
3. Monitor anger and aggressive behavior. Do not minimize such behavior in the hope that it will go away.

Minimizing the extent of angry feelings and aggressive behaviors contributes to unresponsiveness to potential violence.

4. Set clear, consistent, and enforceable limits on behavior, and stress the consequences of not adhering to those behaviors. *Behavioral limits provide structure for the patient and promote consistent responses from the staff.*

5. Emphasize that cognitively aware patients are responsible for the consequences of their aggressive behavior, including legal charges. *Patients may believe that behaviors in the hospital are immune from legal ramification. The majority of states have statutes addressing assaults on health care providers, and most states have made such assaults felonies.*

6. Emphasize that you are setting limits on specific behaviors, not feelings (e.g., "It is okay to be angry with Dennis, but it is not okay to threaten him or yell at him"). *Patients can learn to express feelings safely while recognizing that acting on feelings is not acceptable.*

7. Use a matter-of-fact, neutral approach. Remain calm using a moderate, firm voice and calming hand gestures. *A matter-of-fact approach can help interrupt the cycle of escalating anger.*

8. If anger escalates, let the patient know that you will leave the room for a period of time and will be back when the situation is calmer. Return when the time is up. *When this response is given in a neutral, matter-of-fact manner, the patient's anger is not rewarded. Always return at the time specified and focus communication on neutral topics.*

9. Provide positive feedback for interactive communication, such as non–illness-related topics, by responding to requests and providing emotional support. *This reinforces appropriate communication and behaviors and gives the patient and nurse time to share healthier communication and increase rapport.*

10. Avoid power struggles. *Power struggles are perceived as a challenge and generally lead to escalation of the conflict.*

11. Respond to feelings of anxiety or anger with active listening and validation of distress. *Active listening and validation build trust and allow the patient to feel heard and understood.*

12. Work with the patient to identify triggers for anger. *Recognizing triggers is an important step in a structured violence-prevention strategy.*

13. Identify risk factors for perpetuating violence (e.g., family chaos, other mental or environmental risk factors). *Treating the risk factors (e.g., getting family counseling, finding a job) reduces the family cycle of violence.*

14. Work with the patient to identify what supports are lacking, and problem-solve ways to attain support. *Feeling alone feeds into a sense of powerlessness and anger. Gaining external support promotes a sense of safety.*

15. Teach the patient, and if possible, the family or significant others, the steps in the problem-solving process.
    a. Define the problem
    b. Generate alternative solutions
    c. Select an alternative solution
    d. Implement the solution
    e. Evaluate the results of the solution
    Many people have never learned a systematic and effective approach to dealing with and mastering tough life situations or problems. A concrete method for problem solving empowers the patient.

16. Role-play alternative behaviors that can be used in stressful and overwhelming situations when becoming angry. *Role-playing allows the patient to rehearse alternative ways of handling stressful and angry feelings in a safe environment.*

17. Work with the patient to set behavioral goals. Give positive feedback when goals are reached. *Setting goals and giving positive feedback allow the patient a sense of control while learning goal-setting skills. Achieving self-set goals can enhance a person's sense of self and support new and more effective approaches to feelings of frustration.*

18. Explore outlets for stress and anxiety such as exercising, listening to music, reading, talking to others, attending support groups, and participating in a sport. *Alternative means of channeling emotions may help patients decrease anxiety and stress and allow for more cognitive approaches to their situation (e.g., using a problem-solving approach).*

19. Provide the patient and family with community resources that teach assertiveness training, anger management, and stress-reduction techniques. *Goal-directed and structured activities provide patients and families with continued support in the community.*

Patients With Potential to Harm Self or Others

Risk for Violence

Related to

- Neurological dysfunction
- History of violent behavior
- History of childhood abuse or witnessing family violence
- History of violence against others
- Psychosis (i.e., hallucinations, delusions, disorganized thought)
- Impulsivity
- Rage
- Mania
- Cognitive impairment
- Substance use, intoxication, or withdrawal
- Excitement, irritability, agitation

Desired Outcome The patient will be free from violence.

Assessment/Interventions and *Rationales*

1. Keep environmental stimulation at a minimum during periods of anger and aggressive behavior (e.g., lower lights, keep levels of noise down, ask patients and visitors to leave the area, or have staff take the patient to another area). *Overstimulation can increase the patient's anxiety level, leading to increased agitation or aggressive behaviors.*

2. Keep your voice calm, and speak in a low tone. A high-pitched rapid voice can increase anxiety levels in others. *The opposite is true when the tone of voice is low and calm and the words are spoken slowly.*

3. Call the patient by name and, if necessary, introduce yourself. Orient the patient as needed and explain what you are going to do. *Calling the patient by name helps to establish contact. Orienting and giving information can minimize misrepresentation of nurses' intentions.*

4. Use personal safety precautions:
   a. Leave the door open or use a hallway to talk.
   b. If you sense a potential for violence, alert other staff to stay nearby.
   c. Never turn your back on an angry patient.
   d. Have an exit available.
   e. For home visits: (1) Visit the patient with a colleague if there is concern regarding aggression, and

(2) leave the home immediately if there are signs that the patient's behavior is escalating.
Your safety is always the first priority. Always call in colleagues or other staff if you feel threatened or in physical danger.

5. Nursing and security staff require initial and ongoing training in managing disruptive behavior, including anger deescalation and seclusion and restraint procedures. *Professional training increases safe responses and reduces negative outcomes such as injury.*

6. Document the patient's behaviors and staff interventions during each level of intervention. *Documentation provides direction for future episodes and is essential from a legal standpoint.*

7. When interventions are needed to reduce escalating anger, always use the least restrictive intervention first and then move to more restrictive methods if necessary:
   a. Verbal intervention
   b. Decrease environmental stimulation or suggest a quiet area
   c. Pharmacological interventions
   d. Physical—seclusion or restraint
   Human dignity and autonomy are supported through the least restrictive approach. Use seclusion or restraint only when there is no less restrictive alternative.

8. Encourage the patient to talk about angry feelings and find ways to tolerate or reduce angry and aggressive feelings. *When the patient feels heard and understood and has help with problem-solving alternative options, deescalation of anger and aggression is often possible.*

9. Use empathetic verbal interventions (e.g., "It must be frightening to be here and to be feeling out of control"). *Empathetic verbal intervention is the most effective method of calming an agitated, fearful, anxious patient.*

10. When interpersonal interventions fail to decrease the patient's anger, consider the need for medication. Assessment includes determining whether aggression is acute or chronic. *Often pharmacological interventions can help patients gain control of their behavior and prevent continued escalation of anger and hostile impulses.*

11. Alert other staff and hospital security if anger and aggressive responses are evident and ask for their presence at a distance. *Demonstrating a show of force if*

necessary provides the patient with external support. Maintaining a distance provides the patient with a chance to regain control without a physical confrontation.

12. When interpersonal interventions and pharmalogical interventions fail, physical intervention (i.e., seclusion or restraint) is the final resort. Follow organization protocol. Refer to Box 17.1 for guidelines for the use of restraints. *Protocol tells staff when to restrain, how to restrain, how long before a provider's order is needed, nursing interventions for the patient during the period of restraint or seclusion, how often to check restraints or the patient in seclusion, whom to call, and how often the need for restraints or seclusion must be reevaluated by physician.*

 NURSE, PATIENT, AND FAMILY RESOURCES

Anger Busters.com
www.angerbusters.com

Anger Management
www.mentalhelp.net
Search for "anger management."

Centers for Disease Control and Prevention
www.cdc.gov
Search for "anger" to find multiple articles.

Centers for Medicare and Medicaid Services
www.cms.gov
Search for "seclusion and restraint" for national guidelines

National Anger Management Association
https://namass.org/index.html

CHAPTER 18

Family Violence

Family violence can take the form of emotional, physical, or sexual abuse; neglect; or economic abuse.

- Emotional abuse damages the spirit and may impair the ability to succeed later in life, to feel deeply, or to make emotional contact with others.
- Physical abuse includes emotional abuse in addition to the potential for long-term physical injuries, scarring, pain, and, in some cases, death.
- Sexual abuse in children may result in low self-esteem, self-hatred, emotional instability, and anger and aggression. Interpersonal relationships are impaired by an inability to trust and difficulty in protecting themselves.
- Neglect may result in malnutrition, lack of supervision, failure to thrive, inadequate clothing, shelter, and medical care. Behavioral responses to neglect include apathy, fearfulness, and destructive behavior
- Economic abuse is controlling a person's access to economic resources, making an individual financially dependent. This financial abuse is the greatest barrier to partners leaving abusive situations. Older adults may lose assets, property, and self-agency.

In this chapter we discuss abuse as it occurs in the lifespan. Family violence includes child abuse, intimate partner violence, and older adult abuse.

ASSESSMENT

Sensitivity is required of a nurse who suspects family violence. A person who feels judged or accused of wrongdoing will become defensive. This defensiveness will undermine attempts to change coping strategies in the family. It is better for the nurse to ask about ways of solving disagreements or methods of disciplining children rather than using the word abuse or violence, which appears judgmental and therefore is threatening to the family. It is also important not to assume a person's sexual orientation. Use the term partner when asking about the relationship. Interview guidelines are suggested in box 18.1.

Box 18.1 **Interview Guidelines**

- Conduct the interview in private.
- Be direct, honest, and professional.
- Use language the patient understands.
- Ask the patient to clarify words not understood.
- Be understanding.
- Be attentive.
- Inform the patient if a referral is nessesary to child or adult protective services, and explain the process.
- Assess safety, and help reduce danger.
- Indicate that the patient was at fault

Signs and Symptoms

- Feelings of helplessness or powerlessness
- Repeated emergency room or hospital visits
- Vague complaints, including insomnia, abdominal pain, hyperventilation, headache, or menstrual problems
- Unexplained bruises in various stages of healing
- Injuries (bruises, fractures, scrapes, lacerations) that do not seem to fit the description of the "accident"
- Frightened, withdrawn, depressed, or despondent appearance

Assessment Questions

The nurse uses therapeutic communication techniques to obtain the answers to the following questions. Using your discretion, decide which questions are appropriate to complete your assessment. A general question that can be posed to any victim of family violence is "Tell me about what happened to you." Other questions are based on the relationship between the abused and the perpetrators of violence.

For Children

"Who takes care of you?"

"Have you been taken to the hospital for accidents or injuries?"

"Have you been taken to the hospital for accidents or injuries?"

For Parents

"What arrangement do you make when you have to leave your child alone?"

"How do you discipline your child?"

"When your infant cries for a long time, how do you get your infant to stop?"

"What about your child's behavior bothers you the most?"

"Who helps you with your children?"

"How much time do you have for yourself?"

For Intimate Partners

"How do you and your partner resolve disagreements?"

"Have you been hit, kicked, or otherwise hurt by someone in the past year? By whom?"

"Do you feel safe in your current relationship?"

"Is there a partner from a previous relationship who is making you feel unsafe now?"

For Older Adults

Do you feel safe at home?"

"How do you discipline your child?"

"Has anyone limited your daily activities?"

"Does anyone talk to you in a threatening way?"

"Does anyone hit you?"

"Has anyone asked you for money or asked you to sign contracts you didn't recognize?"

ASSESSMENT GUIDELINES

During your assessment and counseling, maintain an interested and empathetic manner. Retain self-awareness and avoid expressions of anger, shock, or disapproval of the perpetrator or the situation. Assess for the following:

A. Signs and symptoms of family violence
B. Qualities of individuals who are vulnerable for child abuse are listed in Box 18.2

Box 18.2 **Assessing Vulnerability for Child Abuse**

- New parents whose behavior toward the infant is rejecting, hostile, or indifferent.
- Teenage parents, most of whom are children themselves, require special help and guidance in handling the baby and discussing their expectations of the baby and their support systems.
- Parents with intellectual disability, for whom careful, explicit, and repeated instructions on caring for the child and recognizing the infant's needs are indicated.
- Parents who grew up in abusive homes. This is the biggest risk factor for perpetuation of family violence.

C. Physical, sexual, or emotional abuse and neglect and economic maltreatment in the case of older adults
D. Family coping patterns
E. Patient's support system
F. Substance use
G. Suicidal or homicidal ideation
H. Posttrauma syndrome

If the patient is a child or an older adult, identify the protection agency in your state that will need to be notified.

SELF-ASSESSMENT

Working with individuals who experience violence may trigger intense and overwhelming feelings in the nurse, especially in new nurses. Strong negative feelings regarding abuse may cloud your judgment and interfere with objective assessment and intervention. A personal history of abuse may also cause a nurse to identify too closely with the victim. Sharing perceptions and feelings with other professionals can help with feelings of anger, frustration, and the need to rescue.

Nursing Diagnoses

Violence brings with it pain, psychological anguish and physical injury and the potential for death. Therefore *risk for violence* is a major concern for nurses and other members of the health care team. (International Council of Nurses, 2019). This chapter discusses *risk for violence* for the child, intimate partner, and older adult

Within all families in which violence occurs, coping skills are not adequate to handle the emotional and environmental events that trigger the crisis situation. Inadequate coping skills within the family result in members not having their needs met, including the need for safety, security, and sense of self. Therefore there exists *risk for violence* within the family. This nursing diagnosis is discussed with interventions geared toward the abused child, partner, and older adult.

While it is obvious that survivors of family violence require intervention, a second level of nursing care is aimed at the perpetrators. In this chapter we use *impaired family coping to address the support needed to break the cycle of violence. Perpetrators include parents, intimate partners, and older adult caregivers.*

There are many other nursing diagnoses the nurse can address in caring for children and adults who are suffering from abuse at the hands of others. These include *anxiety, fear, impaired family role performance, posttrauma response, powerlessness, caregiver stress, disturbed body image, chronic low and situational low self-esteem*, and impaired *parenting.*

INTERVENTION GUIDELINES

CHILD, INTIMATE PARTNER, AND OLDER ADULT

A. Establish rapport before focusing on the details of the violent experience.
B. Provide reassurance that the patient did nothing wrong.
C. Allow the patient to tell the story without interruptions.
D. If the patient is an adult, provide assurance of confidentiality.
E. If the patient is a child, report abuse to appropriate authorities designated in your state.
F. If the patient is an older adult, check with state laws for reporting information.
G. Establish a safety plan in situations of partner abuse.

FORENSIC ISSUES

A. Follow hospital protocol. Keep your charting detailed, accurate, and up to date.
B. The sexual assault nurse examiner (SANE) has specialized training to carry out evidentiary examinations of victims of sexual assault. The SANE nurse:
   1. Documents verbatim statements of who caused the injury and when it occurred

2. Draws a body map to indicate size, color, shape, areas, and types of injuries with explanation
3. Gathers physical evidence, when possible, of sexual abuse (e.g., vaginal and anal swabs, fingernail scrapings)
4. Obtains permission to take photos

Nursing Care for Family Violence

Survivors of Abuse

Risk for Violence

Related to

- History of rage reaction
- Poor coping skills
- History of or current substance use
- Limited impulse control
- Pathological family dynamics
- History of violence? neglect, or emotional deprivation as a child
- Psychiatric disorders

Abused Child

Desired Outcome The child will be free from violence.

Assessment/Interventions and *Rationales*

1. Use a nonthreatening, nonjudgmental relationship with the parents. *If the parents feel judged or blamed or become defensive, they may take the child and either seek help elsewhere or not seek help at all.*
2. Understand that children do not want to betray their parents. *Even in an intolerable situation, the parents are the most important security the child knows.*
3. Provide for a complete physical assessment of the child. *A complete physical assessment will support essential care and substantiate reporting to the child welfare agency if required.*
4. Use dolls to help tell the child's story. *The child might not know how to articulate what happened or might be afraid of punishment. Using dolls can be an easier way for the child to act out what happened.*

Forensic Issues With an Abused Child

1. Identify your agency and state policies on reporting child abuse. Contact the supervisor or social worker to

implement appropriate reporting. *Health care workers are mandated to report cases of suspected or actual child abuse.*

2. Ensure that proper procedures are followed, and evidence is collected. *If the child is temporarily taken to a safe environment, appropriate evidence helps protect the child's future welfare.*

3. Keep accurate and detailed records of the incident:
   a. Verbatim statements of who caused the injury and when it occurred
   b. Body map to indicate size, color, shape, areas, and types of injuries, along with an explanation
   c. Physical evidence, when possible, of sexual abuse
   d. Photographs (check hospital policy regarding permissions)
   Accurate records can help ensure the child's future safety and court presentation.

4. Conduct a forensic examination of a sexually assaulted child according to specific protocols provided by law enforcement agencies and particular medical facilities. Ideally, SANE nurses, or nurses who have advanced training, will conduct the examination. *The proper collection, handling, and storage of forensic specimens are crucial to the court presentation.*

Abused Partner
Desired Outcome The abused partner will be free from violence.

Assessment/Interventions and *Rationales*
1. Ensure that medical attention is provided to the patient. Ask permission to take photographs. *If the patient wants to file charges, photographs will support the case.*

2. Set up an interview in private and ensure confidentiality. *The patient might be terrified of retribution and further attacks from the partner for telling someone about the abuse.*

3. In a nonthreatening manner, assess the following areas:
   a. Sexual abuse
   b. Physical abuse
   c. Economic abuse
   d. Suicidal or homicidal thoughts
   These are all vital issues in planning care. Sexual abuse often accompanies physical abuse. Economic abuse may deter the individual from leaving. Self-directed or other-directed violence may seem like the only way out.

Box 18.3 **Partner Abuse—Assessing the Level of Violence in the Home**

Does the patient feel safe?
Has there been a recent increase in violence?
Has the patient been choked?
Is there a weapon in the house?
Has the perpetrator used or threatened to use a weapon?
Has the perpetrator threatened to harm the children?
Has the perpetrator threatened to kill the patient?

---

4. Encourage the patient to talk about the incident without interruptions. *Listening, along with attending behaviors, will facilitate full sharing.*
5. Assess for the level of violence in the home (Box 18.3). *Each cycle of violence can become more intense. Danger for the life of the survivor and children increases over time. When the perpetrator chokes the individual, they are in real danger.*
6. Ask about the welfare of the children in the home. *Intimate partner abuse is often accompanied by child abuse.*
7. Assess whether the patient has a safe place to go when violence is escalating. Provide a list of shelters or safe houses with other written information. *When an abused partner makes the decision to leave, the risk of homicide dramatically increases. An emergency shelter can make the difference between life and death.*

Forensic Issues With An Abused Partner
1. Identify whether the patient is interested in pressing charges. If yes, give information on:
   a. Attorneys who specialize in abuse
   b. Nonprofit law firms for low-income individuals and families
   c. Community advocates
      Legal support and advocates who can direct the abused partner to community resources are essential in helping to establish independence.
2. Identify your state laws for documenting and reporting suspected partner abuse. *State laws vary on the process for documenting and reporting domestic violence.*
3. Provide a written plan that includes shelter and referral numbers that can be used during the escalation of

anxiety, before actual violence erupts. *A sense of emergency may be the motivation to leave, and a plan must be in place to keep the patient safe.*

4. Emphasize the following messages:
   a. "No one deserves to be beaten."
   b. "You cannot make anyone hurt you."
   c. "It is not your fault."
      When self-esteem is eroded, people often buy into the myth that they deserved the abuse because they did something wrong, and if they had not done it, then it would not have happened.

5. Encourage patients to reach out to family and friends whom they might have been avoiding or isolated from. *Often survivors of violence are isolated from family and friends due to shame and/or control on the part of their partners who want to isolate them. Rallying support will strengthen the patient's resolve.*

6. Become familiar with therapists in your community with experience working with battered partners. *Psychotherapy with survivors of trauma requires special skills on the part of even an experienced therapist.*

7. If the patient is not ready to act at this time, provide a list of community resources available:
   a. Hotlines
   b. Shelters
   c. Support groups
   d. Community advocates
   e. Social services
      It can take time for patients to make decisions to change their life situation. Survivors of abuse need appropriate information.

See Box 18.4 for a personalized safety plan for when the abused partner is in a relationship and when the relationship is over.

Abused Older Adult
Desired Outcome The older adult will be free from violence.

Assessment/Interventions and *Rationales*

1. Assess the severity of signs and symptoms of abuse and potential for further abuse on a weekly level. *This determines the need for further intervention.*

Box 18.4 **Personalized Safety Plan**

Suggestions for Increasing Safety—In the Relationship

I will have important phone numbers available to my children and myself.

I can tell _____ and _____ about the violence and ask them to call the police if they hear suspicious noises coming from my home.

If I leave my home, I can go (list four places) _____, _____, _____, or _____.

I can leave extra money, car keys, clothes, and copies of documents with _____.

If I leave, I will bring _____ (see checklist below).

To ensure safety and independence, I can: keep change for phone calls with me at all times; open my own savings account; rehearse my escape route with a support person; and review my safety plan on _____ (date).

Suggestions for Increasing Safety—When the Relationship Is Over

I can change the locks; I can install steel or metal doors, a security system, smoke detectors, and an outside lighting system.

I will inform _____ and _____ that my partner no longer lives with me and ask them to call the police if my former partner is observed near my home or my children.

I will tell people who take care of my children the names of those who have permission to pick them up. The people who have permission are: _____, _____, and _____.

I can tell _____ at work about my situation and ask _____ to screen my calls.

I can avoid stores, banks, and _____ that I used when I lived with my abusive partner.

I can obtain a protective order from _____. I can keep it on or near me at all times, as well as have a copy with _____.

If I feel down and ready to return to a potentially abusive situation, I can call _____ for support or attend workshops and support groups to gain support and strengthen my relationships with other people.

Important Phone Numbers

Police _____

Hotline _____

Friends _____

Shelter _____

Continued

Box 18.4 **Personalized Safety Plan—cont'd**

Items to Take Checklist
Identification
Mobile phones and chargers
Birth certificates for me and my children
Social Security cards
School and medical records
Money, bankbooks, credit cards
Keys (house/car/office)
Driver's license and registration
Medications
Change of clothes
Welfare identification
Passports, Green Cards, work permits
Divorce papers
Lease/rental agreement, house deed
Mortgage payment book, current unpaid bills
Insurance papers
Address book
Pictures, jewelry, items of sentimental value
Children's favorite toys and/or blankets

Box 18.5 **Older Adult Abuse/Neglect—Home Assessment**

- House in poor repair
- Inadequate heat, lighting, furniture, cooking utensils
- Presence of garbage or rodents
- Old food in kitchen
- Lack of assistive devices
- Locks on refrigerator
- Blocked stairways
- Older adult lying in urine, feces, or food
- Unpleasant odors

---

2. Assess environmental conditions as factors in the abuse or neglect (Box 18.5). *Assessment identifies the areas in need of intervention and the degree of abuse or neglect.*
3. If abuse is suspected, discuss it with the older adult and caregiver separately. *Talking separately helps attain*

a better understanding of what is happening and minimizes friction among the parties involved.

4. Discuss with the older adult the factors leading to abuse. *Discussing these factors identifies triggers to abusive behaviors and areas for teaching for the perpetrator.*

5. Stress concern for physical safety. *Stressing concern validates that the situation is serious.*

Forensic Issues With An Abused Older Adult

1. Know your state laws regarding older adult abuse. Notify your supervisor, physicians, and social services when a suspected abuse is reported. *Knowing the laws keeps the channels of communication open and emphasizes the need for accurate and detailed records.*

2. If undue influence is suspected, consult with an expert who is experienced in geriatric or forensic psychiatry. *Consulting with an expert can help determine whether the older adult is making medical, legal, or financial decisions based on coercion and manipulations of others to gain control of the older adult's finances, home, or decision making.*

3. Stress that no one has the right to abuse another person. *Often individuals who have been abused begin to believe they deserve the abuse.*

4. Discuss the following with the patient:
   a. Hotline
   b. Crisis unit
   c. Emergency numbers
   Discussing these options with the patient maximizes older adult safety through the use of support systems.

5. Explore with the older adult ways to make changes. *Exploring the various ways to make changes directs the assessment to positive areas.*

6. Assist the older adult in making decisions for future action. *Assisting the older adult lowers feelings of helplessness and identifies realistic options to an abusive situation.*

7. Involve community agencies to help monitor and resources the older adult. *It is best to involve as many agencies as can take a legitimate role in maintaining the older adult's safety.*

Perpetrators of Abuse

Impaired Family Coping
Related to
- Domestic violence
- Inadequate support system
- Family conflict
- Young age, developmental level
- Low socioeconomic status
- Substance or alcohol use
- Psychiatric disorders
- Neurological condition
- Lack of resources
- Lack of knowledge about role skills

Parents Who Abuse
Desired Outcome Parents will demonstrate improved family coping.

Assessment/Interventions and *Rationales*

1. Identify whether the child needs the following:
   a. Hospitalization for treatment and observation
   b. Referral to child protective services
      Immediate safety of the child is foremost. Temporary removal of the child in a volatile situation gives the nurse or counselor time to assess the family situation and coping skills and to rally community resources to decrease family stress.
2. Discuss with parents stresses the family unit is currently facing. Contact the appropriate agencies to help reduce stress:
   a. Economic aid
   b. Job opportunities
   c. Social services
   d. Family service agencies
   e. Social supports
   f. Public health nurse
   g. Day care teacher
   h. School teacher
   i. Social worker
   j. Respite worker
   k. Anger management therapy
   l. Encourage and give referrals for a specialist in family therapy. Family therapy is complex, teaches family members how to develop new strategies,

With the help of outside resources, family stress can be reduced, leading to an improved ability to problem solve.

3. Reinforce the parents' strengths and acknowledge the importance of continued medical care for the child. *Giving parents credit and support for positive parenting skills will encourage growth.*

4. Work with the parents to try safe methods to effectively discipline the child. *Understanding alternatives to abuse increases healthy family functioning while minimizing feelings of frustration and helplessness.*

5. Encourage parents to join a self-help group (e.g., Parents Anonymous, family counseling, group counseling). *Learning new ways of dealing with stress takes time, and support from others acts as an important incentive to change.*

6. Provide written information on hotlines, community supports, and agencies. *External resources reduce isolation and increase support during crisis periods.*

Partners Who Abuse

Desired Outcome The partner who abuses will demonstrate improved family coping.

Assessment/Interventions and *Rationales*

1. If the partner who abuses is motivated, arrange for participation in an anger management program. *Some evidence suggests that a 6- to 8-week structural program that trains patients with anger issues may help to deactivate angry emotional states.*

2. Work with the perpetrator to recognize signs of escalating anger. *Often the perpetrator is unaware of the process leading up to the rage reaction.*

3. Work with the perpetrator to learn ways of channeling anger nonviolently. *Violence is often a learned coping skill. Adaptive skills for dealing with anger must be learned.*

4. Encourage the perpetrator to discuss thoughts and feelings with others who have similar problems. *Discussing these thoughts and feelings minimizes isolation and encourages problem solving.*

5. Refer to self-help groups that are available virtually or in the community (e.g., Batterers Anonymous). *Self-help groups help patients look at their own behaviors among those who have similar problems.*

Provide the number of the National Domestic Violence Hotline, which is 1-800-799-SAFE (7233). *Hotlines provide immediate support for individuals who are beginning to escalate or want to stop the cycle of abuse.*

Older Adult Caregivers Who Abuse

Desired Outcome The perpetrator of older adult abuse will demonstrate improved family coping.

Assessment/Interventions and *Rationales*

1. Research your state laws regarding older adult abuse. *State laws vary regarding documenting and reporting abuse of older adults.*
2. Encourage the perpetrator to verbalize feelings about the older adult and the abusive situation. *The abuser might feel overwhelmed, isolated, and unsupported.*
3. Encourage problem solving when identifying stressful areas. *Encouragement assesses the perpetrator's approach to problem-solving skills and explores alternatives.*
4. Meet with the entire family, and identify stressors and problem areas. *Other family members might not be aware of the strain the perpetrator is under or the lack of safety to the abused family member.*
5. If there are no other family members, notify other community agencies that might help the stabilize the situation:
   a. Meals on Wheels
   b. Day care for seniors
   c. Respite services
   d. Visiting nurse service
      Support minimizes family stress and isolation and increases safety.
6. Initiate referrals for education, psychotherapy, group therapy, and support groups for the older adults and the perpetrator. *Education and therapy for an abusive caregiver may provide tools to deal with stress, develop coping skills, gain social support, and treat underlying mental health conditions such as major depressive disorder and anxiety.*
7. Suggest that family members meet together on a regular basis for problem solving and support. *Meeting will encourage the family to learn to solve problems together.*

Nurse, Patient, and Family Resources

Adult Survivors of Childhood Abuse Anonymous
www.asca12step.org

Child Abuse Prevention—KidsPeace
(800) 334-4KID.
www.kidspeace.org

Childhelp USA
(800) 4-A-CHILD—(800) 422-4453 (hotline)
www.childhelp.org

Institute on Violence, Abuse, and Trauma
www.fvsai.org

National Coalition Against Domestic Violence
www.ncadv.org

National Domestic Violence Hotline
www.thehotline.org
(800) 799-SAFE (hotline)

Rape, Abuse, and Incest National Network (RAINN)
www.rainn.org

Survivors of Incest Anonymous
www.siawso.org

Teen Line
www.teenlineonline.org
(800) TLC-TEEN

CHAPTER 19

Sexual Assault

Sexual assault is a violent crime. It is an act of violence, power, and hate, and sex is the weapon used by the perpetrator. Sexual assault includes fondling or unwanted sexual touch and forcing a victim to perform sexual acts. This type of violence includes child sexual assault, incest, intimate partner sexual violence, sexual assault of men and boys, and drug-facilitated sexual assault.

Sexual violence typically results in severe and long-term trauma. Long-term psychological effects of sexual assault include major depressive disorder, anxiety, fear, and even suicide in many survivors. Victims of incest might experience a negative self-image, major depressive disorder, eating disorders, personality disorders, self-destructive behavior, and substance use.

Rape is an extreme and specific type of sexual assault. The official Federal Bureau of Investigation (FBI) (US Department of Justice, 2013, para 1) definition of rape is, "penetration, no matter how slight, of the vagina or anus with any body part or object, or oral penetration by a sex organ of another person, without the consent of the victim."

It is usually men who rape, and most individuals who are raped are women. However, women may also sexually assault other women. Male-on-male sexual assault is also more prevalent in prisons and in the military than in the general population. A male who is sexually assaulted is more likely to have physical trauma and to have been victimized by several assailants than is a female. Males experience the same devastating severe and long-lasting trauma as females.

Rape-trauma response is closely related to acute stress disorder (ASD) and posttraumatic stress disorder (PTSD) This response also consists of two phases: (1) the acute phase and (2) the long-term reorganization phase. Nurses may encounter a patient right after the sexual assault or weeks, months, or even years after the assault. In either case, the individual will benefit from compassionate and effective nursing interventions.

When available, special care for this population is provided by sexual assault nurse examiners (SANEs). They are forensic nurses who have been certified to work with victims of sexual assault. Functions of the SANE are to perform a physical examination of the survivor, collect forensic evidence, provide expert testimony regarding forensic evidence collected, and support the psychological needs of the survivor.

ASSESSMENT

Signs and Symptoms

Acute Phase (0–2 Weeks)

- Shock, numbness, and disbelief
- Calm and composed
- Severe anxiety
- Tearful, sobbing
- Smiling, laughing
- Disorganization
- Somatic symptoms

Long-Term Reorganization Phase (2 Weeks or More)

- Intrusive thoughts of the rape throughout the day and night
- Flashbacks of the incident (i.e., re-experiencing the traumatic event)
- Dreams with violent content
- Insomnia
- Increased motor activity (e.g., moving, taking trips, changing telephone numbers, staying with friends)
- Mood swings, crying spells, depression
- Fears of:
  - The indoors (if rape occurred indoors)
  - Being outdoors (if rape occurred outdoors)
  - Being alone
  - Crowds
  - Sexual encounters

ASSESSMENT GUIDELINES

Assessment should be done in a nonthreatening manner. Use open-ended questions, broad openings, and general leads. For example, "It must have been very frightening to know that you had no control over what was happening."

A. Assess:
   1. Physical trauma: Document using a body map, and ask permission to take photographs.
   2. Emotional trauma: Document verbatim statements of the patient.
   3. Level of anxiety: If patients are in severe-to-panic levels of anxiety, they will not be able to problem solve or process information.
   4. Support system: Often partners or family members do not understand rape and might not be the best supports at this time.
   5. Community supports (e.g., attorneys, support groups, therapists) who work in the area of sexual assault.

B. Encourage patients to tell their story, but do not pressure them to do so.

INTERVENTION GUIDELINES

A. Follow your institution's protocol for sexual assault.
B. Do not leave the patient alone.
C. Maintain an accepting attitude.
D. Ensure confidentiality.
E. Encourage the patient to talk. Listen empathetically.
F. Emphasize that the patient is not responsible for the rape.

Nursing Care for Sexual Assault

Rape-Trauma Response

Related to
- Sexual assault

Desired Outcome The patient will return to pre-crisis level of functioning.

Assessment/Interventions and *Rationales*

1. Arrange for someone to stay with the patient (e.g., friend, neighbor, or staff member) while the patient is waiting to be treated in the emergency department. *Individuals who are experiencing high levels of anxiety need someone with them until the anxiety level is reduced to moderate or mild.*

2. Approach the patient in a nonjudgmental manner. *Nurses' attitudes can have an important therapeutic effect.*

3. The patient's situation should not be discussed with anyone other than medical personnel involved, unless the patient gives consent. *Confidentiality is crucial from a moral and ethical standpoint, as well as a legal right.*

4. Provide support and anticipate acute and provide support for symptoms such as shock, numbness, disbelief, anxiety, tearfulness, disorganization, and somatic symptoms. *Patients need external support and direction during the acute phase of the rape-trauma response when anxiety levels are high.*

5. Listen and let the patient talk, but do not pressure the patient to talk. *When the patient feels understood and sets the pace of the conversation, the patient feels more in control of the situation. Allowing the patient to set the pace.*

6. If the patient is feeling guilt or shame about the rape, stress that the patient did nothing wrong. *Individuals who are raped patients might feel guilt or shame. Reinforcing that they did nothing wrong can reduce guilt and maintain self-esteem.*

7. Avoid judgmental language. For example, consider the difference between the following words: reported rather than alleged, declined rather than refused, penetration rather than intercourse. *Sensitive word choices support the patient during the crisis phase and as the patient recovers.*

8. Arrange for follow-up support:
   a. Rape counselor
   b. Support group
   c. Group therapy
   d. Individual therapy
   e. Crisis counseling

9. As anxiety resolves, identify the symptoms that patients may experience during the long-term reorganization phase, such as nightmares, phobias, anxiety, depression, insomnia, and somatic symptoms. *Many*

patients think they are going crazy as time goes on and they still are not better. They are often unaware that this is a process that many individuals in their situation have experienced.

Forensic Issues for Sexual Assault Survivors.

1. Assess the patient for signs and symptoms of physical trauma. *The most common injuries are to the face, head, neck, and extremities.* The patient may not realize the extent of the injuries and their treatment may become the priority for itnervention.
2. Make a body map to identify the size, color, and location of injuries. *A body map of injuries provides direction for the treatment team along with legal documentation.*
3. Ask permission to take photographs. *Accurate records and photos can be used as medicolegal evidence for the future.*
4. Carefully explain all procedures before doing them (e.g., "We would like to do a vaginal (or rectal) examination and obtain evidence. Have you had a vaginal (or rectal) examination before?"). *The patient is experiencing high levels of anxiety. Matter-of-fact explanations of what you plan to do and why you are doing it can help reduce fear and anxiety.*
5. Explain the forensic specimens you plan to collect. Inform the patient that they can be used for identification and prosecution of the perpetrator:
   a. Pubic hair
   b. Skin from underneath nails
   c. Semen samples
   d. Blood
      Collecting body fluids and i.e., swabbing for DNA is essential for identifying the perpetrator.
6. Encourage the patient to consider treatment and evaluation for sexually transmittcd diseases before leaving the emergency department. *Many survivors do not follow-up after being seen in the emergency department or crisis center and will not otherwise get protection.*
7. Prescribers offer emergency contraception to women who have been assaulted. Follow through on dispensing the contraception. *Women are at risk for pregnancy.*
8. Carefully document all data:
   a. Verbatim statements
   b. Detailed observations of physical trauma

c. Detailed observations of emotional status
d. Physical examination findings
e. Laboratory test results
   Accurate and detailed documentation supports the patient with crucial legal evidence.

 Nurse, Patient, and Family Resources

Institute on Violence, Abuse, and Trauma
www.ivatcenters.org

Rape, Abuse, and Incest National Network (RAINN)
(800) 656-HOPE (4673)
www.rainn.org
Online chat: online.rainn.org

Survivors of Incest Anonymous (SIA)
www.siawso.org

David Baldwin's Trauma Information Pages
www.trauma-pages.com
Focuses on emotional trauma and traumatic stress

Male Survivor
www.malesurvivor.org

CHAPTER 20

Grieving

Loss is a part of life, and grieving is the response that enables people to accept and reconcile with the loss and adapt to change. Losing a significant other by death is a major life crisis. Long-term relationships bond us to each other deeply, shaping our world and our identity in it. The loss of a loved one can diminish aspects of our own self-concept. Other types of losses include loss of a significant object such as a possession, job, status, home, and parts and processes of one's body. Grief is experienced holistically, affecting us emotionally, cognitively, physically, and spiritually.

A couple of terms related to grief timing are bereavement and mourning. Bereavement, derived from the Old English word *berafian*, poignantly meaning, "to rob," is the period of grieving after a death. Mourning refers to things people do to cope with grief, including shared social expressions of grief such as calling hours, funerals, and bereavement groups. The length of time, degree, and rituals for mourning are often typically determined by cultural, religious, and familial factors.

Grieving is a complex, individual, culturally embedded process of accepting death. It involves experiencing the pain of grief, constructing an identity, and living life in a transformed environment. Depending on many factors, this process can take months to a number of years. Losses transform lives. After a loss, we are never quite the same person again. Yet, over time, people move from pain that defines who they are, to living with the residual pain and integrating the memory of the loved one into their future lives.

Successful grieving is evidenced by the following attributes:
- Accepting the death of a loved one.
- Minimal distressing memories of the deceased.
- An absence of anger over the loss.
- Avoidance of reminders of the deceased no longer occurs.
- A belief that life is worth living without the deceased.

- Increased sense of identity apart from the lost relationship.
- Engaging in activities, pursuing relationships, or planning for the future.

GRIEF VERSUS MAJOR DEPRESSIVE DISORDER

Symptoms of grieving may mirror those of major depressive disorder. Feelings of intense sadness, constant thinking about the loss, insomnia, lack of appetite, and weight loss may be understandable. However, in grief, the predominant feelings are emptiness and loss that occur in waves, sometimes alternating with feelings of acceptance. The depression experienced in major depressive disorder, on the other hand, results in a global inability to experience joy and feelings of guilt and self-loathing.

Prior to the current edition of the *Diagnostic and Statistical Manual of Mental Disorders (DSM)*, clinicians were discouraged from diagnosing an individual with major depressive disorder within 2 months of losing a loved one. This guideline was referred to as the bereavement exclusion. This exclusion was removed from the fifth edition of the manual, the *DSM-5*. The recognition that grieving could, in fact, be complicated by major depressive disorder has resulted in more people being treated for the disorder, thereby alleviating painful depressive symptoms.

PERSISTENT COMPLEX BEREAVEMENT DISORDER

The American Psychiatric Association (APA, 2013) proposed a condition for further study, *persistent complex bereavement disorder*. This disorder would apply to individuals whose bereavement persists beyond 12 months in adults and 6 months in children. In addition to the timing, interference with normal functioning is the hallmark symptom that distinguishes grieving from a disorder. Suicidal ideation and disinterest in living make this bereavement disorder particularly dangerous.

Symptoms of this complicated grieving include preoccupation with thoughts of the deceased person, feelings of emptiness, anger, depression, disbelief, detachment, and rumination. Self-blame may be a prominent symptom. For example, a widow may obsessively blame herself for her spouse not seeking help for chest pain.

THEORY

Kübler-Ross's (1973) groundbreaking work provides a framework for understanding individuals' reactions to dying. Her stage theory was eventually applied to the grieving process as well. Denial, anger, bargaining, depression, and acceptance are used to describe responses to loss.

Although viewing the grieving process as linear—from denial to eventual acceptance—is appealing, grieving is not that simple. In reality, these stages overlap and may be nonsequential. Stroebe and Schut (1999) incorporated the stage–phase models of loss-oriented processes with the restoration of a new lifestyle. This process involves coping with everyday life, building a new identity, and developing new relationships. Table 20.1 summarizes the dual process model.

Assessment

Signs and Symptoms of Anticipatory Grief and Grief

- Anger
- Blame
- Despair
- Preoccupation with the deceased
- Crying
- Detachment
- Disorganization
- Altered activity level

Table 20.1 **Dual Process Model of Coping**

Loss-Oriented Processes	Restoration-Oriented Process
Grief work	Attending to life changes
Intrusion of grief	Distraction from grief
Denial or avoidance of restoration changes	Doing new things
Breaking bonds or ties	Establishing new roles, identities, and relationships

- Disturbed sleep pattern
- Pain
- Panic behavior
- Vegetative signs (e.g., anorexia, insomnia, bowel dysfunction, immobility)

Additional Signs and Symptoms of Dysfunctional Grief

- Prolonged, severe symptoms beyond 12 months in adults and 6 months in children
- Limited response to support
- Profound feelings of hopelessness
- Excessive withdrawal
- Fears of being alone
- Inability to work
- Inability to feel emotion
- Feeling dead or unreal
- Panic attacks
- Self-neglect
- Suicidal ideation
- Maladaptive behaviors: alcohol or substance use, indiscriminate sexual activity, compulsive spending, fugue states, and aggression
- Recurrent nightmares, night terrors, and compulsive reenactments
- Other common expressions of grieving are found in Table 20.2

ASSESSMENT GUIDELINES

A. Identify the patient's perception of the impending loss/loss.
B. Identify the stage of grieving that the patient is experiencing or has experienced (i.e., denial, anger, bargaining, depression, or acceptance).
C. Evaluate whether the individual is at risk for complicated grieving.
D. Evaluate for psychotic symptoms, agitation, increased activity, alcohol or substance use, and extreme vegetative symptoms (e.g., anorexia, insomnia, weight loss, bowel dysfunction, immobility).

Table 20.2 Common Expressions of Grieving

Yearnings	Survivors repeatedly want to reunite with the person who died in some way, and they may even want to die themselves to be with their loved one.
Deep sadness	Waves of deep sadness and regret about the loved one; crying is common.
Other negative emotions	Anger, remorse, and guilt.
Somatic disturbances	Grief commonly results in sleep problems, changes in appetite, digestive difficulties, dry mouth, or fatigue after a loss. Restlessness and agitation may also occur.
Disbelief	It takes people a long time to accept that a loved one has died. People may forget the loved one is gone until some reminder brings the reality back.
Apathy	People often withdraw or disengage when grieving. People may become irritable toward others.
Emotional surges	Although the worst emotions and disturbances diminish with time, the grieving process also involves surges of emotions. Holidays, anniversaries, birthdays, and other significant events can trigger grief reactions.
Vivid memories	Recalling vivid memories of the deceased is common. Images of the deceased—or even the sound of a loved one's voice—may emerge without warning.

E. Consider individuals who do not express significant grief in the context of a major loss as at risk for dysfunctional grief.

F. Always assess for suicide with signs and symptoms of depression.

G. Assess for significant anger and the potential for violence.

H. Assess social support and support available in the community.

I. Determine whether religious or spiritual counseling would be useful.

Nursing Diagnoses

Four specific questions nursing diagnoses are applicable: *anticipatory grief, grief, risk for dysfunctional grief*, and *dysfunctional grief* (International Council of Nurses, 2019). In this chapter, nursing care is presented separately for *anticipatory grief, grief*, and then *dysfunctional grief*. The nursing diagnosis *risk for dysfunctional grief* may be addressed with combined interventions from *grief* and *dysfunctional grief*.

Because nurses are in contact with people and their families experiencing painful losses, other responses may also be the focus of care. During this time, the nurse may need to intervene for *impaired coping, impaired family coping, powerlessness, risk for spiritual distress*, or *spiritual distress*. Furthermore, nursing diagnoses associated with major depressive disorder may be applicable in the care for individuals experiencing grief (see Chapter 7).

INTERVENTION GUIDELINES

A. Listening is the best nursing intervention that a nurse can use. People need to tell their stories, usually over and over, and move through the storyline in their own time.

B. Sincere expression of sympathy such as "I am so sorry for the death of your wife. You must be devastated," shows engagement, interest, and empathy.

C. Avoid clichés and minimizing expressions or questions such as "She is no longer suffering" or "Will you have another child?" These comments are not helpful and may be emotionally painful.

D. Spiritual and religious interventions are important to people with spiritual convictions and religious beliefs. Offer spiritual support and referrals to pastoral counseling (when available) or community resources.

E. Grief support groups are available in the community and virtual settings for every type of loss (e.g., spouse, child, pet), age group, and special conditions (e.g., disease, suicide, casualty of war).

Nursing Care for Anticipatory Grief, Grief, and Dysfunctional Grief

Anticipatory Grief

Related to

- Anticipatory loss of significant object (e.g., possession, job, status, home, parts and processes of body)
- Anticipatory death of a loved one

Desired Outcome The patient will express feelings about the imminent loss and express feeling supported during the process.

Assessment/Interventions and *Rationales*

At the imminent death of a family member:

1. Inform the family of the imminent death of the family member in a private place. *Family members can support each other in an atmosphere in which they can respond and behave naturally.*
2. Provide support, answers to questions, and guidance regarding immediate tasks and information. *Nurses are the constant members of the health care team who have the experience and expertise to provide support during this difficult period.*
3. If only one family member is available, stay with that member until a family member, a friend, or another supportive professional (e.g., hospice worker, clergy) arrives. *The presence and comfort of the nurse during the initial stage of shock can help minimize feelings of acute isolation and anxiety.*

If the family requests to see the dying person:

1. Explain what is happening (e.g., tubes, other medical equipment/treatments) and the patient's condition (e.g., physical deterioration, marks from medical interventions) prior to taking them to the patient's bedside. *Nurses who are experienced in caring for dying patients can prepare loved ones both psychologically and intellectually for the visit.*
2. Support the request to see the dying person. *Individuals may need to say goodbye, ask for forgiveness, or take such actions as keeping a lock of hair. These actions help people face the reality of death.*
3. Remain physically available and reasonably close while the family is with the dying person. *Witnessing the process of death, especially the death of a loved one, is a profound event. The physical presence of a nurse provides support and comfort.*

If angry family members suggest that healthcare professionals have mismanaged the care of the dying:

1. Continue to provide the best care possible for the dying patient. Avoid involvement in angry and painful arguments and power struggles. *Anger is a common initial response to a painful loss. Even small events may be magnified and become the targets of frustration for powerless family members and friends.*

2. Show patience and tact and offer sympathy and warmth. *Shock and disbelief are the first responses to anticipatory grief, and the grieving individuals need ways to protect themselves from the overwhelming reality of loss.*

3. Allow the grieving individual to cry. *Crying helps provide relief from feelings of acute pain and tension.*

4. Provide a place of privacy for grieving. *Privacy facilitates the natural expression of grief and a chance to regain composure.*

Grief

Related to
- Death of a loved one
- Loss of a significant object (e.g., possession, job, status, home, body parts and processes)

Desired Outcome The patient will express positive expectations for the future and report a successful life reorganization.

Assessment/Interventions and *Rationales*

1. Provide your full presence: use appropriate eye contact, listen attentively, and use appropriate touch. *Appropriate eye contact helps the patient know you are there. Listening supports the patient's processing of the loss. Suitable touch can express warmth and nurturance.*

2. Be patient with the grieving individual during times of silence. Do not fill the silence. *Sharing painful feelings followed by periods of silence allows the patient to process thoughts and feelings without being rushed. Listening patiently helps the patient express feelings, even those that are negative.*

3. Avoid euphemisms (i.e., replacing direct words with less direct words) such as, "I am sorry to tell you this,

but James is *declining.* or "You *lost* your husband." The words *death*, *dead*, and *dying* should be used when it's important to be clear about what is happening.

4. Avoid trite and philosophical statements such as "He's no longer suffering"; "You can always have another child"; or "It's better this way." Table 20.3 provides recommendations for communicating with grieving individuals. *Making these statements gives the grieving individual the impression that the experience is not understood and that you are minimizing the feelings and pain.*

Table 20.3 **Communication and Grief**

What Not to Say	What to Say	Rationale
"I know how you feel."	"Your loss must be devastating. I can't imagine how you must be feeling right now."	Unfortunately, you cannot really know how that person feels.
"When my mother died, I cried for months and could hardly eat... [*and proceed with long story*]."	"When I lost my mother, I was in a fog for days. This must be difficult for you right now."	Although it is helpful to know that others have experienced loss, during the acute grief period, the focus should be on the griever. Sharing lengthy stories is not helpful.
After a sudden and unexpected death: "At least he didn't suffer."	"It must have been so shocking to lose your husband so suddenly. Did he have any symptoms?"	No one wants suffering for a loved one, yet sudden deaths are also highly traumatizing. Chances to prepare and say goodbye are lost.
"Have you thought about getting _____ [remarried; pregnant again; another pet, another job]?"	"Your loved one was irreplaceably special."	Grievers are not interested in a replacement. They want their loved one back.

Continued

Table 20.3 **Communication and Grief—cont'd**

What Not to Say	What to Say	Rationale
"She is with [God, in heaven] now."	"I can only imagine how much you are missing her now."	Implying that the loss is a high power's doing may make the griever feel betrayed or punished by God. This statement also assumes that the griever has Christian religious beliefs.
"You can be grateful for the time you had together."	"You were married for 36 years."	This implies that the griever is ungracious. The griever still wants the loved one back.
"Let me know if there is anything I can do for you."	"I would like to take the flowers from the funeral home to your house."	The grieving person is overwhelmed. Suggesting that they find something for you to do is an additional burden. Make a concrete offer of assistance.

5. It is helpful to acknowledge the individual's painful feelings:
   a. "His death will be a terrible loss."
   b. "No one can replace her."
   c. "He will be missed for a long time."
   d. "Your relationship was complicated."
   Verbalizing painful feelings reduces feelings of isolation.
6. Instead of asking what you can do to help, encourage the support of family and friends for the following:
   a. Getting food to the house
   b. Making telephone calls
   c. Driving to the funeral home
   d. Taking care of children or other family members
   Patients who are grieving often cannot identify areas where they need help. Family and friends can help with routine acitivies and matters that may be overwhelming to the grieving individual.
7. Refer the individual who is grieving to a grief, loss, and bereavement support group. *Support groups are helpful for sharing a loss, even when the patient has many friends or family support.*

8. Offer spiritual support and referrals when needed. *Dealing with an illness or catastrophic loss can cause profound spiritual pain.*
9. When the patient is experiencing intense emotions, provide understanding and support. *Empathetic words that reflect acceptance of an individual's feelings promote healing.*

Dysfunctional Grief
Related to
- Lack of support systems
- Preexisting psychiatric disorders
- Death of a significant other
- Other risk factors (e.g., substance use, multiple losses, poor physical health, other mental health risks)
- Violent death of loved one
- Death of child
- Death of a non–socially sanctioned significant other

Desired Outcome Patient will verbalize a realistic appraisal of the deceased and return to a baseline level of functioning.

Assessment/Interventions and *Rationales*
1. Assess for suicidal thoughts or ideation. *Individuals who have severe depression or suicidal thoughts following a loss may require hospitalization and protection from self-neglect and self-harm.*
2. Talk with the grieving individual in realistic terms. Discuss concrete changes that have occurred and how they may affect the person's future. *Discussing the death and how it has and will continue to affect the person's life can help the death become more concrete and real.*
3. If the individual who is grieving has difficulty talking about the death, encourage other means of expression (e.g., keeping a journal, drawing, reading literature about grief). *Talking is usually the most important tool for resolving initial pain. However, any expression of feelings can help the individual to identify, accept, and process the loss.*
4. Explore negative feelings toward the deceased, feelings of guilt, or feelings of resentment. Understanding that negative feelings are normal and experienced by most people can make the patient aware of such feelings and then process them.

5. Encourage the patient to recall memories (happy ones, sad ones, difficult ones), listen actively, and stay silent when appropriate. *Reviewing memories is an important stage in mourning. Being with the grieving individual and sharing painful feelings supports healing.*

6. Encourage the patient to talk to others individually, in small groups, or in community-based bereavement groups. *Talking and listening are the most important activities to activate the mourning process and help resolve grief.*

7. Avoid false reassurances that the grieving individual will recover from the loss. *For some, separation through death is never okay. Even when the grieving process is complete, the person might be deeply missed.*

8. Provide referrals for comprehensive grief and bereavement services. *Complicated grief treatment includes both interpersonal and cognitive–behavior approaches to mitigate the effects of trauma and reduce stress.*

9. Identify the person's religious or spiritual background and determine whether religious or spiritual counseling might be helpful. *For many people, religious and spiritual support, and sharing feelings with a trusted and empathetic religious or spiritual figure are extremely comforting at this time.*

10. Offer written guidelines for coping with overwhelming grief. *When one is grieving, even simple tasks can become monumental, life becomes confusing, and normal routines are often interrupted. These guidelines offer simple reminders and help validate the grieving individual's experience.*

Box 20.1 provides guidelines that can be provided to people who are grieving.

Box 20.1 Caring for Yourself While Grieving

Take the time you need to grieve. The hard work of grief uses psychological energy. Resolution of the "numb state" that occurs after loss requires a few weeks at least. A minimum of 1 year—to cover all the birthdays, anniversaries, and other important dates without your loved one—is expected before you can "learn to live" with your loss.

Continued

Box 20.1 **Caring for Yourself While Grieving—cont'd**

Express your feelings. Remember that anger, anxiety, loneliness, and even guilt are normal reactions and that everyone needs a safe place to express them. Tell your personal story of loss as many times as you need to—this repetition is a helpful and necessary part of the grieving process.

Make a daily structure and stick to it. Although it is hard to do, keeping some semblance of structure makes the first few weeks after a loss easier. Getting through each day helps restore the confidence you need to accept the reality of loss.

At some point, you might want to read books about how others have dealt with loss. They often have helpful suggestions for a person in your situation.

As hard as it is, try to take good care of yourself. Eat well, talk with friends, and get plenty of rest. Make use of exercise. It can help you vent pent-up frustrations.

Expect the unexpected. You may begin to feel a bit better, only to have a brief "emotional collapse." These are expected reactions. You also might dream, visualize, think about, or search for your loved one. This, too, is a part of the grief process.

If you are losing weight, sleeping excessively or intermittently, or still experiencing deep depression after 3 months, seek professional help. If you have or have experienced a psychiatric disorder in the past (e.g., major depressive disorder, substance use), be sure to get the additional support you need.

Nurse, Patient, and Family Resources

American Academy of Hospice and Palliative Medicine
www.aahpm.org

American Association of Retired People (AARP)
www.aarp.org

GriefShare (Support Groups)
www.griefshare.org

Hospice Foundation of America
www.hospicefoundation.org

HOSPICEINFO.org
www.hospiceinfo.org

National Institute on Aging
www.nia.nih.gov

CHAPTER 21

Attention-Deficit/ Hyperactivity Disorder Medications

Children and adults with attention-deficit/hyperactivity disorder (ADHD) show symptoms of inattention, impulsiveness, and hyperactivity. Pharmacotherapy for ADHD includes stimulants and nonstimulants, as well as medications that are used to address symptoms of anger and aggression.

STIMULANTS

Paradoxically, the symptoms of ADHD are treated with stimulant drugs. Responses to these drugs are often dramatic and can quickly increase attention and task-directed behavior while reducing impulsivity, restlessness, and distractibility.

Methylphenidate (Ritalin and other brand names) and mixed amphetamine salts (Adderall) are the most widely used stimulants due to their relative safety and simplicity of use. Not surprisingly, insomnia is a common side effect while taking stimulant medications. Treating with the minimum effective dose is essential. Administering the medication no later than 4 p.m. in the afternoon or lowering the last dose of the day helps. The long-acting versions allow for a morning administration with sustained release of the medication over the course of the day and with a decreased incidence of insomnia. Other common side effects include appetite suppression, headache, abdominal pain, and lethargy.

Among the concerns with the use of stimulant drugs are side effects of agitation, exacerbation (worsening) of psychotic thought processes, hypertension, and growth suppression. As with any controlled substance, there is a risk of misuse such as selling the medication on the street or the use by people for whom the medication was not intended.

NONSTIMULANTS

The US Food and Drug Administration (FDA) approves three nonstimulants for the treatment of ADHD: atomoxetine, guanfacine, and clonidine.

Atomoxetine, sold under the brand name Strattera, is a norepinephrine reuptake inhibitor approved for use in children 6 years and older. Common side effects include gastrointestinal disturbances, urinary retention, fatigue, dizziness, and insomnia. It may also cause liver injury in some patients and a small increase in blood pressure and heart rate. Therapeutic responses develop slowly, and it may take up to 6 weeks for full improvement. This medication is preferable for individuals whose anxiety is increased with stimulants. It is also useful for those with comorbid anxiety, active substance use disorders, or tics.

Ongoing monitoring of vital signs and regular screening of liver function are important when using atomoxetine. Rarely, serious allergic reactions occur. Educate patients and their families on the risks and benefits of treatment before starting this medication. Atomoxetine is used with extreme caution in patients with comorbid major depressive disorder, since its use has been associated with increased suicidal ideation.

Two centrally acting alpha-2 adrenergic agonists, clonidine (Kapvay/Catapres) and guanfacine (Intuniv/Tenex), have FDA approval for the treatment of ADHD. Recommendations for both medications include increasing slowly and not discontinuing abruptly. They may be used alone or in conjunction with other ADHD medications.

Of the two drugs, clonidine causes more side effects: somnolence, fatigue, insomnia, nightmares, irritability, constipation, respiratory symptoms, and dry mouth. Guanfacine's most common side effects include somnolence, lethargy, fatigue, insomnia, nausea, dizziness, hypotension, and abdominal pain.

See Table 21.1 for a summary of the FDA-approved medications used to treat ADHD.

MANAGING AGGRESSIVE BEHAVIORS IN ATTENTION-DEFICIT/ HYPERACTIVITY DISORDER

To control aggressive behaviors, pharmacological agents, including stimulants, mood stabilizers, alpha-adrenergic agonists, and antipsychotics, are used. Stimulants have a dose-dependent effect. Interestingly, low doses stimulate aggressive behaviors, whereas moderate to high doses suppress aggression. Mood stabilizers such as lithium and anticonvulsants reduce aggressive behavior and are recommended for impulsivity, explosive temper, and mood lability.

Due to the side effects of fatigue and somnolence, clonidine and guanfacine are helpful in reducing agitation and rage and in increasing frustration tolerance. Antipsychotic medications have reduced violent behavior, hyperactivity, and social unresponsiveness. However, due to the risk of tardive dyskinesia associated with long-term use, antipsychotic medications are only recommended for severe aggressive behavior.

Table 21.1 **FDA-Approved Drugs for Attention-Deficit/ Hyperactivity Disorder**

Generic and Trade Names	Ages	Duration in Hours	Doses Per Day
Stimulants			
Amphetamine			
Adzenys XR-ODT	6+	12	1
Dyanavel XR	6+	12	1
Evekeo	3+	4-6	2-3
Dexmethylphenidate			
Focalin	6+	4-5	2
Focalin XR	6+	8-12	1
Dextroamphetamine			
Dexedrine	3-16	4-6	2-3
Procentra	3-16	4-6	2-3
Zenzedi	3-16	4-6	2-3
Lisdexamfetamine dimesylate			
Vyvanse	6+	10-12	1

Continued

Table 21.1 **FDA-Approved Drugs for Attention-Deficit/ Hyperactivity Disorder—Cont'd**

Generic and Trade Names	Ages	Duration in Hours	Doses Per Day
Methamphetamine			
Desoxyn	6+	6-8	1-2
Methylphenidate HCl			
Adhansia XR	6+	10-12	1
Aptensio XR	6+	10-12	1
Concerta, Relexxii	6-65	10-12	1
Cotempla XR-ODT	6-17	12	1
Daytrana (patch)	6-17	10-12	1
Jornay PM	6+	10-12	1 (evening)
Metadate ER	6-15	6-8	1-2
Metadate CD	6-15	6-8	1
Methylin ER	6+	6-8	1
Mydayis	13+	Up to 16 h	1
QuilliChew ER	6+	12	1
Quillivant XR	6-17	12	1
Ritalin	6-12	6-8	1-2
Ritalin LA	6-12	7-9	1
Ritalin SR	6-12	6-8	1-2
Mixed salts of a single-entity amphetamine product			
Adderall-XR	6+	10-12	1-2
Nonstimulants			
Atomoxetine			
Straterra	6-65	24	1-2
Clonidine			
Kapvay/Catapres	6-17	24	2
Guanfacine			
Intuniv/Tenex	6-17	24	1

Data from Food and Drug Administration (2019). *FDA online label repository.* https://labels.fda.gov

CHAPTER 22

Antipsychotic Medications

Antipsychotic medications are used to treat psychotic symptoms in disorders such as schizophrenia and bipolar mania. Before the development of antipsychotics, medications such as antihistamines provided sedation but did not reduce psychosis. Individuals with schizophrenia usually spent months or years in state or private hospitals, resulting in emotional and financial costs to patients, families, and society.

In 1951 the first antipsychotic, chlorpromazine, was developed in France for use as a general anesthetic. The following year, its antipsychotic properties were discovered. Chlorpromazine, later sold by the trade name Thorazine, and other antipsychotic drugs at last provided symptom control and allowed most patients to live and be treated in the community.

Antipsychotic agents typically take 2 to 6 weeks to achieve the desired effects. Antipsychotics are not addictive. However, they should be discontinued gradually to minimize a discontinuation syndrome that can include dizziness, nausea, tremors, insomnia, electric shock–like pains, and anxiety. Antipsychotics are unlikely to be lethal in overdose. Liquid preparations and orally disintegrating tablets are available that make it difficult for a person to cheek or palm the medication (i.e., hide the medication in the cheek or palm and then dispose of it).

Some antipsychotics are available in short-acting intramuscular injection form, used primarily for treatment of agitation, emergencies such as aggressiveness, or when a patient refuses court-mandated medication. However, side effects can be intensified and less easily managed when medication is administered directly into the system. The inhaled antipsychotic loxapine (Adasuve) can also reduce agitation, but it requires some patient cooperation.

Two major classifications of antipsychotics are used:

1. First-generation antipsychotics (FGAs) are named based on being the original antipsychotics. They are also known as *typical* antipsychotics. These drugs are traditional dopamine (D_2 receptor) antagonists and include such medications as chlorpromazine (Thorazine) and haloperidol (Haldol).

2. Second-generation antipsychotics (SGAs) were developed subsequent to FGAs. They are also known as *atypical* antipsychotics. These drugs are serotonin (5-HT_{2A} receptor) and dopamine (D_2 receptor) antagonists such as clozapine (Clozaril). Some drugs in this group are antagonists in areas of high dopamine activity but agonists in areas of low dopamine activity, such as aripiprazole (Abilify).

FIRST-GENERATION ANTIPSYCHOTICS

The FGAs primarily reduce positive symptoms, but they have little effect on negative symptoms. Positive symptoms refer to qualities that are there, but should not be. They are hallucinations, delusions, and disorganized thoughts. Negative symptoms refer to qualities that should be there, but are not, such as anhedonia (lack of pleasure), avolition (lack of motivation), and asociality (disinterest in interacting with others).

FGAs are less commonly used now due to their limited effect on negative symptoms and high level of side effects. However, they are effective in treating positive symptoms and are relatively inexpensive. For patients untroubled by their side effects, FGAs remain an appropriate choice.

Drug-Induced Movement Disorders

FGAs are dopamine (D_2) antagonists in both limbic and motor centers. Blockage of D_2 receptors in motor areas can cause extrapyramidal symptoms (EPSs). Acute EPSs include the following symptoms:

- Acute dystonia: Sudden, sustained contraction of one or several muscle groups, usually of the head and neck. Acute dystonia can be frightening and painful, but unless it involves muscles affecting the airway, it is not dangerous. It causes significant anxiety and are treated promptly.

- Akathisia: An inner restlessness or an inability to stay still or remain in one place. Akathisia can be severe and distressing to patients and may be mistaken for anxiety or agitation. These symptoms may lead to administering more of the drug that originally caused the akathisia, making it worse.
- Parkinsonism: Temporary symptoms that look like Parkinson's disease. These symptoms include a tremor, reduced accessory movements (e.g., less arm swinging when walking), gait impairment, reduced facial expressiveness (i.e., facial masking), and slowing of motor behavior (bradykinesia).

EPSs can be extremely distressing. They impact medication adherence, reduce quality of life, impair social relationships, and interfere with daily activities such as driving a car. EPSs can be minimized by lowering doses, and can be prevented by using antipsychotics less likely to cause EPSs. These side effects may diminish over time.

EPSs can also be treated with the addition of other drugs. Anticholinergic medications are useful but carry their own side effects, including dry mouth, constipation, urinary hesitancy, tachycardia, thickening of secretions, and dry skin. Misuse of anticholinergic drugs is also a potential problem because they can produce an enjoyable altered sensorium. Drugs used for dystonia, akathisia, and parkinsonism are listed in Table 22.1.

Tardive dyskinesia is a delayed and persistent drug-induced movement disorder consisting of involuntary rhythmic movements. Tardive dyskinesia develops in about 25% of patients after chronic exposure to dopamine receptor blockers, which leads to hyperactive dopamine signaling. Tardive dyskinesia often persists even after discontinuing the medication. Early symptoms begin in the mouth and facial muscles and may eventually progress to include the fingers, toes, neck, trunk, or pelvis. More common in women, tardive dyskinesia varies from mild to severe. It can be disfiguring or incapacitating.

The National Institute of Mental Health (NIMH) developed the Abnormal Involuntary Movement Scale (AIMS; Fig. 22.1) to identify and track involuntary movements. Using the AIMS is an essential nursing role in caring for individuals using FGAs. This scale is typically administered every 3 to 6 months or as indicated. A positive AIMS examination is a score of 2 in two or more movements or a score of 3 or 4 in a single movement.

Table 22.1 **Medications Used for Drug-Induced Movement Disorders**

Generic (Brand) Name	Indications
Anticholinergic	
Benztropine (Cogentin)	Dystonias, parkinsonism,
Trihexyphenidyl (Artane)	akathisia
Dopaminergic	
Amantadine (Symmetrel)	Parkinsonism
Antihistamine	
Diphenhydramine (Benadryl)	Dystonias, parkinsonism
Beta-Adrenergic Antagonist	
Propranolol (Inderal)	Akathisia
Alpha-Adrenergic Agonist	
Clonidine (Catapres)	Akathisia
Antianxiety Agents	
Clonazepam (Klonopin)	Akathisia, dystonia
Lorazepam (Ativan)	Akathisia, dystonia

Primary prevention of tardive dyskinesia by using the lowest effective dose of antipsychotic medication for the shortest period is recommended. When tardive dyskinesia is detected, reduce or discontinue the medication if possible. Some clinicians recommend switching to clozapine (Clozaril) if tardive dyskinesia develops. The risk of a permanent movement disorder is weighed against the risks of exacerbating psychosis.

Tardive dyskinesia in adults is treated with two drugs: valbenazine (Ingrezza) and deutetrabenazine (Austedo). These are selective vesicular monoamine transporter inhibitors that reduce the severity of abnormal involuntary movements. Individuals can continue to take antipsychotics while on these medications. Adverse effects include sleepiness and QT prolongation, which can result in fainting, seizures, or sudden death. They are contraindicated with congenital or acquired long-QT syndrome or related dysrhythmias. They are used with caution for individuals who drive or operate heavy machinery or do other dangerous activities until it is known how the drug affects them.

Ideally, prior to antipsychotic therapy, patients are screened for undiagnosed movement disorders such as Parkinson's disease. Symptoms of an other underlying disease can be mistaken as drug side effects and go untreated.

ABNORMAL INVOLUNTARY MOVEMENT SCALE (AIMS)

Public Health Service
Alcohol, Drug Abuse, and Mental Health Administration
National Institute of Mental Health

Name: _____
Date: _____
Prescribing Practitioner: _____

Code: 0 = None
1 = Minimal, may be extreme normal
2 = Mild
3 = Moderate
4 = Severe

Instructions: Complete Examination Procedure before making ratings.

Movement ratings: Rate highest severity observed. Rate movements that occur upon activation one *less* than those observed spontaneously. Circle movement as well as code number that applies.		Rater Date	Rater Date	Rater Date	Rater Date
Facial and Oral Movements	1. **Muscles of facial expression** (e.g., movements of forehead, eyebrows, periorbital area, cheeks, including frowning, blinking, smiling, grimacing)	0 1 2 3 4	0 1 2 3 4	0 1 2 3 4	0 1 2 3 4
	2. **Lips and perioral area** (e.g., puckering, pouting, smacking)	0 1 2 3 4	0 1 2 3 4	0 1 2 3 4	0 1 2 3 4
	3. **Jaw** (e.g., biting, clenching, chewing, mouth opening, lateral movement)	0 1 2 3 4	0 1 2 3 4	0 1 2 3 4	0 1 2 3 4
	4. **Tongue:** Rate only increases in movement both in and out of mouth – *not* inability to sustain movement. Darting in and out of mouth.	0 1 2 3 4	0 1 2 3 4	0 1 2 3 4	0 1 2 3 4
Extremity Movements	5. **Upper (arms, wrists, hands, fingers):** Include choreic movements (i.e., rapid, objectively purposeless, irregular, spontaneous) and athetoid movements (i.e., slow, irregular, complex, serpentine). *Do not include tremor* (i.e., repetitive, regular, rhythmic).	0 1 2 3 4	0 1 2 3 4	0 1 2 3 4	0 1 2 3 4
	6. **Lower (legs, knees, ankles, toes)** (e.g., lateral knee movement, foot tapping, heel dropping, foot squirming, inversion and eversion of foot)	0 1 2 3 4	0 1 2 3 4	0 1 2 3 4	0 1 2 3 4
Trunk Movements	7. **Neck, shoulder, hips** (e.g., rocking, twisting, squirming, pelvic gyrations)	0 1 2 3 4	0 1 2 3 4	0 1 2 3 4	0 1 2 3 4
Global Judgments	8. **Severity of abnormal movements overall**	0 1 2 3 4	0 1 2 3 4	0 1 2 3 4	0 1 2 3 4
	9. **Incapacitation due to abnormal movements**	0 1 2 3 4	0 1 2 3 4	0 1 2 3 4	0 1 2 3 4
	10. **Patient's awareness of abnormal movements:** Rate only patient's report. No awareness 0 / Aware, no distress 1 / Aware, mild distress 2 / Aware, moderate distress 3 / Aware, severe distress 4	0 1 2 3 4	0 1 2 3 4	0 1 2 3 4	0 1 2 3 4
Dental Status	11. **Current problems with teeth and/or dentures**	No Yes	No Yes	No Yes	No Yes
	12. **Are dentures usually worn?**	No Yes	No Yes	No Yes	No Yes
	13. **Edentia**	No Yes	No Yes	No Yes	No Yes
	14. **Do movements disappear in sleep?**	No Yes	No Yes	No Yes	No Yes

Fig. 22.1 Abnormal Involuntary Movement Scale (AIMS). Instructions: Rate highest severity observed. Rate movements that occur upon activation as one point *less* than those observed spontaneously. Circle movement as well as code number that applies. Scoring: 0 = Absent, 1 = Minimal, 2 = Mild, 3 = Moderate, 4 = Severe.   *Continued*

Anticholinergic Side Effects

The FGAs cause anticholinergic side effects by blocking muscarinic acetylcholine receptors. Anticholinergic side effects include urinary retention, dilated pupils, reduced visual accommodation (blurred near vision), tachycardia, dry mucous membranes, reduced peristalsis (resulting in constipation, rarely, leading to paralytic ileus and risk of

AIMS Examination Procedure
Either before or after completing the Examination Procedure, observe the patient unobtrusively, at rest (e.g., in waiting room).

The chair to be used in this examination should be a hard, firm one without arms.

1. Ask patient to remove shoes and socks.
2. Ask patient whether there is anything in his or her mouth (e.g., gum, candy) and, if there is, to remove it.
3. Ask patient about the *current* condition of his or her teeth. Ask patient if he or she wears dentures. Do teeth or dentures bother the patient *now*?
4. Ask patient whether he or she notices any movements in mouth, face, hands, or feet. If yes, ask to describe and to what extent they *currently* bother patient or interfere with his or her activities.
5. Have patient sit in chair with hands on knees, legs slightly apart, and feet flat on floor. Look at entire body movements while in this position.
6. Ask patient to sit with hands hanging unsupported: if male, between legs; if female and wearing a dress, hanging over knees. Observe hands and other body areas.
7. Ask patient to open mouth. Observe tongue at rest within mouth. Do this twice.
8. Ask patient to protrude tongue. Observe abnormalities of tongue movement. Do this twice.
9. Ask patient to tap thumb, with each finger, as rapidly as possible for 10 to 15 seconds, separately with right hand, then with left hand. Observe each facial and leg movement.
10. Flex and extend patient's left and right arms (one at a time). Note any rigidity.
11. Ask patient to stand up. Observe in profile. Observe all body areas again, hips included.
12. Ask patient to extend both arms outstretched in front with palms down. Observe trunk, legs, and mouth.
13. Have patient walk a few paces, turn, and walk back to chair. Observe hands and gait. Do this twice.

Fig. 22.1, cont'd

bowel obstruction), and cognitive impairment. Taking multiple medications with anticholinergic side effects increases the risk of anticholinergic toxicity, covered later in this chapter. In general, FGAs have either strong EPS potential or strong anticholinergic potential. That is, when one side effect is prominent, the other is not.

Other First-Generation Antipsychotic Side Effects

FGAs cause sedation, which gradually improves. Orthostatic (postural) hypotension increases the risk of falls when standing suddenly. A reduced seizure threshold increases the risk of seizures. Visual changes such as photosensitivity and cataracts are associated with chlorpromazine (Thorazine) and thioridazine (Mellaril). An increased release of prolactin (hyperprolactinemia) can result in sexual dysfunction (e.g., impotence, anorgasmia, impaired ejaculation), galactorrhea (production of breast milk), gynecomastia (increase in male breast tissue), and amenorrhea (cessation of menses). Weight gain of more than 50 pounds in a year often results in psychological distress and an increased risk of cardiovascular disorders and diabetes mellitus.

Serious side effects are uncommon. However, anticholinergic toxicity, neuroleptic malignant syndrome prolongation of the QT interval, and liver impairment may occur during

FGA therapy. FGAs increase mortality in older adults with major neurocognitive disorders. Food and Drug Administration (FDA)–approved FGAs and specific side effects are listed in Table 22.2.

SECOND-GENERATION ANTIPSYCHOTICS

As is the case with FGAs, the SGAs can cause sedation, sexual dysfunction, seizures, and increased mortality in older adults with major neurocognitive disorders. However, most SGAs are less likely to cause significant EPS, especially tardive dyskinesia. Although they have the same potential side effects as the FGAs, SGA side effects are usually fewer, milder, and better tolerated. Some serious SGA side effects include anticholinergic toxicity, neuroleptic malignant syndrome, and prolongation of the QT interval.

Some SGAs also have antidepressant properties and are FDA approved for adjunctive use in the treatment of major depressive disorder as well as bipolar disorder. As with all antidepressants, they carry a theoretical risk of increased suicidality, particularly in adolescents.

When the first SGA, clozapine (Clozaril), was approved in 1989, it produced dramatic improvement in patients whose treatment had been resistant to FGAs. It also helped to improve negative symptoms. Unfortunately, clozapine causes agranulocytosis, or severe neutropenia, in about 1% of those who take it. Other serious side effects are myocarditis, life-threatening bowel emergencies, new-onset type 2 diabetes, and, rarely, ketoacidosis. Because of these problems, clozapine use has declined in the United States, and many clinicians reserve its use as a last resort. However, it is one of the few drugs with FDA approval for the treatment of suicidality in schizophrenia.

Metabolic Syndrome

All SGAs carry a risk of metabolic syndrome, which includes weight gain (especially in the abdominal area), dyslipidemia, increased blood glucose, and insulin resistance. This metabolic syndrome is a significant concern and increases the risk of diabetes, certain cancers, hypertension, and cardiovascular disease, making its prevention an important role for nurses.

Table 22.2 **FDA-Approved First-Generation Antipsychotics**

Generic (Trade) Name	Specific Side Effects
Chlorpromazine (Thorazine)	NMS, akathisia, EPS, tardive dyskinesia, sedation, weight gain, hypotension, constipation, hyperprolactinemia, photosensitivity
Fluphenazine (Prolixin)	Sedation, weight gain, hyperprolactinemia, NMS, EPS, akathisia, tardive dyskinesia, dystonia
Haloperidol (Haldol)	NMS, akathisia, EPS, tardive dyskinesia, dystonia, sedation, hypotension, constipation, hyperprolactinemia
Loxapine (Loxitane)	NMS, akathisia, EPS, tardive dyskinesia, sedation, hypotension, constipation, hyperprolactinemia, dystonia
Loxapine (Adasuve)	Altered taste, sedation, bronchospasm. Contraindicated with asthma and chronic obstructive pulmonary disease
Molindone (Moban)	NMS, akathisia, EPS, tardive dyskinesia, sedation, constipation, hyperprolactinemia, dystonia
Perphenazine (Trilafon)	NMS, akathisia, EPS, tardive dyskinesia, sedation, weight gain, hypotension, constipation, hyperprolactinemia, dystonia
Thioridazine (Mellaril)	NMS, akathisia, EPS, tardive dyskinesia, pigmentary retinopathy, sedation, weight gain, hypotension, constipation, hyperprolactinemia, dystonia
Thiothixene (Navane)	NMS, akathisia, EPS, tardive dyskinesia, sedation, hypotension, constipation, hyperprolactinemia, dystonia
Trifluoperazine (Stelazine)	NMS, akathisia, EPS, tardive dyskinesia, sedation, hypotension, constipation, hyperprolactinemia, dystonia

EPS, Extrapyramidal symptom; *LAIM*, long-acting intramuscular injection; *NMS*, neuroleptic malignant syndrome; *SAIM*, short-acting intramuscular injection.

A subset of the SGAs is sometimes referred to as third-generation antipsychotics. These drugs are aripiprazole (Abilify), brexpiprazole (Rexulti), and cariprazine (Vraylar). They are dopamine system stabilizers that reduce dopamine activity in some brain regions while increasing it in other brain regions. Aripiprazole and brexpiprazole act as D_2 partial agonists. This means that they attach to the D_2 receptor without fully activating it, reducing the effective level of dopamine activity. Cariprazine is a partial agonist more on D_3 than D_2 receptors, which may help improve cognitive symptoms.

FDA-approved SGAs and specific side effects are listed in Table 22.3.

Table 22.4 summarizes side effects of antipsychotic medication and the nursing care that is associated with these side effects.

Serious Antipsychotic Side Effects

Rare but serious and potentially fatal side effects of antipsychotic drugs include anticholinergic toxicity, neuroleptic malignant syndrome, agranulocytosis. Prolongation of the QT interval, and liver impairment. It is important for nurses who work in psychiatric settings, primary care, and emergency services to be aware of and monitor for the early signs and symptoms of these side effects. Patients and their families are also taught how to recognize and respond to dangerous side effects.

Anticholinergic toxicity is a potentially life-threatening condition caused by antipsychotics or other medications with anticholinergic effects, including many antiparkinsonian drugs. Older adults and those taking multiple anticholinergic drugs are at greatest risk. Symptoms include autonomic nervous system instability, dilated pupils, urinary retention, and delirium with altered mental status. Mental status changes can include hallucinations and may be mistaken for a worsening of the patient's psychosis. Individuals whose psychosis is inexplicably worsening should be evaluated for anticholinergic toxicity.

Neuroleptic malignant syndrome occurs in about 0.2% to 1% of patients who have taken FGAs. This side effect is less likely with SGAs. Its symptoms are reduced consciousness and responsiveness, increased muscle tone (generalized muscular rigidity), and autonomic dysfunction. A fever in excess of 103°F (39°C) is the most telling symptom. Caused by excessive dopamine receptor blockade, Neuroleptic malignant syndrome is an emergency that is fatal in about 6% of cases. It usually occurs early in therapy but has also occurred 20 years into treatment. Early detection, discontinuation of the antipsychotic, management of fluid balance, temperature reduction, and monitoring for complications such as deep vein thrombosis and rhabdomyolysis (protein in the blood from muscle breakdown, which can cause organ failure) are essential.

Table 22.3 **FDA-Approved Second- and Third-Generation Antipsychotics**

Generic (Trade) Name	Specific Side Effects
Aripiprazole (Abilify) Aripiprazole (Abilify Discmelt)	Dizziness, insomnia, akathisia, activation, nausea, vomiting, sedation
Aripiprazole (Abilify Maintena) Aripiprazole lauroxil (Aristada, Aristada Initio)	Akathisia, injection site pain, sedation
Asenapine (Saphris, Secuado)	Risk of diabetes and dyslipidemia, EPS, hyperprolactinemia, sedation weight gain, akathisia, NMS, tardive dyskinesia, oral hypoesthesia/tongue numbing (sublingual tablet), application site reaction (patch)
Brexpiprazole (Rexulti)	Headache, EPS, dyspepsia
Cariprazine Vraylar)	EPS, insomnia, nausea, sedation
Clozapine (Clozaril, Versacloz) Clozapine (FazaClo)	Risk of diabetes and dyslipidemia, increased salivation, sweating, agranulocytosis, sedation, weight gain, constipation, hypotension, seizures
Iloperidone (Fanapt)	Risk of diabetes and dyslipidemia, EPS, hyperprolactinemia, sedation, weight gain, akathisia, NMS, tardive dyskinesia
Lumateperone (Caplyta)	Risk of diabetes and dyslipidemia, weight gain, complete blood counts in patients with preexisting low white blood cell count or history of leukopenia or neutropenia, tardive dyskinesia, sedation
Lurasidone (Latuda)	Risk of diabetes and dyslipidemia, EPS, hyperprolactinemia, sedation, weight gain, akathisia, NMS, tardive dyskinesia
Olanzapine (Zyprexa) Olanzapine (Zyprexa Zydis)	Risk of diabetes and dyslipidemia, sedation, weight gain, hyperprolactinemia, constipation, hypotension, seizures
Olanzapine (Zyprexa Relprevv)	Postinjection delirium/sedation syndrome

Table 22.3 **FDA-Approved Second- and Third-Generation Antipsychotics—cont'd**

Generic (Trade) Name	Specific Side Effects
Paliperidone (Invega) Paliperidone (Invega Sustenna, Invega Trinza)	Risk of diabetes and dyslipidemia, EPS, hyperprolactinemia, sedation, weight gain, tachycardia, headache
Quetiapine (Seroquel, Seroquel XR)	Risk of diabetes and dyslipidemia, dizziness, sedation, weight gain, constipation, hypotension
Risperidone (Risperdal) Risperidone (Risperdal Consta) Risperidone (Perseris) Risperidone (Risperdal M-Tab)	Risk of diabetes and dyslipidemia, EPS, hyperprolactinemia, sedation, weight gain, akathisia, NMS, tardive dyskinesia
Ziprasidone (Geodon)	Activating, sedation, hypotension, akathisia

EPS, Extrapyramidal symptom; *FDA*, Food and Drug Administration; *LAIM*, long-acting intramuscular injection; *NMS*, neuroleptic malignant syndrome; *SAIM*, short-acting intramuscular injection; *SQ*, subcutaneous.

Table 22.4 **Antipsychotic Medication Side Effects and Nursing Care**

Side Effect	Nursing Care
Extrapyramidal Symptoms (EPSs)	
Acute dystonic reactions	
Acute painful contractions of tongue, face, neck, and back (usually tongue and jaw first)	Monitor and ensure open airway. Administer antiparkinsonian agent (intramuscular for faster response).
Spasm of the muscles causing backward arching of the head, neck (torticollis), and spine	Consider diphenhydramine hydrochloride (Benadryl) 25–50 mg intramuscularly or intravenously.
Eyes roll back (oculogyric crisis)	Provide prophylactic oral antiparkinsonian agent as ordered.
Laryngeal dystonia could threaten airway (rare)	Provide reassurance and presence for the patient.

Continued

Table 22.4 **Antipsychotic Medication Side Effects and Nursing Care**—cont'd

Side Effect	Nursing Care
Akathisia	
Motor restlessness (e.g., pacing, unable to stand still or stay in one location, rocking while seated or shifting from one foot to the other while standing)	Distinguish akathisia (i.e., inability to sit still, generalized muscle restlessness) from anxious repetitive movement (usually involves only the extremities). Ask specific questions such as "do you feel anxious about something?" Consult prescriber regarding possible medication change. Provide propranolol (Inderal), lorazepam (Ativan), or diazepam (Valium) as ordered. Encourage relaxation exercises. Monitor for suicidality in severe cases.
Parkinsonism	
Masklike face, stiff and stooped posture, shuffling gait, drooling, tremor, "pill-rolling" finger movements, dysphagia, or reduction in spontaneous swallowing	Administer antiparkinsonian agent such as trihexyphenidyl (Artane) or benztropine (Cogentin), as ordered. If intolerable, consult prescriber regarding dose reduction or medication change. Provide towel or handkerchief to wipe excess saliva. Provide education regarding how to reduce fall risk.
Tardive Dyskinesia	
Face: protruding or writhing tongue; blowing, smacking, licking; facial distortion Limbs: Chorea: rapid, purposeless, and irregular movements Athetoid: slow, complex, and serpentine movements Trunk: neck and shoulder movements, hip jerks and rocking, or twisting pelvic thrusts	Screen with the AIMs scale at least every 3 months. Discuss reconsidering medication choice or lowering dose with the provider. Teach the patient that purposeful muscle movement overrides and masks involuntary tardive movements. Discussing Teach the patient ways to conceal involuntary movements such as holding one hand with the other. Administer valbenazine (Ingrezza) or deutetrabenazine (Austedo) as ordered.

Table 22.4 **Antipsychotic Medication Side Effects and Nursing Care—cont'd**

Side Effect	Nursing Care
Hypotension and Orthostatic (Postural) Hypotension	
When standing, systolic rises, diastolic decreases, and pulse increases	Monitor both lying (or sitting) and standing blood pressure and pulse.
	Hold dose and consult prescriber if systolic pressure is <80 mm Hg when standing.
	Advise the patient to arise slowly to reduce dizziness and to hold on to railings or furniture while rising.
	If lying down, instruct the patient to the patient move slowly to sitting position and pause until dizziness passes before standing.
	Share that this side effect usually subsides in 1–2 weeks.
	Promote adequate hydration.
Anticholinergic	
Dry mouth	Encourage ice chips or frequent sips of water.
	Suggest the use of sugarless candy or gum to stimulate salivation.
	Encourage the use of xylitol-containing moisture supplements or other saliva substitutes.
	Provide education on agents that increase mouth dryness including caffeine, alcohol, tobacco, antihistamines, and decongestants.
	Discuss the use of pilocarpine (Salagen) or cevimeline (Evoxac) to stimulate saliva production with the provider.
	Promote dental hygiene and regular dental care.
Urinary retention and hesitancy	Assess for distended bladder.
	Suggest running water and a warm moist towel on abdomen. Catheterization may be necessary.

Continued

Table 22.4 **Antipsychotic Medication Side Effects and Nursing Care—cont'd**

Side Effect	Nursing Care
Constipation	Encourage adequate fluid and fiber intake.
	Promote physical activity.
	Consider stool softeners, laxatives, or dietary laxatives (e.g., prune juice).
Blurred vision	Inform the patient that blurred vision may improve in 1–2 weeks.
	Encourage the use of reading or magnifying glasses.
	If intolerable, consult prescriber regarding medication change.
Dry eyes	Encourage the use of artificial tears.
Sexual dysfunction	Discuss the use of an alternative medication with the provider.
	Suggest artificial lubricants for vaginal dryness.
Metabolic Syndrome	
Weight gain, dyslipidemia (abnormal lipid levels), increased insulin resistance leading to increased risk of cardiovascular disease, diabetes, and other medical conditions	Minimize weight gain through proper nutrition and physical activity:
	Monitor and report weight and blood pressure.
	Monitor and report labs for fasting lipids and blood glucose.
	Help the patient to identify low-calorie snacks.
	Engage the patient in regular physical activity.
	Help the patient to identify and pursue physical activities such as walking or cycling.
	Provide education on the importance of regular medical evaluation and care to identify symptoms of this syndrome.
	Metformin and liraglutide have been used off-label to reduce diabetes in patients with metabolic syndrome.

Drug-induced agranulocytosis, or severe neutropenia, is most often associated with clozapine (Clozaril), but is also possible with most other antipsychotics. This is an acute condition involving a dangerously low white blood cell count, which increases the risk of a serious infection. While neutropenia is defined by an absolute neutrophil count (ANC) of less than 500/µL, agranulocytosis is characterized by an ANC of less than 100/µL. Left untreated, this life-threatening condition leads to death, most commonly through bacterial infection of the blood, or septicemia. Monitoring for neutropenia is done as part of the complete blood count through an ANC. Symptoms of agranulocytosis include signs of infection (e.g., fever, chills, and sore throat) or increased susceptibility to infection.

Prolongation of the QT interval is a delay of ventricular repolarization. This condition may result in tachycardia, fainting, seizures, and even sudden death. The FGAs chlorpromazine (Thorazine), haloperidol (Haldol), and thioridazine (Mellaril) may cause this cardiac emergency. SGAs iloperidone (Fanapt), quetiapine (Seroquel), risperidone (Risperdal), and ziprasidone (Geodon) can also prolong the QT interval. It is recommended to evaluate all patients for existing QT prolongation with an electrocardiogram before beginning antipsychotic therapy.

Liver impairment may also occur, particularly with FGAs. SGAs also lead to serum enzyme elevations but rarely with injury or jaundice. Liver impairment usually occurs in the first weeks of therapy. Signs of liver problems include jaundice, abdominal pain, ascites, vomiting, lower extremity edema, dark urine, pale or tar-colored stool, and easy bruising. The patient may complain of itchy skin, chronic fatigue, nausea, and decreased appetite. This makes monitoring of liver function values essential.

Table 22.5 summarizes dangerous side effects of antipsychotics and nursing care to respond to these side effects.

Long-Acting Injectable Antipsychotics

Some antipsychotics are available in long-acting injectable (LAI) formulations that only need to be administered every 2 to 4 weeks or even months (Table 22.6). Some require special administration protocols. When less frequent medication administration is necessary,

Table 22.5 **Serious Side Effects of Antipsychotics and Associated Nursing Care**

Side Effect	Nursing Care
Anticholinergic Toxicity	
Potentially life-threatening medical emergency	Hold all medications.
	Contact prescriber immediately.
Reduced or absent peristalsis (can lead to bowel obstruction); urinary retention; mydriasis (pupillary dilation); hyperpyrexia without diaphoresis (hot dry skin); delirium with tachycardia, unstable vital signs, agitation, disorientation, hallucinations, reduced responsiveness; worsening of psychotic symptoms; seizure; repetitive motor movements.	Implement emergency cooling measures as ordered (cooling blanket, alcohol, or ice bath). Use urinary catheterization as needed. Administer a benzodiazepine or other sedation as ordered. Physostigmine may reverse the anticholinergic toxicity. Evaluate for anticholinergic toxicity any time psychosis seems to be worsening.
Neuroleptic Malignant Syndrome (NMS)	
Rare but dangerous. Acute, life-threatening medical emergency.	Hold all medications. Contact prescriber immediately.
Early detection increases patient's chance of survival.	Transfer to a critical care unit. If in community, contact 911 for transport to an emergency department.
Hyperpyrexia (fever) over 103°F is most diagnostic symptom.	Administer bromocriptine (Parlodel) and dantrolene (Dantrium) to relieve muscle rigidity and reduce the heat (fever) generated by muscle contractions as ordered.
Severe muscle rigidity, dysphasia, flexor–extensor posturing, reduced or absent speech and movement, decreased responsiveness.	Implement emergency cooling measures as ordered (cooling blanket, alcohol, or ice bath).
Autonomic dysfunction: hypertension, tachycardia, diaphoresis, incontinence.	Maintain hydration with oral or intravenous fluids. Monitor and correct electrolyte imbalance.
Delirium, stupor, coma.	Monitor and report cardiac dysrhythmias. Small doses of heparin may be ordered and administrered to decrease possibility of pulmonary emboli.

Table 22.5 **Serious Side Effects of Antipsychotics and Associated Nursing Care—cont'd**

Side Effect	Nursing Care
Agranulocytosis *Potentially fatal blood dyscrasia* Symptoms include reduced neutrophil counts and increased frequency and severity of infections. Any symptoms suggesting infection (e.g., sore throat, fever, malaise, body aches) should be carefully evaluated.	Monitor for neutropenia weekly for 6 months, then twice monthly for 6 more months, then monthly. If neutropenia develops, hold drug and consult prescriber. Moderate neutropenia (absolute neutrophil count [ANC] < 500 µL) and severe neutropenia (ANC <100 µL) results in treatment interruption. In some cases, clozapine may be reinstituted once the ANC returns to normal. Provide temporary reverse isolation may be initiated. Provide education regarding signs of infection reporting these symptoms promptly to the prescriber.
Prolongation of the QT Interval *Medical emergency, potentially fatal* Prolongation increases the risk of ventricular tachyarrhythmias, which may lead to syncope, cardiac arrest, or sudden death. Tachycardia, irregular pulse, fainting. Seizures may occur because of erratic heartbeats resulting in brain oxygen deprivation.	Evaluate all patients for existing QT prolongation with electrocardiogram, as ordered, before beginning antipsychotic therapy. Monitor pulse for tachycardia and irregularities. Recognize that fainting and seizures in a person taking antipsychotics are signs of impending cardiac arrest. Consider life-saving emergency intervention.

Table 22.6 Long-Acting Injectable Antipsychotics

Generic (Trade) Name	Nursing Considerations
Aripiprazole[b] (Abilify Maintena)	Every 4 weeks Deltoid or gluteal site. Shake vigorously just before administering.
Aripiprazole lauroxil[b] (Aristada)	Every 4, 6, or 8 weeks Deltoid for lowest strength or gluteal site. Shake vigorously just before administering.
Aripiprazole lauroxil (Aristada Initio[b])	One-time injection Deltoid or gluteal site. One-time initiation dose combined with a 30 mg dose of aripiprazole and a selected dose of Aristada.
Fluphenazine decanoate[a] (generic only)	Every 2–3 weeks Viscous, deltoid, or gluteal site. Z-track method.
Haloperidol decanoate[a] (Haldol Decanoate)	Every 4 weeks Viscous, deltoid, or gluteal site. Z-track method.
Olanzapine pamoate[b] (Zyprexa Relprevv)	Every 2–4 weeks Must monitor the patient for excess sedation for 3 hours postinjection. Gluteal site only. Shake vigorously just before administering.
Paliperidone palmitate[b] (Invega Sustenna)	Every 4 weeks When initiating, the first two injections must be given deltoid on days 1 and 8. Deltoid or gluteal site afterward. Shake vigorously just before administering.
Paliperidone palmitate[b] (Invega Trinza)	Every 12 weeks Must be treated with once-monthly paliperidone for at least 4 months before transitioning to this preparation. Deltoid or gluteal site.
Risperidone microspheres[b] (Risperdal Consta)	Every 2 weeks Deltoid or gluteal site. Shake vigorously just before administering.

Table 22.6 **Long-Acting Injectable Antipsychotics—cont'd**

Generic (Trade) Name	Nursing Considerations
Risperidone[b] (Perseris)	Every 4 weeks Subcutaneous in abdomen only. Lump on abdomen will decrease in size over time. Do not rub or massage injection site.

[a]First generation.
[b]Second generation.
Data from manufacturer's product insert and Burchum, J., & Rosenthal, L. (2019). *Lehne's pharmacology for nursing care* (10th ed.). Elsevier.

adherence is improved and conflict about taking medications is reduced. The downsides of LAIs are a lack of dosing flexibility and that patients may feel like they have less control or feel coerced into treatment.

CHAPTER 23

Mood-Stabilizers

Mood stabilizers are a class of drugs used to treat symptoms associated with bipolar disorder. The original intent of the term mood stabilizer was to indicate that these drugs were effective in the treatment of both mania and depression. However, while most all of the medications in this category are effective in treating mania, not all of them effectively treat depression.

Table 23.1 summarizes medications used for the treatment of bipolar disorder.

LITHIUM

In 1970, lithium was given U.S. Food and Drug Administration (FDA) approval for the treatment of acute mania, and in 1974 for maintenance therapy in bipolar disorder. Until the mid-1990s, lithium was the only drug approved for both acute and maintenance treatment. Lithium is sold as Eskalith, Eskalith CR, and Lithobid.

Lithium is a soft natural silvery metal, and most of the lithium in the United States is derived from dry lake beds in South America. Lithium is found in variable amounts in vegetables, grains, spices, and drinking water. Trace amounts are present in most rocks, and weather moves them into the soil, ground and standing water, and even into the public water supply. Geographical areas with high levels of lithium in public drinking water are associated with lower suicide rates (Memon et al., 2020).

Lithium is particularly effective in reducing the following:
- Elation, grandiosity, and expansiveness
- Flight of ideas
- Irritability and manipulation
- Anxiety
- Self-injurious behavior

Table 23.1 **FDA-Approved Drugs for Bipolar Disorder**

Generic (Trade) Name	Bipolar Depression	Acute Mania	Bipolar Maintenance
Mood Stabilizers			
Lithium (Eskalith, Eskalith CR, Lithobid)	—	FDA approved	FDA approved
Anticonvulsant Mood Stabilizers			
Carbamazepine (Equetro)	—	FDA approved	—
Divalproex sodium delayed release (Depakote), divalproex sodium extended release (Depakote ER)	—	FDA approved	—
Lamotrigine (Lamictal)	—	—	FDA approved
First-Generation Antipsychotics			
Chlorpromazine (Thorazine)	—	FDA approved	—
Loxapine (Adasuve) orally inhaled	—	FDA approved for [a]bipolar I acute agitation	—
Second-Generation Antipsychotics			
Aripiprazole (Abilify)	—	FDA approved	FDA approved
Aripiprazole (Abilify Maintena)	—	—	FDA approved
Asenapine (Saphris)	—	FDA approved	FDA approved[b]
Cariprazine (Vraylar)	FDA approved	FDA approved	—
Lurasidone (Latuda)	FDA approved	—	—
Olanzapine (Zyprexa)	—	FDA approved	FDA approved

Continued

Table 23.1 **FDA-Approved Drugs for Bipolar Disorder—cont'd**

Generic (Trade) Name	Bipolar Depression	Acute Mania	Bipolar Maintenance
Quetiapine (Seroquel, Seroquel XR)	FDA approved	FDA approved	FDA approved
Risperidone (Risperdal)	—	FDA approved	—
Risperidone (Risperdal Consta)		—	FDA approved
Ziprasidone (Geodon)	—	FDA approved	FDA approved
Combination Second-Generation Antipsychotic and Antidepressant			
Olanzapine (Zyprexa) + fluoxetine (Prozac) = Symbyax	FDA approved	—	—

[a]Bipolar I acute agitation
[b]Bipolar I mixed episode
From U.S. Food and Drug Administration (2016). FDA online label repository. Retrieved from http://labels.fda.gov/

To a lesser extent, lithium controls the following:
- Insomnia
- Psychomotor agitation
- Threatening or assaultive behavior
- Distractibility
- Paranoia
- Hypersexuality

Lithium's antimanic effect usually takes 7 to 14 days to achieve. Therefore, during the initial stages of treatment, other medications such as a second-generation antipsychotic may be given to help decrease psychomotor activity, aggressive behaviors, and prevent exhaustion.

A narrow range exists between the therapeutic dose and toxic dose of lithium. The lithium level is drawn every 2 to 3 days after beginning lithium therapy and after any dosage change, until the therapeutic level has been reached. Blood levels are then checked every 3 to 6 months. Initially, levels should be from 0.8 to 1.2 mEq/L during acute manic states. Maintenance blood levels are lower ranging from 0.6 to 0.8 mEq/L. To prevent serious toxicity, lithium levels should not exceed 1.5 mEq/L. Lithium side effects, signs of toxicity, and interventions are listed in Table 23.2.

Lithium treatment is associated with a decline in renal function and thyroid function, and with hypercalcemia. Women younger than 60 years and people with lithium concentrations higher than median are at greatest risk. Individuals need baseline measures of renal, thyroid, and parathyroid function and regular long-term monitoring.

Lithium therapy is generally contraindicated in patients with cardiovascular disease, brain damage, renal disease, thyroid disease, or myasthenia gravis. Whenever possible, lithium is not given to women who are pregnant because it may harm the fetus. There is controversy regarding the use of lithium in breastfeeding mothers. Some sources list lithium as a contraindication in breastfeeding, while other sources do not, particularly if the infant is older than 2 months. The amount of lithium excreted into breast milk and absorbed by the infant varies widely, but it is generally considered low. If lithium therapy is continued during breastfeeding, maternal, and sometimes infant, serum levels are monitored closely. Lithium use is also contraindicated in children younger than 12 years.

A fine hand tremor, polyuria, and mild thirst may occur early in therapy for the acute manic phase and may persist throughout treatment. Transient and mild nausea and general discomfort may also appear during the first few days of lithium administration. Because lithium is a salt, patients are advised to maintain balanced hydration by drinking an adequate amount of water and consuming a normal level of dietary salt. Dehydration from exercise, heat, vomiting, or diarrhea may result in toxic levels of lithium in the bloodstream. Patient and family teaching is provided in Box 23.1.

ANTICONVULSANTS

Anticonvulsant drugs, or antiepileptics, were developed to treat convulsions associated with epilepsy. Providers observed that patients treated with anticonvulsants in early epilepsy trials experienced improvements in mood. These findings prompted investigations into the possible effects of anticonvulsant use in psychiatry. Anticonvulsant medications are now commonly used to treat acute bipolar depression, acute mania, and/or bipolar maintenance. They generally share several characteristics including:

Table 23.2 **Lithium Side Effects, Signs of Toxicity, and Interventions**

Side Effects and Signs of Lithium Toxicity		Interventions
Expected Side Effects	<1.5 mEq/L Nausea, vomiting, diarrhea, thirst, polyuria, (producing too much urine) polydipsia (abnormal thirst), lethargy, sedation, and fine hand tremor. Renal toxicity, goiter, and hypothyroidism may occur with long-term use.	Symptoms often subside during treatment. Doses should be kept low. Kidney function and thyroid levels should be assessed before treatment and then on an annual basis.
Early Signs of Toxicity	1.5–2.0 mEq/L Gastrointestinal upset, coarse hand tremor, confusion, hyperirritability of muscles, electroencephalographic changes, sedation, and incoordination.	Medication should be withheld, blood lithium levels measured, and dosage reevaluated.
Advanced Signs of Toxicity	2.0–2.5 mEq/L Ataxia, giddiness, serious electroencephalographic changes, blurred vision, clonic movements, large output of dilute urine, seizures, stupor, severe hypotension, and coma. Death is usually secondary to pulmonary complications.	Hospitalization is indicated. The drug is stopped, and excretion is hastened. Whole bowel irrigation may be done to prevent further absorption of lithium.
Severe Toxicity	2.0–2.5 mEq/L Convulsions, oliguria (producing no or small amounts of urine), and death can occur.	In addition to the previously listed interventions, hemodialysis may be necessary.

Data from Burchum, J. R., & Rosenthal, L. D. (2019). *Lehne's pharmacology for nursing care* (10th ed.). Elsevier Saunders.

Box 23.1 **Patient and Family Teaching: Lithium Therapy**

Give the patient and the patient's family the following information, both verbally and in written form, and encourage them to ask questions

- Lithium is a mood stabilizer and helps prevent relapse. It is important to continue taking the drug even after the current episode subsides.
- Lithium is not addictive.
- Lithium blood levels are monitored until a therapeutic level is reached. More frequent testing of blood levels will be needed initially, then once every 3 to 6 months after that.
- Fluid and sodium balance are important since lithium is a salt.
  - Maintain a consistent fluid intake of six 12-oz glasses of fluid a day (1500–3000 mL). High fluid intake leads to lower levels of lithium and less therapeutic effect. Lower fluid intake leads to higher lithium levels, which could produce toxicity.
  - Aim for consistency in sodium intake. Like fluid, high sodium intake leads to lower levels of lithium and less therapeutic effect. Low sodium intake leads to higher lithium levels, which could produce toxicity.
  - Stop taking lithium if you experience excessive diarrhea, vomiting, or sweating. All of these symptoms can lead to dehydration and increase blood lithium to toxic levels. Inform your care provider if you have any of these problems.
- Lithium levels may be increased while taking angiotensin-converting enzyme (ACE) inhibitors, angiotensin receptor blockers, thiazide diuretics, and nonsteroidal anti-inflammatory drugs. Let your prescriber know if you are taking any of these medications.
- Talk to your prescriber about having renal (kidney), thyroid, and parathyroid function checked periodically due to potential side effects.
- Do not take over-the-counter medicines without checking with your prescriber. Even nonsteroidal anti-inflammatory drugs (e.g., ibuprofen, naproxen) may increase serum lithium levels, diminish renal lithium clearance, and possibly induce lithium toxicity.
- Take lithium with meals to prevent stomach irritation.
- In the first week, you may gain up to 5 pounds of water weight. Additional weight gain may occur, particularly

Continued

> ## Box 23.1 **Patient and Family Teaching: Lithium Therapy—cont'd**
>
> in women. Discuss how much weight gain is acceptable with your prescriber.
> - Groups are available to provide support for people with bipolar disorder and their friends, family, and caregivers. A local self-help group is [provide name and phone number]. Online support groups are available and may be specific to the population being served such as veterans, young adults, older adults, and minorities.

- Superior in treating patients with rapid cycling bipolar disorders
- Effective in diminishing impulsive and aggressive behavior in patients without psychosis.
- Beneficial in controlling mania within 2 weeks and depressive symptoms within 3 weeks or earlier
- More effective when there is no family history of bipolar disorder
- Helpful in cases of alcohol and benzodiazepine withdrawal

Valproate

Valproate, available as divalproex (Depakote), and valproic acid have FDA approval for treating acute mania. This group of drugs is one of the most widely prescribed mood stabilizers in psychiatry. Valproate and valproic acid are first-line mood stabilizers. They work quickly, and most people tolerate them well. It takes about a week for sufficient serum level of the drug to be reached. Patients typically experience symptom reduction within 1 to 4 days after reaching the adequate serum level.

Common side effects of valproate include gastrointestinal irritation, nausea, diarrhea, vomiting, weakness, sedation, tremor, weight gain, and hair loss. The FDA features a black box warning for several adverse responses. Box 23.2 contains the actual warning on the valproic acid label The warning is essentially identical on the divalproex label. Hepatotoxicity is the first warning. Although rare, it is important to monitor liver function. Low platelets (thrombocytopenia) may also occur, so platelet counts and coagulation studies are also monitored.

> ### Box 23.2 **FDA Black Box Warning for Valproic Acid**
>
> Warning: Life-Threatening Adverse Reactions
>   See full prescribing information for complete boxed warning.
> - Hepatotoxicity, including fatalities, usually during first 6 months of treatment. Children under the age of 2 years are at considerably higher risk of fatal hepatotoxicity. Monitor patients closely, and perform liver function tests prior to therapy and at frequent intervals thereafter.
> - Teratogenicity, including neural tube defects.
> - Pancreatitis, including fatal hemorrhagic cases.

From U.S. Food and Drug Administration. (2008). Approved label – FDA. Retrieved from https://www.accessdata.fda.gov/drugsatfda_docs/label/2009/022152s002lbl.pdf

Another warning on the FDA label is the risk of valproate use in pregnancy due to teratogenicity (i.e., a drug that interferes with the development of the fetus). Before taking this medication, pregnancy screening is recommended and patients should use birth control to prevent pregnancy while taking it. Fetal valproate syndrome is the result of exposure to valproate during the first three months of pregnancy. It includes neural tube defects such as spina bifida, distinctive facial features, congenital heart defects, and musculoskeletal abnormalities. There have been rare, spontaneous reports of polycystic ovary disease associated with these drugs.

Pancreatitis, including fatal hemorrhagic cases, has been reported while using valproate. Symptoms of pancreatitis include abdominal pain or tenderness, vomiting, abdominal distention, fever, and chills. There is no correlation between serum level of the drug nor length of time on therapy and the onset of symptoms. After successful management of pancreatitis, the reintroduction of valproate is avoided.

Carbamazepine

Carbamazepine (Equetro) is indicated as a second-line treatment for acute mania and mixed states. It seems to work better for mania with rapid cycling, paranoia, and anger than in mania with euphoria and hyperactivity., paranoia, and anger

Liver enzymes are monitored at least weekly for the first 8 weeks of treatment. Carbamazepine can increase drug metabolizing enzymes which can speed up its own metabolism. Liver function studies are also important because this drug can cause hepatitis. The FDA provides a black box warning for aplastic anemia and agranulocytosis. Pretreatment hematological testing is recommended along with periodic complete blood counts. Carbamazepine is discontinued if significant bone marrow suppression is detected.

Carbamazepine also carries a black box warning for serious dermatologic reactions. These include toxic epidermal necrolysis and Stevens-Johnson syndrome. Both conditions result in erythema and death of the epidermis and mucous membranes, resulting in serious exfoliation and possible sepsis. Involvement of the mucous membranes can result in gastrointestinal hemorrhage, respiratory failure, ocular abnormalities, and genitourinary complications. These reactions occur in up to 6 per 10,000 new users who are of Western European descent. The risk in some people of Asian descent is 10 times higher because of an inherited variation of the HLA-B gene. At-risk individuals are screened for this gene before beginning treatment with carbamazepine.

Lamotrigine

Lamotrigine (Lamictal) is an FDA-approved maintenance therapy medication. Patients usually tolerate lamotrigine well. It is more effective in lengthening the time between depressive episodes. The most common side effects are dizziness, ataxia, somnolence, headache, diplopia, blurred vision, and nausea.

Like carbamazepine, the FDA provides a black box warning for life-threatening rashes such as Stevens-Johnson syndrome and toxic epidermal necrolysis. About 1 in 10 patients develop a rash within 8 weeks of starting treatment with lamotrigine. Even though usually benign, the medication is discontinued if a rash occurs. Instruct patients to seek immediate medical attention if a rash appears.

SECOND-GENERATION ANTIPSYCHOTICS

Many of the second-generation antipsychotics are FDA approved for acute mania. In addition to showing sedative properties during the early phase of treatment thereby decreasing insomnia, anxiety, and agitation, the second-generation antipsychotics seem to have mood-stabilizing properties.

Second-generation antipsychotics may also cause serious side effects. These side effects stem from a tendency toward weight gain that may lead to insulin resistance, diabetes, dyslipidemia, and cardiovascular impairment. See Chapter 22 for a more complete discussion of antipsychotic medications and their side effects.

Benzodiazepines

Though not considered a core treatment in bipolar disorder, some benzodiazepines (e.g., clonazepam [Klonopin] and lorazepam [Ativan]) can rapidly help control manic symptoms such as restlessness, agitation, or insomnia until mood-stabilizing drugs take effect. These drugs are used for a limited time in treatment-resistant mania.

BIPOLAR DEPRESSION

Treatment of bipolar depression with a common antidepressant alone may increase the risk of bringing on a manic episode. This risk is significantly reduced when the antidepressant is combined with a mood stabilizer.

Specific medications are indicated for bipolar depression. The second-generation antipsychotics lurasidone (Latuda), quetiapine (Seroquel), and cariprazine (Vraylar) have FDA approval for the treatment of bipolar depression. Symbyax is another drug with approval for this type of depression. It is a combination of medication consisting of the second-generation olanzapine (Zyprexa) and the selective serotonin reuptake inhibitor fluoxetine (Prozac).

CHAPTER 24

Antidepressants

Major depressive disorder is the most common psychiatric disorder, affecting nearly 14.5% of people at least once in a lifetime. Symptoms of depression include a long-lasting depressed mood along with feelings of guilt, anxiety, and recurrent thoughts of death and suicide. The monoamine hypothesis, which suggests a deficiency or imbalance in the monoamine neurotransmitters, such as serotonin, dopamine, and norepinephrine at the synaptic gap, as the cause of depression, was developed in the 1950s. Most currently used antidepressants are considered to act based on the monoamine hypothesis and continue to provide a basis for pharmacotherapy.

One concern regarding the monoamine hypothesis is that it fails to explain why antidepressants have a latent, or delayed, response. We know that antidepressants work fairly rapidly at improving the amount or balance of monoamines. However, antidepressants generally need 2 to 4 weeks or more for therapeutic effects on depressive symptoms. Another problem with antidepressant pharmacotherapy is that up to 30% of individuals do not respond to medications. Delayed responses and lack of response to antidepressants suggest that we may need alternate hypotheses to understand the pathophysiology of depression. Research into alternate hypotheses of depression will lead to the development of new medications for major depressive disorder.

ANTIDEPRESSANT MEDICATIONS

Antidepressant medications can positively impact poor self-concept, social withdrawal, vegetative signs of depression, and activity level. Target symptoms include the following:
- Sleep disturbance (decreased or increased)
- Appetite disturbance (decreased or increased)
- Fatigue
- Decreased or absent libido

- Psychomotor retardation or agitation
- Diurnal (i.e., daily cycle) variations in mood (often worse in the morning)
- Impaired concentration or memory
- Anhedonia (inability to experience pleasure)
- Feelings of guilt and self-loathing

A drawback of antidepressant drugs is that improvement in mood may take 2 to 4 weeks or longer. If a patient has acute suicidal ideation, a somatic treatment such as electroconvulsive therapy (discussed in Chapter 30) may be a reliable and effective alternative.

The goal of antidepressant therapy is the complete remission of symptoms. Often, the first antidepressant prescribed is not the one that will ultimately bring about remission. Aggressive treatment helps in finding the proper treatment. Opinions vary regarding an adequate drug trial for the treatment of depression, but 6 weeks is often used in clinical trials.

Individuals who experience a first depressive episode are usually maintained on an antidepressant for 6 to 12 months after symptoms of depression remit. The individual along with the clinician then determine whether or not to continue pharmacotherapy. The risk of relapse after antidepressant medication discontinuation is high but is not uniform. Some people may have multiple episodes of depression or may have a chronic form of depression and benefit from indefinite antidepressant therapy.

Antidepressants may precipitate a manic episode with bipolar disorder. Patients often receive a mood-stabilizing drug along with an antidepressant to reduce the possibility of this event.

CHOOSING AN ANTIDEPRESSANT

Antidepressants generally work to increase the availability of one or more of the neurotransmitters—serotonin, norepinephrine, and dopamine. In clinical trials, antidepressants demonstrate similar efficacy (i.e., the ability to produce the desired result). However, each of the antidepressants has different adverse effects, costs, safety profiles, and maintenance considerations. Selection of the appropriate antidepressant is based on the following considerations:

- Symptom profile of the patient
- Side effect profile (e.g., sexual dysfunction, weight gain)

- Ease of administration
- History of past response
- Safety and medical considerations

Advanced practice providers such as psychiatric–mental health nurse practitioners and psychiatrists may use drug–gene testing to support medication decisions. One genetic test is based on drug metabolism. The human body uses cytochrome P450 (CYP) enzymes to process medications. These P450 enzymes include the CYP2D6 enzyme, which catalyzes the metabolism of many antidepressant medications. Polymorphisms on CYP2D6 impact the way an individual may respond to a new drug. Genetic testing can help to determine the quality of drug metabolism. People fall into one of the four categories:

1. Poor metabolizers are missing an enzyme, resulting in slow processing of certain drugs. This can cause the medication to build up and increase the likelihood of side effects. The medication may still be used, but at lower doses.
2. Intermediate metabolizers have reduced enzyme function, resulting in suboptimal processing of certain drugs, which can increase side effects and drug interactions.
3. Normal metabolizers (commonly referred to as extensive metabolizers) are more likely to benefit from treatment and experience fewer side effects than those who do not process the medication as well.
4. Ultra-rapid metabolizers process medications too quickly (i.e., before they have a chance to work properly). Individuals in this category will require higher-than-usual doses of medications.

DISCONTINUING AN ANTIDEPRESSANT

An underrecognized problem may occur with abrupt discontinuation of antidepressant medications. This withdrawal reaction, known as discontinuation syndrome, occurs at a high rate—about 20%—in patients after taking medication for at least 6 weeks. Symptoms include flu-like aching, insomnia, nausea, imbalance, sensory disturbances, and hyperarousal. These symptoms tend to last 1 or 2 weeks or are eliminated quickly if the drug is restarted.

The syndrome is more common with longer duration of treatment and with drugs with a shorter half-life. All approved antidepressant drugs carry the potential for this problem. It is important for nurses to be aware of this syndrome and provide education on how to prevent it, such as slow tapering off of the antidepressant.

ANTIDEPRESSANT CLASSIFICATION

This chapter reviews several classifications of antidepressants, beginning with the most commonly prescribed groups. Table 24.1 provides an overview of antidepressants used in the United States and discussed in this chapter.

Selective Serotonin Reuptake Inhibitors

The selective serotonin reuptake inhibitors (SSRIs) selectively block the neuronal uptake of serotonin. This blockage increases the availability of serotonin in the synaptic cleft. Some SSRIs tend to be more activating, while others tend to be more sedating. The choice of drug depends, in part, on the patient's symptoms.

The first SSRI to be introduced was fluoxetine (Prozac) in 1987. This drug proved to be extremely popular and effective. Within 2 years of its introduction, pharmacies were filling 65,000 fluoxetine prescriptions per month in the United States alone. By 2018, that number rose to 25,619,277.

Indications

SSRIs are commonly the first-line treatment for treating major depressive disorder. In addition to their use in treating depressive disorders, the SSRIs are prescribed for anxiety disorders. Generalized anxiety disorder, panic disorder, social anxiety disorder, and obsessive–compulsive disorder are all treated with US Food and Drug Administration (FDA)–approved SSRIs. Fluoxetine (Prozac) has FDA approval for bulimia nervosa. Fluoxetine, sertraline (Zoloft), and controlled-release paroxetine (Paxil CR) have FDA approval for the treatment of premenstrual dysphoric disorder. Another paroxetine, Brisdelle, is used to treat moderate to severe vasomotor symptoms (e.g., hot flashes, night sweats) associated with menopause.

Table 24.1 **FDA-Approved Drugs for Major Depressive Disorder**

Generic (Trade) Name	Side Effects	Warnings
Selective Serotonin Reuptake Inhibitors (SSRIs)		
Citalopram (Celexa) Escitalopram (Lexapro) Fluoxetine (Prozac, Prozac Weekly) Paroxetine (Paxil, Paxil CR, Pexeva) Sertraline (Zoloft)	Agitation, insomnia, headache, nausea and vomiting, sexual dysfunction, hyponatremia	Discontinuation syndrome—dizziness, insomnia, nervousness, irritability, nausea, and agitation— may occur with abrupt withdrawal (depending on half-life); taper slowly.
Serotonin Norepinephrine Reuptake Inhibitors (SNRIs)		
Desvenlafaxine (Pristiq)	Nausea, headache, dizziness, insomnia, diarrhea, dry mouth, sweating, constipation	Neonates with *in utero* exposure may require respiratory support and tube feeding.
Duloxetine (Cymbalta, Drizalma)	Nausea, dry mouth, insomnia, somnolence, constipation, reduced appetite, fatigue, sweating, blurred vision	It may reduce pain associated with depression, approved for fibromyalgia, pain of diabetic peripheral neuropathy, and chronic musculoskeletal pain.
Levomilnacipran (Fetzima)	Nausea, orthostatic hypotension, constipation, sweating, increased heart rate, palpitations, difficulty urinating, decreased appetite, sexual dysfunction	It may cause urinary hesitancy.

Drug	Side Effects	Notes/Warnings
Venlafaxine (Effexor, Effexor XR)	Hypertension, nausea, insomnia, dry mouth, sedation, sweating, agitation, headache, sexual dysfunction	Monitor blood pressure, especially at higher doses and with a history of hypertension. Discontinuation syndrome.
Serotonin Antagonists and Reuptake Inhibitors (SARIs)		
Nefazodone	Sedation, hepatotoxicity, dizziness, hypotension, paresthesia	Life-threatening liver failure is possible but rare; priapism of the penis or clitoris is a rare but serious side effect.
Trazodone	Severe sedation, hypotension, nausea	Risk of prolonged erections and priapism. Palpitations, ventricular premature beats, serotonin syndrome.
Vilazodone (Viibryd)	Diarrhea, nausea, vomiting, dry mouth, dizziness, insomnia	
Serotonin Modulator and Stimulator		
Vortioxetine (Trintellix)	Constipation, nausea, vomiting	Hyponatremia, rare induction of manic states, serotonin syndrome.
Norepinephrine Dopamine Reuptake Inhibitor (NDRI)		
Bupropion (Wellbutrin, Aplenzin XL, Forfivo XL)	Agitation, insomnia, headache, nausea, and vomiting; sexual dysfunction is rare.	High doses increase seizure risk, especially in individuals who are predisposed to them.
Noradrenergic and Specific Serotonergic Antidepressant (NaSSA)		
Mirtazapine (Remeron)	Weight gain/appetite stimulation, sedation, dizziness, and headache. Sexual dysfunction is rare.	Somnolence is exaggerated by alcohol, benzodiazepines, and other central nervous system depressants.

Continued

Table 24.1 **FDA-Approved Drugs for Major Depressive Disorder—cont'd**

Generic (Trade) Name	Side Effects	Warnings
Tricyclic Antidepressants (TCAs)		
Amitriptyline	Dry mouth, constipation, urinary retention, blurred vision, hypotension, cardiac toxicity, sedation	Lethal in overdose; use cautiously in older adults and in patients with cardiac disorders, elevated intraocular pressure, urinary retention, hyperthyroidism, seizure disorders, and liver or kidney dysfunction.
Amoxapine		
Desipramine (Norpramin)		
Doxepin (Sinequan)		
Imipramine (Tofranil)		
Maprotiline		
Nortriptyline (Aventyl, Pamelor)		
Protriptyline (Vivactil)		
Trimipramine (Surmontil)		
Monoamine Oxidase Inhibitors (MAOIs)		
Isocarboxazid (Marplan)	Insomnia, nausea, agitation, and confusion; hypertensive crisis	It is contradicted with most antidepressants. Tyramine-rich food may result in a hypertensive crisis. There are many drug and dietary interactions.
Phenelzine (Nardil)		
Selegiline (Emsam transdermal patch)		
Tranylcypromine (Parnate)		

N-Methyl-D-Aspartate (NMDA) Receptor Antagonist

Esketamine (Spravato)

Dissociation, dizziness, nausea, sedation, vertigo, hypoesthesia (loss of sensation), anxiety, lethargy, increased blood pressure, vomiting, and feeling drunk

Monitor for sedation, dissociation, and hypertension for 2 hours when using the nasal spray.
It is a controlled substance schedule III.
It is extremely expensive.
It is available only through an FDA Risk Evaluation and Mitigation Strategy (REMS) program.

Gamma-Aminobutyric Acid (GABA) A Receptor Positive Modulator

Brexanolone (Zulresso)

Sedation/somnolence, dry mouth, loss of consciousness, and flushing/hot flush

IV infusion over 60 hours.
There is a risk of excessive sedation or sudden loss of consciousness during administration.
Controlled substance schedule IV.
Patients must be accompanied during interaction with children.
It is available only through an FDA REMS program.

From US Food and Drug Administration. *FDA online label repository.* www.labels.fda.gov

Common Adverse Reactions

Medications that enhance synaptic serotonin within the central nervous system (CNS) may result in agitation, anxiety, sleep disturbance, tremor, sexual dysfunction (primarily anorgasmia), or tension headache. Autonomic nervous system reactions such as a dry mouth, sweating, weight change, mild nausea, and loose stools may also be experienced with the SSRIs.

Potential Toxic Effect

A rare and life-threatening event associated with SSRIs, and with any of the antidepressants that increase serotonin, is serotonin syndrome. This syndrome is related to overactivation of the central serotonin receptors caused by either too high a dose or interaction with other drugs. These other drugs include the following:

- Antimigraine medications, such as lasmiditan and triptans, (almotriptan, naratriptan, and sumatriptan)
- Pain medications, such as opioid pain medications including codeine, fentanyl, hydrocodone, meperidine, oxycodone, and tramadol
- Lithium, a mood stabilizer
- Amphetamines in overdose
- Illicit drugs, including lysergic acid diethylamide (LSD), ecstasy, and cocaine.
- Herbal supplements, including St. John's wort, ginseng, and nutmeg
- Cough and cold medications containing dextromethorphan
- Antinausea medications such as granisetron, metoclopramide, droperidol, and ondansetron
- Linezolid, an antibiotic
- Skeletal muscle relaxants such as cyclobenzaprine and metaxalone

Symptoms of serotonin syndrome are abdominal pain, diarrhea, sweating, fever, tachycardia, elevated blood pressure, altered mental state (delirium), myoclonus (muscle spasms), increased motor activity, irritability, hostility, and mood change. Severe manifestations are hyperpyrexia (excessively high fever), cardiovascular shock, and death.

The risk of this syndrome seems to be greatest when an SSRI is administered in combination with a second serotonin-enhancing agent, especially monoamine oxidase inhibitors (MAOIs). SSRIs are discontinued for 2 to 5 weeks

---

Box 24.1 **Signs of Serotonin Syndrome and Treatments**

Signs
- Hyperactivity or restlessness
- Tachycardia → cardiovascular shock
- Fever → hyperpyrexia
- Elevated blood pressure
- Altered mental states (delirium)
- Irrationality, mood swings, hostility
- Seizures → status epilepticus
- Myoclonus, incoordination, tonic rigidity
- Abdominal pain, diarrhea, bloating
- Apnea → death

Treatments
- Discontinue serotonergic medications
- Initiate symptom management:
  - Serotonin receptor blockade with cyproheptadine, methysergide, propranolol
  - Cooling blankets
  - Dantrolene, diazepam (Valium) for muscle rigidity or rigors
  - Anticonvulsants
  - Artificial ventilation
  - Induction of paralysis

---

before starting an MAOI. Box 24.1 lists the signs of serotonin syndrome and provides a summary of emergency treatments.

Serotonin Norepinephrine Reuptake Inhibitors

Serotonin norepinephrine reuptake inhibitors (SNRIs) inhibit the reuptake of both serotonin and norepinephrine. The SNRIs include venlafaxine (Effexor), desvenlafaxine (Pristiq), duloxetine (Cymbalta), and levomilnacipran (Fetzima). All are FDA approved and are first-line treatments of major depressive disorder, and several have indications for anxiety disorders. Another SNRI, milnacipran (Savella), is indicated only for fibromyalgia.

The SNRIs have a similar side effect profile to the SSRIs, but SNRIs are more likely to cause excessive sweating. In addition, SNRIs cause dose-dependent increases in blood pressure and heart rate due to their norepinephrine reuptake blockade. Monitor blood pressure and heart rate at baseline and periodically thereafter, particularly at dose changes.

Venlafaxine is a serotonergic agent at lower therapeutic doses, and norepinephrine reuptake blockage only occurs at higher doses (i.e., over 150 mg/day). Of the SNRIs, venlafaxine is the most likely to produce discontinuation syndrome (i.e., flu-like symptoms, insomnia, nausea, dizziness, paresthesia, anxiety).

Desvenlafaxine (Pristiq) is the primary active metabolite of venlafaxine. When an individual takes venlafaxine, it will eventually be metabolized into desvenlafaxine. Therefore the mechanism of action and side effects of the two antidepressants are similar. Nausea is a prominent side effect of this drug.

Duloxetine (Cymbalta) is an SNRI that has FDA approval for both major depressive disorder and generalized anxiety disorder. It is also approved for treating diabetic peripheral neuropathy, fibromyalgia, and chronic musculoskeletal pain.

Levomilnacipran (Fetzima) is the most noradrenergic SNRI. It causes urinary hesitancy in up to 6% of patients secondary to the actions of norepinephrine on the genitourinary tract. Levomilnacipran is the most selective for norepinephrine reuptake of all of the SNRIs.

Serotonin Antagonist and Reuptake Inhibitors

Nefazodone (Serzone) and trazodone (Desyrel) belong to the serotonin antagonist and reuptake inhibitor, or SARI, class of antidepressants. Both medications inhibit neuronal uptake of serotonin and antagonize $5\text{-}HT_{2A}$ receptors. Nefazodone also inhibits norepinephrine reuptake. Common side effects include sedation, headache, nausea, dizziness, and blurred vision.

Nefazodone is not commonly prescribed. Sexual dysfunction is minimal with its use, but it is associated with rare, life-threatening liver failure. Avoid nefazodone in patients with preexisting liver impairment. Nefazodone is also contraindicated with several medications due to its inhibition of CYP3A4, a common drug-metabolizing enzyme.

Trazodone is FDA-approved for major depressive disorder, but it is most commonly prescribed off-label as a hypnotic. Due to its sedating effects, it is prescribed at bedtime for insomnia.

Trazodone is a potent α1 receptor antagonist, which contributes to dizziness and orthostatic hypotension. Educate patients to rise slowly when awakening to avoid falls.

Potent α1 antagonists with little anticholinergic activity, such as trazodone, can cause priapism, a painful prolonged erection caused by the inability for detumescence (subsidence of erection).

Vilazodone (Viibryd) enhances serotonin neurotransmission via 5-HT$_{1A}$ receptor partial agonism (similar to buspirone) and neuronal inhibition of serotonin reuptake (similar to SSRIs). Weight gain is not associated with this drug, and sexual side effects are limited. Patients are instructed to take this antidepressant with food for better bioavailability and avoid nighttime doses to prevent sleep disruption. Common side effects include diarrhea, nausea, insomnia, and vomiting. Vilazodone should be used with caution in people taking medications that affect coagulation because it can increase the risk of bleeding. The decision to use vilazodone in pregnant or nursing women should consider the potential risks to the fetus or baby versus the benefit to the mother.

Serotonin Modulator and Stimulator

Vortioxetine (Trintellix) has a similar side effect and contraindication profile to vilazodone. Nausea is the most common reason identified for discontinuing vortioxetine treatment. Constipation and vomiting have also been reported.

Norepinephrine and Dopamine Reuptake Inhibitor

Bupropion (Wellbutrin) is a norepinephrine and dopamine reuptake inhibitor (NDRI). It is also FDA-approved for smoking cessation as Zyban. With no serotonergic activities, it carries a lower risk of sexual dysfunction than most other antidepressants. Side effects include insomnia, tremor, anorexia, and weight loss. Contraindications include seizure disorders or eating disorders, or the abrupt discontinuation of alcohol or sedatives (including benzodiazepines) secondary to the increased risk of seizures.

Noradrenergic and Specific Serotonergic Antidepressant

Mirtazapine (Remeron) is a noradrenergic and specific serotonergic antidepressant (NaSSA). Mirtazapine enhances norepinephrine and serotonin neurotransmission by antagonizing both presynaptic α2 receptors and post-synaptic 5-HT2 and 5-HT3 receptors. This drug provides both antianxiety and antidepressant effects with minimal sexual dysfunction, limited gastrointestinal symptoms, and improved sleep. Common side effects are sedation, appetite stimulation, and weight gain. This drug is used with caution in patients with renal and hepatic insufficiency.

Tricyclic Antidepressants

The tricyclic antidepressants (TCAs) inhibit the reuptake of norepinephrine and serotonin by the presynaptic neurons in the CNS. They also block the actions of acetylcholine, and some TCAs also affect histamine.

The first TCAs were imipramine (Tofranil) and amitriptyline (formerly sold as Elavil). These TCAs were introduced in the early 1960s.

Positive effects on some symptoms of depression, such as insomnia and anorexia, may be experienced within 10 to 14 days. Full effects may not be seen for 4 to 8 weeks.

Indications

Most TCAs are indicated for the treatment of major depressive disorder. Side effect profiles are considered when choosing a particular TCA. A stimulating TCA, such as desipramine (Norpramin) or protriptyline (Vivactil), may be best for a patient who is lethargic and fatigued. If a more sedating effect is needed for agitation or restlessness, drugs such as amitriptyline and doxepin (Sinequan) may be more appropriate choices. Regardless of which TCA is given, the initial dose should always be low and be increased gradually.

Common Adverse Reactions

Many of the side effects of TCAs are due to their secondary pharmacological actions. The TCAs antagonize several receptors, including H1, α1, and M1, and these receptor effects are responsible for several side effects. By blocking H1 receptors in the brain, sedation and weight gain occur. Blockade of α1 receptors on blood vessels results in vasodilation and the side effects of dizziness and orthostatic hypotension. The effects of acetylcholine are blunted by M1 receptor blockade, and this leads to anticholinergic effects such as blurred vision, dry mouth, tachycardia, urinary retention, and constipation. In older adults, anticholinergic activity causes memory difficulties or confusion.

Administering the total daily dose of TCA at night is beneficial for two reasons. First, most TCAs have sedative effects and thereby aid sleep. Second, the minor side effects occur while the individual is sleeping, which increases adherence to drug therapy.

Toxicity/Overdose

TCA overdose carries a risk of death from cardiac conduction abnormalities: dysrhythmias, tachycardia, myocardial infarction, and heart block. Initial symptoms are CNS stimulation, including hyperpyrexia, delirium, hypertension, hallucinations, seizure, hyperreflexia, and parkinsonian symptoms. This phase is followed by CNS depression. Immediate medical care is essential with TCA overdose. The TCAs are used cautiously in patients with suicidal history or ideation because they are lethal in overdoses.

Contraindications

People who have recently had a myocardial infarction or other cardiovascular problems, those with narrow-angle glaucoma or a history of seizures, and women who are pregnant are not typically treated with TCAs except with extreme caution and careful monitoring. TCAs are contraindicated for use with MAOIs.

Monoamine Oxidase Inhibitors

The enzyme monoamine oxidase is responsible for inactivating, or breaking down, monoamine neurotransmitters in the brain such as norepinephrine, serotonin, dopamine, and tyramine. When a person takes an MAOI, fewer amines get deactivated, resulting in an increase of the mood-elevating neurotransmitters.

Indications

MAOIs are considered third-line antidepressants due to their significant drug interactions and dietary restrictions. MAOIs with FDA approval are phenelzine (Nardil), tranylcypromine (Parnate), and isocarboxazid (Marplan). A transdermal patch, selegiline (EMSAM), does not require strict dietary restrictions at its lowest dose.

Common Adverse Reactions

Some common and troublesome long-term side effects of the MAOIs are orthostatic hypotension, weight gain, edema, change in cardiac rate and rhythm, constipation, urinary hesitancy, sexual dysfunction, vertigo, overactivity, muscle twitching, insomnia, weakness, and fatigue. Hypomania and mania may be activated with MAOIs.

Potential Toxic Effects

Inhibiting MAO results in the inability to break down tyramine sufficiently. Individuals who take MAOIs and eat tyramine-rich foods are at risk for a hypertensive crisis. This crisis results in severe hypertension that can lead to such events as a cerebrovascular accident, intracranial hemorrhage, and death. Blood pressure is monitored during treatment with these drugs. Also, a reduction or elimination of foods and drugs that contain high amounts of tyramine is essential (Table 24.2).

The hypertensive crisis usually occurs within 15 to 90 minutes of ingestion of the offending substance. Early symptoms include irritability, anxiety, flushing, sweating, and a severe headache. The patient then becomes anxious and restless, and he or she develops a fever. Eventually, the fever becomes severe, seizures ensue, and coma or death is possible.

When a hypertensive crisis is suspected, immediate medical attention is crucial. If ingestion is recent, gastric lavage and charcoal may be helpful. Pyrexia is treated with hypothermic blankets or ice packs. Fluid therapy is essential, particularly with hyperthermia. A short-acting antihypertensive agent such as nitroprusside, nitroglycerine, or phentolamine may be used. Intravenous benzodiazepines are useful for agitation and seizure control.

Table 24.3 identifies common side effects and toxic effects of the MAOIs.

Contraindications

The use of MAOIs may be contraindicated with the following:

Table 24.2 **Safe and Unsafe Foods With Monoamine Oxidase Inhibitors**

Unsafe Foods (High Tyramine Content)	Safe Foods (Little or No Tyramine)
Vegetables and beans	
Avocados, especially if overripe; fermented bean curd; fermented soybean; soybean paste; snow peas, broad beans (fava beans) and their pods	Most fresh, frozen, canned, or dried vegetables, leafy salad greens, lentils, and beans; most veggie burgers that contain no soy product
Fruits	
Dried fruits (e.g., figs); overripe fruit	Most fresh, frozen, or canned fruits and fruit juices
Meats	
Meats that are fermented, smoked, or otherwise aged; spoiled meats; liver, unless very fresh; fermented meats (e.g., pepperoni, salami)	Fresh meats that are known to be fresh (exercise caution in restaurants where meat may not be fresh)
Fish	
Dried or cured fish; fish that is fermented, smoked, or otherwise aged; spoiled fish	Fish that is known to be fresh; vacuum-packed fish, if eaten promptly or refrigerated only briefly after opening
Milk, milk products	
Practically all cheeses	Milk, yogurt, cottage cheese, cream cheese
Breads, cereals, and crackers	
Yeast extract (e.g., Marmite, Bovril); sourdough bread; crackers and breads that contain aged cheese	Commercial yeast breads, hot and cold cereals, most crackers
Beer, wine	
Beer that contains yeast (e.g., draft or homemade beer), red wine, sherry, liqueurs, vermouth	Majority of canned and bottled
Other foods	
Protein dietary supplements; soups (may contain protein extract); shrimp paste; soy sauce	

Continued

Table 24.2 **Safe and Unsafe Foods With Monoamine Oxidase Inhibitors—cont'd**

Unsafe Foods (High Tyramine Content)	Safe Foods (Little or No Tyramine)
Foods That Contain Other Nontyramine Vasopressors	
Chocolate	
It contains phenylethylamine, a pressor agent; large amounts can cause a reaction.	
Fava beans	
They contain dopamine, a pressor agent; reactions are most likely with overripe beans.	
Ginseng	
Headache, tremulousness, and mania-like reactions have occurred.	
Caffeine	
Caffeine is a weak pressor agent; large amounts may cause a reaction.	

Table 24.3 **Adverse Reactions to and Toxic Effects of Monoamine Oxidase Inhibitors**

Adverse Reactions	Comments
Hypotension Sedation, weakness, fatigue Insomnia Changes in cardiac rhythm Muscle cramps Anorgasmia or sexual impotence Urinary hesitancy or constipation Weight gain	Hypotension is an expected side effect. Orthostatic blood pressures should be taken—first lying down, then sitting or standing after 1–2 minutes. This may be a dangerous side effect, especially in older adults who may fall and sustain injuries as a result of dizziness from the blood pressure drop.
Toxic Effects	**Comments**

Hypertensive crisis:
  Severe headache
  Tachycardia, palpitations
  Hypertension
  Nausea and vomiting
	Transport the individual to the emergency department—monitor blood pressure.
	Agents that may be given are 5-mg intravenous phentolamine or sublingual nifedipine to promote vasodilation.
	Individuals may be prescribed a 10-mg nifedipine capsule to carry in case of emergency.

- Cerebrovascular disease
- Hypertension and congestive heart failure
- Liver disease
- Consumption of foods containing tyramine, L-trypto-phan, and dopamine
- Use of certain medications
- Recurrent or severe headaches
- Surgery in the previous 10 to 14 days
- Younger than 16 years old

MISCELLANEOUS ANTIDEPRESSANTS

Two novel medications with FDA approval in 2019 are esketamine (Spravato) and brexanolone (Zulresso). They represent potential new directions for the pharmacological management of major depressive disorder.

Esketamine (Spravato)

Esketamine is a derivative of ketamine, the hallucino-genic and anesthetic party and date-rape drug. It is novel with regard to mechanism of action and dosage form. Esketamine is an antagonist of the *N*-methyl-D-aspartate (NMDA) receptor. Glutamate stimulates NMDA receptors. Esketamine alleviates depression by directly antagonizing the effects of glutamate. It is unknown how NMDA receptor antagonism improves depression.

Like ketamine, esketamine is a controlled US Drug Enforcement Administration (DEA) schedule III substance with the potential for misuse. Esketamine is FDA-approved for treatment-resistant depression, defined as two failed antidepressant trials, and for patients with major depressive disorder with acute suicidal ideation or behavior. It is used in conjunction with an oral antidepressant.

Esketamine is only available through the Spravato Risk Evaluation and Mitigation Strategies (REMS) and is not intended for home use. Pharmacies and health care settings that dispense esketamine are required to be certified in its use. Patients are formally enrolled in the Spravato REMS to receive treatment in an outpatient health care setting.

Administration occurs under the direct supervision of a health care provider. Patients are monitored for disso-ciation and sedation for at least 2 hours after each session. Blood pressure is assessed before and after administration for hypertension. The therapeutic benefit is evaluated after the treatment to determine the need for continued use.

Esketamine is available only as an intranasal spray. Patients require education on its administration. The device, which looks similar to a nasal spray, is not primed (i.e., do not pump it prior to use). Patients are instructed to blow their noses before the first spray only and to recline their head at a 45-degree angle for administration. Afterward, patients rest for 5 minutes between devices if multiple devices are required to achieve the desired dose.

In clinical studies, many individuals felt relief within four hours of taking the drug. Sessions occur twice a week for four weeks, one dose during weeks five through eight, and one or two doses a week after that.

Common side effects include dissociation, dizziness, nausea, sedation, vertigo, hypoesthesia, anxiety, lethargy, increased blood pressure, vomiting, and feeling drunk. Increases in blood pressure may put patients with cardio-vascular and cerebrovascular conditions at an increased risk of associated adverse effects. Cognitive impairment such as inattention, decreased judgment, slowed reaction speed, and impaired motor skills requires that patients do not drive or operate machinery until the next day after a restful sleep. Esketamine may result in embryo–fetal toxic-ity. Discuss pregnancy prevention in females with repro-ductive potential.

Cost may be prohibitive. Depending on the number of sessions and the dose, esketamine treatment cost is roughly between $600 to $900 per session. Treatment may include up to three devices administered on the same day. The pharmaceutical company that produces esketamine suggests that insurance may cover the cost. The company also advertises that they will provide support in finding programs to help individuals pay.

Brexanolone (Zulresso)

Brexanolone is the first medication to receive FDA approval for postpartum depression. The pharmacology of brexano-lone is not fully known, but it appears to interact with GABA type A receptors. It is a neuroactive steroid and identical to a metabolite of progesterone, called allopreg-nanolone. Brexanolone is a DEA schedule IV substance with limited potential for misuse.

Like esketamine, this drug is available only through a REMS program to mitigate the risk of harm resulting from excessive sedation and loss of consciousness. Pharmacies and healthcare settings that dispense brexanolone are required to be certified. All patients who use this therapy are included in a national registry to identify risks and to support its safe use.

Brexanolone is administered over a total of 60 hours (2.5 days) through continuous intravenous infusion. Patients are at risk of excessive sedation and sudden loss of consciousness during the administration. The infusion is stopped if excessive sedation occurs. The infusion may then be resumed at the same or a lower dose. Patients are monitored for hypoxia using continuous pulse oximetry equipped with an alarm. Mothers are accompanied during interactions with their children, for support if excessive sedation and sudden loss of consciousness occur.

The most common side effects are sedation/somnolence, dry mouth, loss of consciousness, and flushing/hot flash. Brexanolone is discontinued if postpartum depression becomes worse or if new suicidal thoughts and behaviors occur. Improved symptoms are noticeable within a few hours and last at least a month.

Like esketamine, the cost of brexanolone may be a barrier to its use. This financial limitation is unfortunate given that low-income women are at the greatest risk for postpartum depression. The pharmaceutical company that produces this drug does advertise financial support and guidance.

ANTIDEPRESSANT USE IN SPECIAL POPULATIONS

Use of Antidepressants by Pregnant Women

Antidepressants cross the placenta. The decision to treat severe depression, particularly with suicidal ideation, must weigh the risks versus the benefits. If antidepressant therapy is used during pregnancy, it is typically a single medication (monotherapy) at the lowest effective dose, especially during the first trimester. SSRIs are considered an option with the exception of paroxetine (Paxil), which has a small association with fetal heart defects.

Antidepressant Use by Children and Adolescents

Although antidepressant medications undoubtedly help children and adolescents with depression, there has been some concern that they may actually induce suicidal behavior in young people. The FDA adopted a black box label warning, the most serious type of warning in prescription drug labeling. The label states that antidepressants may increase the risk of suicidal thinking and behavior in some children and adolescents with major depressive disorder.

Young people taking SSRIs are closely monitored for worsening depression, emergence of suicidal thinking or behavior, or unusual changes in behavior such as agitation. This close monitoring is recommended during the first 4 weeks of treatment and during dose changes.

Use of Antidepressants by Older Adults

Polypharmacy and the normal metabolic processes of aging contribute to concerns about prescribing antidepressants for older adults. While SSRIs are a first-line treatment for older adults, they have the potential for side effects. Other options include tricyclic antidepressants, mirtazapine (Remeron), bupropion (Wellbutrin), and venlafaxine (Effexor). Starting doses are recommended to be half the lowest adult dose, with dose adjustments occurring no more frequently than every 7 days ("start low and go slow").

CHAPTER 25

Antianxiety Medications

Anxiety disorders result in chronic fears and thoughts that are distressing and interfere with everyday living. However, these disorders are treatable in most cases. Pharmacotherapy is an important adjunct to use with other therapies, especially cognitive–behavioral therapy (CBT). Several classes of medications have been found to be effective in the treatment of anxiety disorders.

- Selective serotonin reuptake inhibitors (SSRIs) are the first-line treatment for all anxiety disorders, especially panic disorders.
- Serotonin norepinephrine reuptake inhibitors (SNRIs) are also used as first-line treatment for anxiety disorders.
- Antianxiety agents such as benzodiazepines are effective but are only recommended to be used short term. These medications are not recommended for use by patients with substance use disorders.
- Buspirone (BuSpar) can be used for long-term management of generalized anxiety disorder. It has little abuse potential making it useful for individuals who may have substance use problems.

Table 25.1 summarizes medications approved by the US Food and Drug Administration (FDA) for the treatment of anxiety disorders.

ANTIDEPRESSANTS

SSRIs are considered a first line of treatment in most anxiety and obsessive–compulsive-related disorders. These SSRIs include paroxetine (Paxil), fluoxetine (Prozac), escitalopram (Lexapro), fluvoxamine (Luvox), and sertraline (Zoloft). Some of these antidepressants exert more of an activating effect than others and may actually increase anxiety initially. Fluoxetine and sertraline tend to be the most activating.

Table 25.1 **FDA-Approved Drugs for the Treatment of Anxiety Disorders**

	Generalized Anxiety Disorder	Panic Disorder	Social Anxiety Disorder
Selective serotonin reuptake inhibitors	Escitalopram (Lexapro) Paroxetine (Paxil)	Fluoxetine (Prozac) Paroxetine (Paxil) Sertraline (Zoloft)	Paroxetine (Paxil) Sertraline (Zoloft)
Serotonin–norepinephrine reuptake inhibitors	Venlafaxine (Effexor) Duloxetine[a] (Cymbalta)	Venlafaxine (Effexor)	Venlafaxine (Effexor)
Benzodiazepines	Alprazolam (Xanax) Chlordiazepoxide (Librium) Clorazepate (Tranxene) Diazepam (Valium) Lorazepam (Ativan) Oxazepam (Serax)	Alprazolam (Xanax) Clonazepam (Klonopin)	
Other	BBuspirone (BuSpar)		

[a]Approved for children and adolescents aged 7 to 17 years
From US Food and Drug Administration. (2020). *FDA label online repository.* www.labels.fda.gov

Paroxetine tends to have a more calming effect than the other SSRIs. Antidepressants have the secondary benefit of treating comorbid depressive disorders.

Venlafaxine (Effexor), an SNRI, is another first line of defense used in the treatment of several anxiety disorders. Another SNRI, duloxetine (Cymbalta), is effective in the treatment of generalized anxiety disorder.

Monoamine oxidase inhibitors (MAOIs) are reserved for treatment-resistant conditions. A life-threatening hypertensive crisis could occur if the patient does not follow dietary restrictions of avoiding tyramine-containing foods. Patients are given specific dietary instructions. The risk of hypertensive crisis also makes the use of MAOIs contraindicated in patients with comorbid substance use disorders. See Chapter 24 for more information about the MAOIs and other antidepressant medications.

ANTIANXIETY DRUGS

Antianxiety drugs are often used to treat the somatic and psychological symptoms of anxiety disorders. Benzodiazepines are most commonly used because they have a quick onset of action. When moderate or severe anxiety is reduced, patients are better able to participate in treatment of their underlying problems. However, due to the potential for misuse, these medications are used only for short periods of time, or until other medications or treatments reduce symptoms.

An important nursing intervention is to monitor for side effects of benzodiazepines, including sedation, ataxia, and decreased cognitive function. Paradoxical reactions—reactions that are the exact opposite of intended responses—sometimes occur. Symptoms such as anxiety, agitation, talkativeness, and loss of impulse control may occur when using this classification of medications. They are not recommended for older adult patients because of the risk of delirium, falls, and fractures. The decision to use benzodiazepines during pregnancy is made by weighing the risk of fetal exposure versus the risk of an untreated anxiety disorder (US Department of Health and Human Services, 2012). Benzodiazepines are sometimes used during breastfeeding if the anxiety is severe. Of the benzodiazepines, lorazepam (Ativan) is preferred, because it has not been shown to have adverse effects in infants, most likely due to its shorter half-life.

These medications require tapering if used long term to avoid withdrawal effects. Tapering can last weeks to months depending on the circumstance, namely the dose and half-life of the drug and duration of therapy. Because these drugs are depressants, rebound hyperactivity occurs with sudden removal of the substance. Hence, autonomic hyperactivity, tremor, insomnia, psychomotor agitation, anxiety, and grand mal seizures can occur. Benzodiazepine withdrawal is unusual in that symptoms tend to wax and wane from day to day and week to week.

Buspirone (BuSpar) is an alternative antianxiety medication that has little misuse potential and is not a controlled substance. Buspirone takes 2 to 4 weeks to reach its full effects. This medication may be used for long-term treatment and is taken on a regular schedule.

OTHER CLASSES OF MEDICATIONS

Other classes of medications used to treat anxiety disorders include beta-blockers, anticonvulsants, antihistamines, and antipsychotics. These agents are often added if the first course of treatment is ineffective. Beta-blockers block the receptors that, when stimulated, cause the heart to beat faster and have been used to treat social anxiety disorder. Medications such as propranolol (Inderal) reduce physical manifestations of anxiety by slowing the heart rate and reducing blushing.

Anticonvulsants have shown benefits in the management of generalized anxiety disorder and social anxiety disorder. Gabapentin (Neurontin) and pregabalin (Lyrica), for example, are commonly prescribed.

Antihistamines can be a safe, nonaddictive alternative to benzodiazepines. They may be helpful in treating patients with concurrent substance use disorders. Hydroxyzine (Vistaril) is an effective short-term (up to 4 months) antianxiety agent. A commonly used antihistamine, diphenhydramine (Benadryl), can be used to treat sleep loss associated with anxiety based on its significant sedative properties.

The antihistamines are also anticholinergics, that is, they block the binding of acetylcholine to neural receptors. Anticholinergic side effects, including dry mouth, constipation, and cognitive effects, need to be monitored. These drugs are avoided or used with caution in older adults because the body's production of acetylcholine diminishes with age.

Antipsychotic medications are effective in treating more severe symptoms of anxiety disorders, especially for individuals with schizophrenia or schizoaffective disorder. The risks of metabolic side effects, as well as the consequences of the dopamine blockade, significantly reduce the use of antipsychotics for anxiety disorders. The FDA has not approved any antipsychotics for these disorders.

HERBAL THERAPY AND INTEGRATIVE APPROACHES

Herbal therapy and dietary supplements are commonly used, but they are not subject to the same rigorous testing as prescription medications. Also, herbs and dietary supplements may not be uniformly prepared or dosed, and there is no guarantee of bioequivalence of the active compound among preparations. Problems that can occur with the use of psychotropic herbs include toxic side effects and herb–drug interactions.

Since the use of herbal products has become more mainstream, the importance of better oversight of safety has been heightened. Despite these concerns, the American Association of Poison Control continues to show that most major classes of prescribed medications have significantly more adverse effects and fatalities than vitamins, dietary supplements, herbs, and homeopathic remedies (Gummin et al., 2018). In 2017 the number one cause of poisoning was pharmaceutical in 2314 (86.3%) of the 2682 fatalities.

While the majority of herbal supplements are safe, some herbs may have negative effects on certain individuals and interactions with other medications. One example is kava (or kava-kava), which is derived from the roots of *Piper methysticum*, a South American plant used as a sedative with antianxiety effects. Kava supplements have been found to exert a small effect on reducing anxiety.

In 2010 the FDA issued a warning regarding a correlation between use of kava and a risk of liver damage. Kava is known to dramatically inhibit a liver enzyme (P450) necessary for the metabolism of many medications. This inhibition could result in liver failure, especially when taken along with alcohol or other medications such as central nervous system depressants (antianxiety agents fall into this category). Long-term use of high doses of kava has also been associated with dry, scaly skin or yellowing of the skin.

Valerian is a perennial flowering plant that is used for conditions related to anxiety and psychological stress, but it is most commonly used for insomnia and anxiety. Although it has proven effective for insomnia, there is insufficient scientific evidence to rate its safety. Unlike kava, valerian is considered safe for most people when used in medicinal amounts on a short-term basis. Some side effects of valerian are headaches, excitability, uneasiness, and even insomnia.

German chamomile is an herb whose flowers are used to make a supplement that has been used for generalized anxiety disorder. There have been reports of allergic reactions, including rare cases of anaphylaxis, in response to chamomile products. Allergies to other ragweed plant species seem to predispose people to such reactions.

Essential oils that are either inhaled or massaged into the skin may also reduce anxiety and stress. Table 25.2 provides an overview of anxiety- and stress-relieving oils.

Table 25.2 **Essential Oils Used in Mental Health–Related Concerns**

Essential Oil	Use
Clary sage	Relaxing, relieving anxiety/stress
Ginger	Emotionally and physically warming
Lavender	Calming, decreases anxiety
Lemon	Antistress
Mandarin	Calming
Neroli	Relieves and decreases anxiety
Roman chamomile	Relieving anxiety/stress
Rose	Relieves and decreases anxiety/stress
Vetiver	Calming, grounding

From National Association of Holistic Aromatherapy. (2019). *Most commonly used essential oils.* www.naha.org/explore-aromatherapy/about-aromatherapy/most-commonly-used-essential-oils

ANXIETY TREATMENT IN SPECIAL POPULATIONS

Anxiety Treatment in Children

A few drugs are approved specifically for anxiety disorders in children and adolescents. The SNRI duloxetine (Cymbalta) has FDA approval for children aged 7 to 17 years for generalized anxiety disorder. The FDA has approved four medications for use in children with obsessive–compulsive disorder. They are clomipramine (Anafranil), fluoxetine (Prozac), fluvoxamine (Luvox), and sertraline (Zoloft). Medications approved for other age groups are still prescribed off-label. For example, SSRIs are used to treat generalized anxiety disorder, panic disorder, and social anxiety disorder, all with good results.

Anxiety Treatment in Older Adults

Anxiety disorders occur at the same rate in older adults as in younger people. The most common anxiety disorder in this population is generalized anxiety disorder. The treatment adage of "start low and go slow" is important due to changes in drug absorption and action in the aging body. Medications such as antidepressants are begun with one-half or one-quarter of the usual starting dose and increased slowly.

CHAPTER 26

Sleep–Wake Medications

Sleep is central to life. An essential function, sleep recharges the mind and allows it to function properly. Sleep is impacted and implicated in virtually every psychiatric disorder and condition. This chapter begins with a discussion of medications used to promote sleep for individuals with insomnia. On the opposite side of the sleep spectrum is narcolepsy, a chronic sleep disorder characterized by overwhelming daytime drowsiness and sudden attacks of sleep. Pharmacotherapy for this disorder is also discussed.

INSOMNIA

Insomnia is characterized by dissatisfaction with quantity or quality of sleep. It is the most common sleep disorder affecting nearly half of all adults. Females are more frequently impacted by insomnia, as are older adults.

Table 26.1 provides an overview of US Food and Drug Administration (FDA)–approved medications for insomnia. All drugs in this table are US Drug Enforcement Administration (DEA) schedule IV drugs, with the exception of ramelteon (Rozerem) and doxepin (Silenor).

Over-the-counter, herbal, and dietary sleep aids are briefly discussed. Other classifications of drugs are used off-label without specific FDA approval to promote sleep. These drugs include antidepressants, anticonvulsants, and antihistamines. Second-generation antipsychotics also improve sleep in people using them for other problems such as schizophrenia.

BENZODIAZEPINES

Benzodiazepines have antianxiety, hypnotic (sleep-inducing), anticonvulsant, amnestic (loss of memory), and muscle relaxant properties. Benzodiazepines potentiate, or

Table 26.1 **FDA-Approved Drugs for Insomnia**

Generic (Trade) Name	Onset of Action (min)	Duration of Action	Use in Insomnia	
			DFA	DMS
Benzodiazepines				
Estazolam	<60	Intermediate	✓	✓
Flurazepam (Dalmane)[a]	30–60	Long	✓	✓
Quazepam (Doral)[a]	20–45	Long	✓	✓
Temazepam (Restoril)	45–60	Intermediate	—	✓
Triazolam (Halcion)	15–30	Short	✓	—
Nonbenzodiazepine Receptor Agonists				
Eszopiclone (Lunesta)	60	Intermediate	✓	✓
Zaleplon (Sonata)	15–30	Ultra short	✓	—
Zolpidem immediate release (Ambien)	30	Short	✓	—
Immediate release (Intermezzo)[b]	30	Short	—	✓
Extended release (Ambien CR)	30	Intermediate	✓	✓
Melatonin Receptor Agonist				
Ramelteon (Rozerem)	30	Short	✓	—
Orexin Receptor Antagonists				
Lemborexant (Dayvigo)	15–20	Intermediate	✓	✓
Suvorexant (Belsomra)	30	Intermediate	✓	✓
Tricyclic Antidepressant				
Doxepin (Silenor)	>60	Intermediate	—	✓

DFA, Difficulty falling asleep; *DMS*, difficulty maintaining sleep.
[a]Generally not recommended due to its long duration of action.
[b]A sublingual tablet taken in the middle of the night when there are at least 4 hours left to sleep.
From US Food and Drug Administration. (2020). *Drugs@FDA: FDA-approved drugs*. https://www.accessdata.fda.gov/scripts/cder/daf/

promote, the activity of gamma-aminobutyric acid (GABA) by binding to a specific site on the GABA receptor complex. This binding results in an increased frequency of chloride channel opening causing membrane hyperpolarization, which reduces the cellular excitation. If cellular excitation is decreased, the result is a calming effect.

All benzodiazepines cause sedation at higher therapeutic doses. Several benzodiazepines are FDA-approved for treatment of insomnia with a predominantly hypnotic effect: estazolam, flurazepam (Dalmane), temazepam (Restoril), quazepam (Doral), and triazolam (Halcion).

Nurses caution patients about taking benzodiazepines while engaging in activities requiring mental alertness, such as driving a car or operating machinery, due to sedation, ataxia, and slowed reflexes. Central nervous system (CNS) depressants such as alcohol intensify these effects. In older adults, benzodiazepine use is associated with falls, bone fractures, and delirium, and these medications are avoided.

This class of drugs is categorized as schedule IV by the DEA. Craving, tolerance, and withdrawal can develop even when taken for their intended indication. Chapter 12 provides a discussion of sedative-, hypnotic-, and anxiolytic-related substance use disorders.

When used alone, these drugs rarely inhibit the brain to the degree of respiratory depression and death. However, when combined with other CNS depressants such as alcohol and opiates, they may lead to a coma or fatal overdose.

SHORT-ACTING SEDATIVE-HYPNOTIC SLEEP AGENTS

Nonbenzodiazepine receptor agonists, or Z-hypnotics, include eszopiclone (Lunesta), zaleplon (Sonata), and zolpidem (Ambien). Zolpidem comes in two additional types. Intermezzo is an immediate-release drug and is used to help people fall back to sleep if they wake in the middle of the night. Ambien CR has two separate layers, one that dissolves quickly and promotes falling asleep, and the other dissolves more slowly to help in continuing sleep.

They possess hypnotic and amnestic effects without the antianxiety, anticonvulsant, or muscle relaxant effects of benzodiazepines. This is due to their selectivity for $GABA_A$ receptors containing an alpha-1 subunit. Similar to benzodiazepines, nonbenzodiazepine receptor agonists can cause sedation, ataxia, and harmful effects in older people, including falls, bone fractures, and delirium. They are controlled substances but seem to cause less tolerance and dependence than benzodiazepines. Nevertheless, exercise caution or consider alternatives for patients with substance use disorders. Eszopiclone can cause an unpleasant, bitter taste upon awakening in about one-third of patients.

Compared to benzodiazepines, the nonbenzodiazepines generally have shorter half-lives and no active metabolites. Zaleplon has the shortest half-life, approximately 1 hour, and helps patients to fall asleep, whereas eszopiclone has a half-life of approximately 6 hours and will also assist patients with staying asleep. Zolpidem metabolism occurs more slowly in women than in men, resulting in higher blood levels in female patients. Based on this finding, the FDA lowered the starting dose for all zolpidem products for female patients.

The FDA has issued warnings on all approved hypnotic medications regarding complex sleep-related behaviors. These behaviors include sleepwalking, driving, cooking, or eating. Activities occur while the patient is not fully awake, and patients may have no memory of engaging in them. While these events are rare, the use of other CNS depressants, including alcohol, may increase this risk.

MELATONIN RECEPTOR AGONIST

Melatonin (MT) is a hormone that is excreted by the pineal gland at night as part of the normal circadian rhythm. Ramelteon (Rozerem) is an MT receptor agonist and acts similarly to endogenous MT. It has a high selectivity and potency at the MT_1 receptor site—which regulates sleepiness—and at the MT_2 receptor site—which regulates circadian rhythms.

This medication is not classified as a scheduled substance and lacks misuse potential. Side effects include headache and dizziness. Ramelteon may decrease testosterone and increase prolactin levels, possibly causing a decreased interest in sex or problems with fertility. Ramelteon and fluvoxamine, a selective serotonin reuptake inhibitor (SSRI), interact and use together is contraindicated.

OREXIN RECEPTOR ANTAGONISTS

Orexins (OXs), neuropeptides produced in the hypothalamus, promote wakefulness. OXs naturally bind to OX_1 and OX_2 receptors. Suvorexant (Belsomra) and lemborexant (Dayvigo) are OX receptor antagonists FDA-approved for insomnia characterized by difficulty falling asleep or staying asleep. OX-containing neurons appear to be diminished in narcolepsy. Therefore suvorexant and lemborexant, OX blockers, are contraindicated in patients with narcolepsy. Rare side effects of sleep paralysis, hallucinations upon waking or falling asleep, or cataplexy-like symptoms (loss of muscle tone prompted by strong emotions, such as laughter or surprise) have occurred with use. OX receptor antagonists are controlled substances, so they are used with caution in patients with substance use disorders.

TRICYCLIC ANTIDEPRESSANT

A low-dose formulation of the tricyclic antidepressant doxepin under the brand name. Silenor is FDA-approved for the treatment of insomnia characterized by difficulty staying asleep. It does not decrease time to sleep onset. Doxepin has a high affinity for the H_1 receptor, making it a selective H_1 antagonist in low doses. This affinity results in sedating properties.

Silenor is not recommended for use in patients with severe urinary retention or glaucoma, or those taking monoamine oxidase inhibitors (MAOIs). Because it is not a controlled substance, this medication does not carry misuse potential.

OVER-THE-COUNTER SLEEP AIDS

Individuals use a variety of over-the-counter sleep aids to get a good night's sleep. Many of these drugs contain diphenhydramine (Benadryl), an antihistamine commonly used for allergy symptoms. One of its side effects is drowsiness, making this a popular option as a sleep aid. These sleep aids can cause unwanted sleepiness in the morning, difficulty urinating, and confusion and delirium. Some of the over-the-counter products that contain diphenhydramine include the following:

- Excedrin PM
- Nytol

- Tylenol PM
- ZzzQuil

Another active sleep-promoting antihistamine ingredient is doxylamine, which is found in Unisom. Common side effects include dry mouth, ataxia, urinary retention, drowsiness, and memory problems. Severe consequences of taking this drug in high doses include hallucinations, psychosis, and an increased sensitivity to external stimuli.

Antihistamines are also anticholinergics, that is, they block the binding of acetylcholine to neural cholinergic receptors. Anticholinergic side effects, including dry mouth, constipation, and cognitive effects, should be monitored. These drugs are avoided or used with caution in older adults because the body's production of acetylcholine diminishes with age. Older adults taking anticholinergic drugs are at risk for brain atrophy, deliriium, and clinical decline. Therefore their use is strongly discouraged in this population.

Over-the-counter drugs work best when used for mild and infrequent insomnia. Despite "nonhabit-forming" labels, there is still reason for concern. Most over-the-counter sleep aids result in habituation and, therefore, are not recommended to be used longer than 2 weeks.

HERBAL AND DIETARY SUPPLEMENTS FOR INSOMNIA

Valerian is a tall, flowering plant native to Asia and Europe. Its roots are used as a dietary supplement for insomnia, anxiety, and other conditions such as depression and menopause symptoms. The evidence for its efficacy in treating insomnia is insufficient. No information is available about the long-term safety of valerian or its safety in children younger than 3 years, pregnant women, or nursing mothers. Mild side effects could include morning fatigue, headaches, dizziness, and upset stomach.

Melatonin is a hormone that is produced by the pineal gland in the brain that plays a role in sleep. The production and release of melatonin are closely tied to light. In response to darkness, the pineal gland initiates production of melatonin, but light exposure slows or halts that production. Dietary supplements containing melatonin are used for sleep disorders, such as jet lag, dysfunction with the body's internal clocks, and night shift work sleep problems. In the

US, melatonin is considered a dietary supplement and not a drug, therefore it is less strictly regulated by the FDA.

German chamomile, nicknamed "sleep tea," is a traditional herbal remedy for insomnia. Its use for a variety of conditions including gastrointestinal conditions (e.g., upset stomach, gas, diarrhea), skin conditions, and mouth sores dates back to ancient Greece, Egypt, and Rome (National Center for Complementary and Integrative Health, 2020).

The flowering tops of the plant are used for teas, extracts, and topical ointments. Sedative effects may be due to the flavonoid apigenin that binds to benzodiazepine receptors in the brain. However, no empirical studies support chamomile's medical use other than being a relaxing drink before bedtime. Rare serious allergic reactions, including anaphylaxis, which may be related to allergies to other plants such as ragweed, have been reported. Drug interactions with warfarin, cyclosporine, and other medications may occur.

NARCOLEPSY

Individuals with narcolepsy have an uncontrollable urge to sleep. Overwhelming daytime drowsiness and sudden attacks of sleep significantly impair functioning. Narcolepsy may also be characterized by the disturbing and dangerous symptom of cataplexy. Cataplexy is a bilateral loss of muscle tone similar to the sleep paralysis experienced during rapid-eye-movement (REM) sleep. It may lead to slurred speech and buckling knees, or in more severe cases, complete paralysis.

Treatment for narcolepsy includes naps, exercise, and a balanced diet. Medications with FDA approval for excessive daytime sleepiness include CNS stimulants such as modafinil (Provigil), armodafinil (Nuvigil), methylphenidate, and amphetamine. The CNS depressants sodium oxybate (Xyrem), and calcium, magnesium, potassium, and sodium oxybate (Xywav) are indicated for the treatment of both excessive daytime sleepiness and cataplexy in patients with narcolepsy. Another nonstimulant medication, pitolisant (Wakixis), is also indicated for both excessive daytime sleepiness and cataplexy in patients with narcolepsy. A nonstimulant, noncontrolled substance solriamfetol (Sunosi) was recently introduced to improve wakefulness in patients with narcolepsy.

Modafinil (Provigil) is indicated to improve wakefulness and reduce sleepiness in adult patients with narcolepsy, sleep apnea, and shift work disorder. It is a nonamphetamine, DEA schedule IV–controlled substance with a moderate risk for misuse. Modafinil first thing in the morning with or without food. Common side effects include headache, nausea, nervousness, rhinitis, diarrhea, back pain, anxiety, insomnia, dizziness, and dyspepsia. A serious rash, including Stevens-Johnson syndrome and toxic epidermal necrolysis, has been reported. Individuals are instructed to discontinue modafinil at the first sign of rash, unless the rash is clearly not drug related.

Armodafinil (Nuvigil) is a longer-lasting isomer of modafinil that results in higher plasma concentration later in the day. This difference in pharmacokinetic profile may result in improved wakefulness throughout the day compared with modafinil. Otherwise, there is no difference in safety or efficacy between the two medications. Armodafinil is a DEA schedule IV–controlled substance. It is recommended to be taken early in the day with or without food. Common side effects include headache, nausea, dizziness, and insomnia. Rare cases of serious or life-threatening rash have been reported. Patients are instructed to discontinue aromodafinil if a rash appears.

Methylphenidate (Ritalin) is a CNS stimulant indicated in the treatment of narcolepsy and also commonly prescribed for attention-deficit/hyperactivity disorder (ADHD). Methylphenidate has a high potential for misuse and is a DEA schedule II substance. Immediate-release formulations are generally taken two or three times a day, preferably 30 to 45 minutes before meals. Side effects commonly experienced are tachycardia, palpitations, headache, insomnia, anxiety, hyperhidrosis (excessive sweating), weight loss, decreased appetite, dry mouth, nausea, and abdominal pain. Serious problems secondary to methylphenidate use include hypertension, tachycardia, myocardial infarction, and stroke. This medication is also associated with exacerbation (worsening) of psychiatric disorders such as bipolar mania or psychosis, and potentiating new manic symptoms or psychosis.

Like methylphenidate, **amphetamine (Adderall)** is a CNS stimulant indicated for use in narcolepsy and ADHD. It is also a DEA schedule II–controlled substance with a high potential for misuse. Immediate-release versions of this medication are taken two or three times a day with or without food. Side effects include stomachache, decreased appetite, and nervousness.

Sodium oxybate (Xyrem) is a CNS depressant with FDA approval for both excessive daytime sleepiness and cataplexy in individuals 7 years of age and older with narcolepsy. It helps to restore normal sleep architecture at night, especially slow-wave sleep, which in turn may improve daytime alertness. Sodium oxybate is a sodium salt of gamma-hydroxybutyrate (GHB), a schedule I–controlled substance, also known as a date rape drug. Sodium oxybate is a DEA schedule III medication with low-moderate misuse potential. It can only be prescribed under an FDA program called a Risk Evaluation and Mitigation Strategy (REMS), with prescription only by certified prescribers, and dispensed only to an patient enrolled by a certified pharmacy.

Zyrem should be taken 2 hours after eating while in bed and lying down after dosing. Patients need to set an alarm to wake them 3 hours after the first dose. The second dose is then taken, and a deep sleep should follow. The most common side effects of sodium oxybate in adults are nausea, dizziness, vomiting, somnolence, enuresis (bedwetting), and tremor. In children, the most common adverse reactions were enuresis, nausea, headache, vomiting, weight loss, decreased appetite, and dizziness.

CNS depression for the first 6 hours after dosing contraindicates hazardous activities requiring mental alertness. This medication may also increase depression and suicidality, and it is important to monitor patients carefully. Due to its high sodium content, patients are monitored for heart failure, hypertension, or impaired renal function. Sodium oxybate is contraindicated with concurrent use of sleep medications and alcohol.

Xywav is a **calcium, magnesium, potassium, and sodium oxybate** oral medication used for the treatment of cataplexy and excessive daytime sleepiness in individuals with narcolepsy. It is also the first and only medication approved for idiopathic hypersomnia. Xywav is closely related to Xyrem, although it contains 92% less sodium. Like sodium oxybate, Xywav is approved for children as young as 7, is a schedule III–controlled substance, requires two doses of an oral solution, and requires an REMS protocol for prescribing and dispensing. In patients transitioning from sodium oxybate to Xywav, the dose should be identical.

Common side effects in adults include headache, nausea, dizziness, decreased appetite, parasomnia, diarrhea, hyperhidrosis (excessive sweating), anxiety, and vomiting. Common side effects in children include enuresis, nausea, headache, vomiting, weight loss, decreased appetite, and dizziness.

Pitolisant (Wakix) is a nonstimulant histamine-3 (H_3) receptor antagonist/inverse agonist medication with FDA approval for excessive daytime sleepiness in narcolepsy and cataplexy. Pitolisant is a H_3 receptor antagonist/inverse agonist is not scheduled as a controlled substance by the DEA. Pitolisant is taken once a day in the morning. It is contraindicated in patients with hepatic impairment and has the potential to prolong the QT interval. Its use is not recommended in patients with end-stage renal disease. Common side effects include insomnia, nausea, and anxiety.

Solriamfetol (Sunosi) is a nonstimulant dopamine and norepinephrine reuptake inhibitor. Since both dopamine and norepinephrine are wakefulness neurotransmitters, individuals taking this medication experience less sleepiness. Solriamfetol is indicated to improve wakefulness in adults with excessive daytime sleepiness associated with narcolepsy and obstructive sleep apnea. Like pitolisant, Solriamfetol is not classified as a controlled substance. It is contraindicated with use of MAOIs. Sunosi is administered once daily upon wakening. Common side effects include headache, nausea, decreased appetite, insomnia, and anxiety. Monitor blood pressure and heart rate in patients receiving solriamfetol.

CHAPTER 27

Medications for Substance Use Disorders

Pharmacotherapy for substance use disorders is generally aimed at acute intoxication and overdose, withdraw from the substance, and assisting with abstinence from the substance. The term for using medication along with counseling and behavioral therapies to treat substance use disorders is medication-assisted treatment (MAT). Medication is used to normalize brain chemistry, reduce the euphoric effects of alcohol and substances, address physiological cravings, and assist with the body's return to normal functioning.

ALCOHOL

Alcohol Overdose

An alcohol overdose occurs after drinking more than the body can safely process. Blood alcohol levels can continue to rise even when a person is no longer drinking due to continued absorption from the stomach and intestines. Symptoms of alcohol poisoning are listed in Box 27.1

The patient is at risk for death with an alcohol overdose, making it dangerous to assume that the patient will be able to "sleep it off." Medical care includes managing breathing problems with an artificial airway if necessary, monitoring cardiac status, administering fluids to increase hydration and blood glucose, and flushing the stomach to clear the body of alcohol. Heated blankets may be used to manage hypothermia.

Alcohol Withdrawal

Alcohol is a central nervous system depressant.

Box 27.1 **Signs of Alcohol Poisoning**

- Vomiting
- Dulled responses, such as no gag reflex (can result in choking and asphyxiation)
- Slow respirations (i.e., fewer than 8 breaths per minute)
- Irregular breathing (i.e., 10 seconds or more between breaths)
- Hypothermia (i.e., low body temperature)
- Bluish, pale, clammy skin
- Mental confusion, stupor, coma, or inability to wake up
- Seizures

Two neurotransmitters are involved:
1. Alcohol affects gamma-aminobutyric acid (GABA), a major inhibitory (calming) neurotransmitter in the brain. GABA receptors contain alcohol-specific binding sites that become less sensitive with chronic exposure to ethanol. Reduction or cessation of alcohol from chronically elevated concentrations results in decreased inhibitory tone.
2. Glutamate is a major excitatory (stimulating) amino acid neurotransmitter. Chronic alcohol use results in an increase of the number of glutamate receptors in an attempt to maintain a normal state of arousal. Reduction or cessation of alcohol results in unregulated excess excitation.

Mild alcohol withdrawal begins 6 to 8 hours after alcohol cessation and is characterized by tremulousness (the "shakes"), increased blood pressure and pulse, insomnia, anxiety, panic, twitching, sweating, and nausea. Moderate alcohol withdrawal usually occurs 24 to 36 hours after the cessation of alcohol intake. Symptoms include intense anxiety, tremors, insomnia, seizures, hallucinations, hypertension, and racing pulse. Benzodiazepines such as chlordiazepoxide (Librium) are useful in reducing mild to moderate symptoms of alcohol withdrawal.

Psychotic and perceptual symptoms may begin in 8 to 10 hours. If a patient is undergoing withdrawal to the point of psychosis, it is considered a medical emergency due to the risks of unconsciousness, seizures, and delirium. Benzodiazepines such as lorazepam (Ativan) can be given either orally or intramuscularly and tapered over the next 5 to 7 days.

Withdrawal seizures may occur within 12 to 24 hours after alcohol cessation. These seizures are generalized and tonic-clonic. Additional seizures may occur within hours of the first seizure. Diazepam (Valium) given intravenously is a common treatment for withdrawal seizures.

Alcohol withdrawal delirium, also known as *delirium tremens (DTs)*, is a medical emergency that can result in death in 20% of untreated patients, usually as a result of medical problems such as pneumonia, renal disease, hepatic insufficiency, or heart failure (Sadock et al., 2015). Alcohol withdrawal delirium may happen anytime in the first 72 hours. Autonomic hyperactivity may result in tachycardia, diaphoresis, fever, anxiety, insomnia, and hypertension. Delusions and visual and tactile hallucinations are common in alcohol withdrawal delirium.

Delusions and hallucinations may result in unpredictable behaviors as patients try to protect themselves from what they believe are genuine dangers. All patients are at risk for this condition after cessation of heavy drinking for 3 days and are a danger to themselves and others. However, it is rare to see this syndrome in individuals in good physical health. Serious physical illness such as hepatitis or pancreatitis increases the likelihood of alcohol withdrawal delirium.

Prevention of alcohol withdrawal delirium is the goal. Oral diazepam (Valium) may be useful in the symptomatic relief of acute agitation, tremor, impending or acute DTs, and hallucinosis. Chlordiazepoxide (Librium) is also used to relieve symptoms. However, once delirium appears, intravenous lorazepam (Ativan) is used to treat these severe symptoms.

Seclusion may be necessary. Dehydration, often exacerbated by diaphoresis and fever, can be corrected with oral or intravenous fluids.

Wernicke-Korsakoff Syndrome

People with long-term heavy use of alcohol may experience short-term memory disturbances. One memory-reducing problem is Wernicke's encephalopathy, an acute and reversible condition. A more severe form of this problem is Korsakoff's syndrome, a chronic condition with a low recovery rate (about 20%). The two conditions are a result of a thiamine deficiency, which may be caused by poor nutrition or by malabsorption of nutrients.

Along with memory disturbances, symptoms of Wernicke's encephalopathy are an altered gait, vestibular (balance) dysfunction, confusion, and ocular motility abnormalities (horizontal nystagmus, lateral orbital palsy, and gaze palsy). Sluggish reaction to light and unequal pupil size are also symptoms. Wernicke's encephalopathy responds rapidly to large doses of intravenous thiamine two to three times daily for 1 or 2 weeks. Treatment of Korsakoff's syndrome is thiamine for 3 to 12 months. Although patients with Korsakoff's syndrome may never fully recover, cognitive improvement may occur with thiamine and nutritional support.

Alcohol Relapse Prevention

For many years, disulfiram (Antabuse) was the only medication available for long-term treatment of alcohol use disorder. Its use was limited due to adverse side effects. Now there are two primary medications to prevent cravings in people recovering from alcohol use disorder. These medications are naltrexone (ReVia, Vivitrol) and acamprosate (Campral).

Disulfiram

Disulfiram (Antabuse) was first approved by the US Food and Drug Administration (FDA) for alcohol misuse. In recent years, its use has become less common due to its disabling side effects. Disulfiram was an aversion-based treatment—people taking disulfiram become extremely sick if they drink alcohol. Normally, metabolism of ethanol goes from oxidation by alcohol dehydrogenase to the formation of acetaldehyde, which is further metabolized to acetyl-coenzyme A by aldehyde dehydrogenase. Disulfiram is an aldehyde dehydrogenase inhibitor. Inhibition of this enzyme results in an accumulation of acetaldehyde in the blood. Elimination of the drug from the body takes 1 to 2 weeks.

Disulfiram was thought to motivate individuals to avoid alcohol out of a fear of experiencing unpleasant symptoms, similar to a severe hangover. These symptoms include nausea, throbbing headache, vomiting, hypertension, flushing, sweating, thirst, dyspnea, tachycardia, chest pain, vertigo, and blurred vision. The reaction happens rapidly and may last up to 2 hours.

Severe and life-threatening reactions occur with greater amounts of alcohol. These reactions are respiratory depression, cardiovascular collapse, arrhythmias, myocardial infarction, acute congestive heart failure, unconsciousness, convulsions, and death.

In the absence of alcohol, disulfiram is well tolerated. Common side effects include fatigue, dermatitis, impotence, optic neuritis, and cognitive changes. It may exacerbate psychosis. Disulfiram is associated with a low rate of serum aminotransferase elevations and may cause severe and even fatal liver injury. Because of this rare complication, this drug is given at low doses and is used less widely than alternative medications.

Disulfiram is contraindicated in patients with myocardial disease or coronary occlusion, psychoses, or pregnancy and in those with high levels of impulsivity and suicidality. Disulfiram is not recommended for patients who are taking metronidazole, paraldehyde, and alcohol-containing products such as cough syrups or using aftershave.

Naltrexone

Naltrexone is used once abstinence has been achieved. It is an opiate antagonist widely used for both alcohol and opioid use disorder. Naltrexone competitively binds to opioid receptors. Naltrexone reduces the pleasure associated with drinking and reduces the cravings to use. This drug is available in an oral form (ReVia) and a long-acting injectable form (Vivitrol).

This medication is well tolerated by most people recovering from alcohol use disorder, and most people will not experience serious side effects after the first few days. Common side effects include nausea, headache, dizziness, nervousness, fatigue, insomnia, vomiting, anxiety, and somnolence. For Vivitrol, injection site reactions are a possibility. Hepatitis and liver dysfunction have been associated with the use of naltrexone.

It is important that the patients is opioid free for 7 to 10 days before initiating this therapy. No opiates, even codeine-containing cough syrups, can be taken along with naltrexone. Most patients will use naltrexone for the first few months of sobriety, during which time the cravings to use are strongest.

Intramuscular injection is not used with patients whose body mass precludes the use of a 2-inch needle. Subcutaneous injections may cause a severe injection site reaction.

Acamprosate

Acamprosate (Campral) works like naltrexone to reduce the intensity of cravings in individuals who have quit drinking. Its mechanism of action is to counteract the imbalance between the excitatory glutamatergic and inhibitory GABA activity. This stabilization allows the brain to recover slowly while reducing some of the discomforts of withdrawal symptoms.

Along with reducing alcohol cravings, acamprosate also seems to help people sleep better during recovery. Improved sleep is significant in alcohol use disorder, because since insomnia is a major contributor to relapse.

Common side effects are usually mild and transient. They include headache, diarrhea, flatulence, abdominal pain, paresthesia, and skin reactions. Acamprosate may be discontinued abruptly without symptoms and is not addictive. Acamprosate is contraindicated with renal impairment.

Table 27.1 identifies medications used in the treatment of alcohol withdrawal and relapse prevention.

CANNABIS

Abstinence and support are the main principles of treatment for cannabis use disorder. Hospitalization or outpatient care may be required. Individual, family, and group therapies can provide support. Antianxiety medication may be useful for short-term relief of withdrawal symptoms. Patients with underlying anxiety and depression may respond to antidepressant therapy.

OPIOIDS

Opioid Overdose

Overdose is common among people who misuse illicit substances such as heroin or pain medications such as oxycodone, hydrocodone, and morphine. An opioid overdose is a medical emergency. Signs of opioid overdose are listed in Box 27.2.

It is recommended to administer naloxone in any patient with signs of opioid overdose, or in whom this is suspected. It is a safe drug that produces no clinical effects individuals who are intoxicated. Treatment for an opioid overdose begins with promoting breathing by aspirating secretions, inserting an airway, using mechanical ventilation, and providing oxygen. In the absence of medical equipment, rescue breathing is recommended.

Table 27.1 **Common Medications Used for Alcohol Use Disorder**

Generic (Trade) Name	Uses	Notes
Benzodiazepines: Lorazepam (Ativan) Chlordiazepoxide (Librium) D Diazepam (Valium)	Withdrawal	Sedation, decreased anxiety and blood pressure. Use CIWA-AR scale to assess dose according to agency policies. Assess for seizures that could lead to delirium tremens (DTs). If not treated, this can lead to coma and ultimately death.
Anticonvulsants: Carbamazepine (Tegretol) phenobarbital (Luminal)	Withdrawal	Although still used, other medications are more effective and safer. Assess for seizures that could lead to delirium tremens. If not treated, coma and death may result.
Clonidine (Catapres)	Mild to moderate withdrawal	Alpha-agonist antihypertensive agent. Give every 4–6 hours as needed. Side effects include dizziness, hypotension, fatigue, and headache.
Disulfiram (Antabuse)	Maintenance, relapse prevention, aversion therapy	Alcohol use may result in intense nausea and vomiting, headache, diaphoresis (sweating), flushed skin, dyspnea (respiratory difficulties), and confusion. Avoid all alcohol and substances such as cough syrup and mouthwash containing alcohol.

Continued

Table 27.1 **Common Medications Used for Alcohol Use Disorder—cont'd**

Generic (Trade) Name	Uses	Notes
Naltrexone (ReVia, Vivitrol)	Withdrawal, relapse prevention, decreases pleasurable feelings and cravings	Oral or long-acting (once a month) injectable form. Nausea usually goes away after first month. Headache and sedation may occur. There is pain at the injection site; the patient needs to be opiate free 10 days before initiation of medication.
Acamprosate calcium (Campral)	Relapse prevention, decreases cravings	Tablets are taken three times a day. Side effects include diarrhea, gastrointestinal upset, appetite loss, dizziness, anxiety, and difficulty sleeping. It is contraindicated in patients with renal impairment.

CIWA-AR, Clinical Institute Withdrawal Assessment for Alcohol–Revised.
From Substance Abuse and Mental Health Services Administration and National Institute on Alcohol Abuse and Alcoholism. (2015). *Medication for the treatment of alcohol use disorder: A brief guide. HHS Publication No. (SMA) 15-4907.* Author.

Box 27.2 **Signs of Opioid Overdose**

- Extreme sleepiness
- Unresponsive to verbal stimuli or sternal rub
- Fingernails or lips turning blue/purple
- Slow pulse and/or low blood pressure
- Slow to shallow breathing in a patient who cannot be awakened
- Respiratory death rattle—exhalation with a distinct, labored sound from the throat
- Hallmark symptoms: coma, pinpoint pupils, respiratory depression

Table 27.2 **Methods of Naloxone Delivery**

Brand Name	Delivery Method	Notes
Narcan	Subcutaneous, intramuscular, intravenous	Most rapid onset of action is intravenous administration
Narcan Nasal Spray	Intranasal	Prefilled device that requires no assembly Delivers a single dose into one nostril Two doses per package
Evzio Auto-Injector	Intramuscular or subcutaneous	Hand-held automatic injection into outer thigh Device provides verbal instruction on how to deliver the medication

Naloxone, a specific opioid antagonist, can be given by intranasal spray, intramuscularly, subcutaneously, or intravenously. The most rapid onset of action is by intravenous administration, which is recommended in emergency situations. The smallest effective dose that maintains spontaneous normal respiratory drive is used. Too much naloxone may produce withdrawal symptoms. Duration of action for naloxone is short compared with many opioids (20 to 90 minutes), so repeated administration may be required.

Naloxone usually results in a rapid response of increased respirations and pupillary dilation within 3 to 5 minutes. Methods of naloxone delivery are listed in Table 27.2.

Patients are monitored for recurrence of opioid toxicity for at least 4 hours after naloxone use. Patients who have taken overdoses of long-acting opioids are monitored for a longer period of time.

Opioid Withdrawal and Relapse Prevention

The principles of opioid detoxification/withdrawal are to:
1. Substitute a longer-acting, pharmacologically equivalent drug.
2. Stabilize the patient on the substituted drug.
3. Gradually withdraw the substituted drug.

The following drugs are opioid agonists, partial agonists, and antagonists. Agonists and partial agonists are used for medically supervised withdrawal and maintenance purposes. Antagonists are used to accelerate detoxification and then to prevent relapse.

Methadone

Methadone (Dolophine, Methadose) is a synthetic narcotic opioid used to decrease the painful symptoms of opiate withdrawal and also for maintenance of abstinence. Methadone is a full opioid agonist that tricks the brain by activating opioid receptors and reducing craving. It also blocks the euphoric effects of other opiate drugs such as heroin, morphine, and codeine, as well as semisynthetic opioids like oxycodone and hydrocodone.

Methadone is a US Drug Enforcement Administration (DEA) schedule II drug with high misuse potential. It can only be dispensed through an opioid treatment program certified by a government substance use agency. Duration of methadone therapy can be fairly long. In pregnant individuals, a low dose of methadone may be the safest course. Neonatal withdrawal is usually mild and can be managed with morphine.

Some serious side effects may result from methadone. Patients are instructed to seek medical care if they experience difficulty breathing. Feeling lightheaded, faint, chest pain, and a pounding heartbeat may be symptoms of QT prolongation, a serious cardiac arrhythmia. Hives, rash, or swelling of the face, lips, tongue, or throat could also be serious symptoms. Report hallucinations or confusion to a care provider.

Alpha Agonists

Two alpha-agonist antihypertensives are often used to reduce the symptoms of opioid withdrawal. Clonidine (Catapres) works by blocking neurotransmitters that trigger sympathetic nervous system activity. It eases sweating, hot flashes, watery eyes, and restlessness. This drug also decreases anxiety and may even shorten the detox process.

Lofexidine (Lucemyra) has FDA approval for the mitigation of opioid withdrawal symptoms during abrupt discontinuation. It enables people to withdraw at home in a few days rather than a week.

Buprenorphine

Buprenorphine reduces or eliminates withdrawal symptoms and drug craving without dangerous side effects of heroin and other opioids. It is used to help people reduce or stop their use of heroin or other opiates such as pain relievers like morphine. Buprenorphine both blocks and activates opiate receptors and is known as a partial opioid agonist.

A DEA schedule III drug, buprenorphine, can be prescribed by providers who have completed special education. Some buprenorphine products also contain naloxone. The naloxone in the combined formulation causes a withdrawal reaction if it is intravenously injected, thereby deterring misuse.

Side effects of buprenorphine include nausea, vomiting, constipation, muscle aches and cramps, insomnia, irritability, and fever. This drug is used only after abstaining from opioids for 12 to 24 hours and in the early stages of opioid withdrawal. It can bring on acute withdrawal for patients not in the early stages of withdrawal and who have other opioids in their bloodstream. Long-acting formulations are available. Buprenorphine (Sublocade) is subcutaneously administered into the abdomen once a month. Buprenorphine (Probuphine) implants are used for 6 months.

Naltrexone

Naltrexone is an opioid antagonist that prevents intoxication. Naltrexone is available as ReVia, a tablet form of the drug. A long-acting injectable version, Vivitrol, is given once a month. If a person using naltrexone relapses and uses the misused drug, naltrexone blocks the euphoric and sedative effects.

Side effects of naltrexone include gastrointestinal (GI) distress, muscle cramps, dizziness, sedation, and appetite disturbances. Injection site reactions are common. About 70% of users experience reactions that range from pain, swelling, and bruising to more serious complications like cellulitis, induration, and, more rarely, abscess and necrosis.

Table 27.3 identifies medications used in the treatment of opioid use disorder.

HALLUCINOGENS

Treatment for hallucinogen intoxication includes reassurance that the symptoms are caused by the drug and that the symptoms will subside. Patient and provider safety are essential goals. Physical restraint may be necessary. In severe cases, an antipsychotic such as haloperidol (Haldol)

Table 27.3 **FDA-Approved Medications for Opioid Use Disorder**

Medication and Action	Form	Use
Methadone (opioid agonist)		Withdrawal and maintenance treatment
• Dolophine	Tablet	
• Methadose	Tablet, oral concentrate	
Buprenorphine (partial opioid agonist)		Withdrawal and maintenance treatment
• Subutex (buprenorphine)	Sublingual tablet	
• Bunavail (buprenorphine and naloxone)	Buccal film	
• Suboxone (buprenorphine and naloxone)	Sublingual tablets or sublingual film	
• Zubsolv (buprenorphine and naloxone)	Sublingual tablet	
• Sublocade (buprenorphine XR)	Long-acting injectable	Maintenance treatment
• Probuphine (buprenorphine)	Implanted rods	
Naltrexone (opioid antagonist)		Relapse prevention
• ReVia	Tablet	
• Vivitrol	Long-acting injectable	

FDA, Food and Drug Administration.

or a benzodiazepine such as diazepam (Valium) can be used in the short term.

Patients who have ingested phencyclidine (PCP) cannot be talked down and may require restraint. A calming medication such as a benzodiazepine may be administered intramuscularly or intravenously. Mechanical cooling may be necessary for severe hyperthermia.

INHALANTS

Inhalant intoxication usually does not require any treatment. However, serious and potentially fatal responses such as coma, cardiac arrhythmias, or bronchospasm do happen. A psychotic response can be induced by inhalant intoxication.

SEDATIVES, HYPNOTICS, AND BENZODIAZEPINES

Like alcohol, repeated sedative, hypnotic, and benzodiazepine use results in repeated dampening of the central nervous system, causing rebound hyperactivity. Symptoms such as autonomic hyperactivity, tremor, insomnia, psychomotor agitation, anxiety, and grand mal seizures occur. The degree and timing of the withdrawal syndrome depend on the specific substance. Half-life is an important predictor of withdrawal time.

Gradual reduction of these substances will prevent seizures and other withdrawal symptoms. Benzodiazepine withdrawal can be supported by using a long-acting barbiturate such as phenobarbital.

AMPHETAMINES

Depending on the amphetamine used, specific drugs are used short term to treat withdrawal symptoms. Antipsychotics may be prescribed for a few days. If there is no psychosis, diazepam (Valium) is useful in treating agitation and hyperactivity. Once the patient has been withdrawn from the amphetamine, depression can be treated with antidepressants.

TOBACCO

Withdrawal from and treatment for tobacco use disorder are facilitated by nicotine replacement therapies. This highly successful nicotine replacement is available in the form of gum, lozenges, nasal sprays, inhalers, and patches.

Instruct patients who use the gum that continuously chewing the gum may cause gastrointestinal upset. Patients should chew a few times until they feel a tingling sensation in their mouth. The gum is then placed between the cheek and gums until the tingling almost stops and then start chewing again. This process is repeated until the tingling stops in about 30 minutes. Non-nicotine therapy options include the antidepressant bupropion sustained-release (Zyban), which reduces the cravings for nicotine. Varenicline (Chantix) is a nicotinic receptor partial agonist that mimics the effects of nicotine, thereby reducing cravings and withdrawal. It also partially blocks the nicotine receptors, which blunts the effect of nicotine if smoking is resumed.

CHAPTER 28

Neurocognitive Medications

Six medications have US Food and Drug Administration (FDA) approval for the treatment of Alzheimer's disease (AD). They are:
- Cholinesterase inhibitors: donepezil (Aricept), rivastigmine (Exelon), and galantamine (Razadyne)
- An *N*-methyl-ᴅ-aspartate (NMDA) receptor antagonist: memantine (Namenda)
- NMDA receptor antagonist/cholinesterase inhibitor: memantine/donepezil (Namzaric)
- An amyloid beta-directed antibody: aducanumab (Aduhelm)

With the exception of aducanumab, which was introduced in 2021, these medications have been widely used and have demonstrated statistically significant effects compared with placebos. However, they produce only a marginal improvement in cognition and functioning, and the benefits of these medications diminish after 1 to 2 years. Considering the potential side effects, which double in people older than 85 years, their use should be carefully weighed against the potential benefits.

Other medications are used to treat behavioral manifestations of major neurocognitive disorders, including AD. They will be discussed following the presentation of specific neurocognitive medications.

CHOLINESTERASE INHIBITORS

Because a deficiency of neural acetylcholine has been linked to AD, some medications aim to prevent its breakdown. These drugs function by inhibiting cholinesterase from breaking down acetylcholine into its components of acetate and choline. This allows for an increase in the availability and duration of action of acetylcholine, which leads to temporary improvement of some symptoms of AD.

The first FDA-approved cholinesterase inhibitor was tacrine (Cognex) in 1993 for the treatment of mild to moderate symptoms of AD. Tacrine was withdrawn from the market in 2012 due to a high frequency of side effects, including gastrointestinal effects, elevated liver transaminase levels, and liver toxicity.

Currently used cholinesterase inhibitors include donepezil (Aricept), rivastigmine (Exelon), and galantamine (Razadyne). The cholinesterase inhibitors are indicated for the mild to moderate stages of AD. Donepezil is FDA-approved for severe AD.

The most common side effects are gastrointestinal. These side effects are usually temporary, and a lower dose minimizes them. These medications are taken with food to reduce this side effect. Donepezil is available in a tablet form and as an orally disintegrating tablet (ODT) that should not be crushed. Rivastigmine is provided in both a capsule form and an oral solution. Talantamine is available in a tablet, a capsule, and as an oral solution.

Cholinesterase inhibitors can also rarely cause bradycardia and incontinence due to their cholinergic-enhancing properties. They are used with caution when patients are taking nonsteroidal anti-inflammatory drugs (NSAIDs) due to the combined potential for gastrointestinal bleeding and ulceration.

The rivastigmine transdermal system (Exelon Patch) is applied once a day, making it useful for people who have trouble swallowing pills. The upper or lower back is recommended as the site of application because the patch is less likely to be removed by the individual. With this nonoral delivery method, there is no food requirement. It can cause skin irritation and should be discontinued if the irritation extends beyond the size of the patch.

N-METHYL-D-ASPARTATE RECEPTOR ANTAGONIST

Memantine (Namenda) was approved for use with AD in 2003. It is indicated for treatment of moderate to severe dementia. This medication is typically added after trying the cholinesterase inhibitors.

Memantine regulates the activity of glutamate, which is present in higher levels with AD. Too much glutamate sticks to receptors, allowing too much calcium to move into neurons, which causes damage. Memantine occupies the same receptors, blocking glutamate, thereby preventing excessive calcium movement into the brain cells.

Memantine tablets can be taken with or without food. After using memantine twice a day, patients may be switched to long-acting memantine XR for once-a-day dosing. These capsules can be swallowed intact or opened and sprinkled on food such as applesauce. They should not be divided, chewed, or crushed.

Common side effects of memantine include headache, constipation, and dizziness. Memantine XR may cause constipation. In clinical trials, the most common reason for drug discontinuation was dizziness.

NMDA Receptor Antagonist/Cholinesterase Inhibitor

Memantine XR is combined with donepezil to form the combination medication Namzaric. It is FDA-approved for moderate to severe symptoms of AD. Candidates for this medication are individuals who have been tolerating the separate forms of the drugs in combination. Namzaric is dosed once a day in the evening. The capsules can be taken with or without food, whole or sprinkled on food such as applesauce. They should not be divided, chewed, or crushed.

The most common side effects are those seen individually with the two separate medications. For memantine, they are headaches, diarrhea, and dizziness; for donepezil, they are diarrhea, anorexia, vomiting, nausea, and dizziness.

Amyloid Beta-Directed Antibody

Aducanumab (Aduhelm) is a monoclonal antibody directed against aggregated soluble and insoluble forms of amyloid beta to reduce its build-up. Aducanumab received FDA approval in 2021 under an accelerated approval pathway. This pathway requires the marketer to perform a follow-up study to determine the efficacy of the medication. This accelerated conditional approval is used for serious or life-threatening illnesses that provide a therapeutic advantage over existing treatments. The first new Alzheimer's drug since 2003, it is also the first potentially disease-modifiable drug.

Aducanumab is indicated for the treatment of Alzheimer's disease with no specification of the stage. It is available only in an intravenous infusion, which is delivered in one hour. The medication is titrated (i.e., increased dosage) every four weeks and at least 21 days apart.

Patients are given a brain magnetic resonance imaging (MRI) prior to initiating the treatment and before the 7th and 12th infusions. The MRIs are used to detect amyloid-related imaging abnormalities (ARIA). ARIA-E refers to edema with symptoms of headaches, changes in mental state, confusion, vomiting, nausea, tremor and gait disturbances. ARIA-H refers to microhemorrhages with accompanying symptoms of headache, one-sided weakness, vomiting, seizures, decreased level of consciousness, and neck stiffness. Superficial siderosis is another ARIA-H related problem caused by hemosiderin deposits in the subpial layers of the brain and spinal cord. The hemosiderin deposition results from recurrent bleeding into the subarachnoid space. Other side effects of include falls, diarrhea, and confusion.

Aducanumab's approval was controversial. While the drug has proven highly effective at reducing the beta-amyloid plaques, there is question of whether it actually slows the progression of Alzheimer's disease when it reduces the plaques. Also, the cost of the medication is over $50,000 a year and insurance eligibility is also in question (Cohen, 2021).

Medications approved by the FDA for treatment of AD are described in Table 28.1.

MEDICATIONS FOR BEHAVIORAL SYMPTOMS OF ALZHEIMER'S DISEASE

Most people with dementia will experience behavioral symptoms that reduce their quality of life, are distressing to them and their caregivers, and may lead to placement in a residential care facility. Some of the troubling behaviors are psychotic symptoms (e.g., hallucinations, paranoid delusions), severe mood swings, wandering, anxiety, agitation, and verbal or physical aggression.

Medications are often prescribed, but these medications are associated with risk of mortality, mostly from

Table 28.1 **FDA-Approved Drugs for Alzheimer's Disease**

Generic (Trade)	Stages of AD	Side Effects
Cholinesterase Inhibitors		
Donepezil (Aricept, Aricept ODT)	Mild, moderate, severe	Nausea, diarrhea, cramps, fatigue, anorexia
Rivastigmine (Exelon, Exelon Patch)	Mild, moderate	Oral: Nausea, vomiting, anorexia, indigestion, weakness. Patch: Nausea, vomiting, diarrhea, application site erythema
Galantamine (Razadyne, Razadyne ER)	Mild, moderate	Nausea, vomiting, diarrhea, dizziness, headache, decreased appetite, weight loss
_N_-Methyl-d-Aspartate (NMDA) Receptor Antagonist		
Memantine (Namenda, Namenda XR)	Moderate, severe	Headaches, confusion, constipation, and dizziness XR: Diarrhea
NMDA Receptor Antagonist/Cholinesterase Inhibitor		
Memantine/ donepezil (Namzaric)	Moderate, severe	See side effects listed under memantine and donepezil
Amyloid Beta-Directed Antibody		
Aducanumab (Aduhelm)	Unspecified	Amyloid Related Imaging Abnormalities (ARIA) including cerebral edema and microhemorrhages; headaches, superficial siderosis, and falls

From US Food and Drug Administration. (various dates). *Drugs*. http://www.fda.gov/Drugs/.

cardiovascular and infectious causes. As a result, in 2008, the FDA emphasized that the use of antipsychotics for dementia-related psychosis is an unapproved indication. Therefore any use of antipsychotics in this population is considered off-label. Drug classifications that are used off-label include antidepressants, antipsychotics, antianxiety agents, and anticonvulsants. Of these, antipsychotics have been used most often. It is recommended to use these medications with extreme caution.

A rule of thumb with older adults is to start low and go slow. Another is to use the smallest dose for the shortest duration possible and discontinue if they are not effective. In addition, because people with dementia are at high risk of developing delirium, additional medications should be used with caution.

CHAPTER 29

Psychotherapeutic Models

Nurses prepared at the undergraduate level are qualified to provide counseling, support, and education to their patients. Registered nurses and nursing students promote the stabilization of symptoms and the reinforcement of healthy behaviors and interactions in the context of a therapeutic relationship.

Psychiatric–mental health advanced practice registered nurses are prepared to provide a more complex form of counseling known as psychotherapy. Psychotherapy, informally referred to as "talk therapy," is a term for a variety of treatment techniques that help individuals identify and change negative feelings, thoughts, and behavior.

Most of the therapies in this chapter require advanced education for their application and for third-party reimbursement. Yet it is important for nurses working and training in a psychiatric setting to be familiar with the types of therapies available. Among the benefits of becoming familiar with these therapies is the ability to do the following:

1. Use basic concepts of the models as interventions, such as recognizing negative thought patterns, a technique used in cognitive–behavioral therapy, or taking part in reward system economies when working with children and adolescents as used in behavioral therapy.

2. Understand the therapy being recommended or being provided for your patient, and being able to discuss the proposed therapy or the work currently being done.

This chapter offers snapshots of some of the most common and popular psychotherapies. Most of these therapies are provided for individuals, families, and groups. They include the following:

- Cognitive–behavioral therapy (CBT)
- Dialectical behavioral therapy (DBT)
- Mindfulness-based approaches
  - Mindfulness-based stress reduction (MBSR)
  - Mindfulness-based cognitive therapy (MBCT)
- Eye movement and desensitization and reprocessing (EMDR) therapy
- Exposure and response prevention (ERP) therapy
- Interpersonal therapy
- Behavioral therapy
  - Modeling
  - Operant conditioning
  - Systematic desensitization
  - Aversion
  - Biofeedback
- Acceptance and commitment therapy
- Motivational interviewing
- Milieu therapy
- Group therapy

COGNITIVE–BEHAVIORAL THERAPY

CBT is an active, time-limited, and structured approach. This evidence-based therapy is used to treat psychiatric disorders such as major depressive disorder, anxiety, and phobias. It is based on the underlying theoretical principle that feelings and behaviors are largely determined by the way people think about the world and their place in it (Beck, 1979). Cognitions (verbal or pictorial events in their streams of consciousness) are based on attitudes or assumptions developed from previous experiences. These cognitions may be fairly accurate or distorted.

People have schemas, or unique assumptions, about themselves, others, and the world in general. For example, if a man has the schema, "The only person I can trust is myself," he will have expectations that everyone else has questionable motives, is dishonest, and will eventually hurt him. Other negative schemas include incompetence, abandonment, evilness, and vulnerability. People are typically not aware of such cognitive biases.

Rapid, unthinking responses based on schemas are known as automatic thoughts. These responses are particularly intense and common in psychiatric disorders such as depression and anxiety. Often automatic thoughts, or cognitive distortions, are irrational and lead to false assumptions and misinterpretations. For example, if a woman interprets all experiences in terms of whether she is competent and adequate, her thinking may be dominated by the cognitive distortion, "Unless I do everything perfectly, I'm a failure." Consequently, that person reacts to situations in terms of adequacy, even when these situations are unrelated to whether she is personally competent. Table 29.1 describes common cognitive distortions.

Therapeutic techniques are designed to identify, reality test, and correct distorted thinking and the dysfunctional beliefs underlying them. Individuals are taught to challenge their negative thoughts and substitute them with positive, rational thoughts. They learn to recognize when thinking is based on distortions and misconceptions.

Homework assignments play an important role in CBT. A particularly useful technique is a four-column thought diary to record the precipitating event or situation, the resulting automatic thought, and the following feelings and behaviors. Finally, a challenge to the negative thoughts based on rational evidence and thinking is listed in the last column. Table 29.2 illustrates an entry in a thought diary.

DIALECTICAL BEHAVIOR THERAPY

Dialectical behavior therapy (DBT) is an evidence-based therapy developed to treat borderline personality disorder (Linehan, 1993). Research supports the use of DBT with individuals experiencing comorbid personality disorders (such as obsessive–compulsive personality disorder) and other psychiatric disorders (such as major depressive disorder, generalized anxiety disorder, substance use disorders, and eating disorders).

DBT combines cognitive and behavioral techniques with mindfulness, which emphasizes being aware of thoughts and actively shaping them. The goals of DBT are to increase the patient's ability to manage distress, improve interpersonal effectiveness skills, and enhance the therapist's effectiveness in working with this population.

Table 29.1 **Common Cognitive Distortions**

Distortion, Definition and Example	Example
All-or-nothing thinking: Thinking in black and white, reducing complex outcomes into absolutes	Although Kennady earned the second-highest score in the state's cheerleading competition, she consistently referred to herself as "a loser."
Overgeneralization: Using a bad outcome (or a few bad outcomes) as evidence that nothing will ever go right again	Andrew had a minor traffic accident. He is reluctant to drive and says, "I shouldn't be allowed on the road."
Labeling: A form of generalization in which a characteristic or event becomes definitive and results in an overly harsh label for self or others	"Because I failed the advanced statistics examination, I am a failure. I might as well give up. I will look for an easier major."
Mental filter: Focusing on a negative detail or bad event and allowing it to taint everything else	Anne's boss evaluated her work as exemplary and gave her a few suggestions for improvement. She obsessed about the suggestions and ignored the rest.
Disqualifying the positive: Maintaining a negative view by rejecting information that supports a positive view as being irrelevant, inaccurate, or accidental	"I've just been offered the job I thought I always wanted. There must have been no other applicants."
Jumping to conclusions: Making a negative interpretation despite the fact that there is little or no supporting evidence	"My fiancé, Juan, didn't call me for 3 hours, which proves he doesn't love me anymore."
a. Mind-reading: Inferring negative thoughts, responses, and motives of others	Isabel is giving a presentation and a man in the audience is sleeping. She panics, "I must be boring."
b. Fortune-telling error: Anticipating that things will turn out badly as an established fact	"I'll ask her out, but I know she won't have a good time."

Table 29.1 **Common Cognitive Distortions—cont'd**

Distortion, Definition and Example	Example
Magnification or minimization: Exaggerating the importance of something (such as a personal failure or the success of others) or reducing the importance of something (such as a personal success or the failure of others)	"I'm alone on a Saturday night because no one likes me. When other people are alone, it's because they want to be."
Catastrophizing: An extreme form of magnification in which the worst case scenario is assumed to be a probable outcome	"If I don't make a good impression on the boss at the company picnic, she will fire me."
Emotional reasoning: Drawing a conclusion based on an emotional state	"I'm nervous about the examination. I must not be prepared. If I were, I wouldn't be afraid."
"Should" and "must" statements: Rigid self-directives that presume an unrealistic amount of control over external events	Renee believes that a patient with diabetes has high blood sugar today because she is not a very good nurse and that her patients should always get better.
Personalization: Assuming responsibility for an external event or situation that was likely outside personal control	"I'm sorry your party wasn't more fun. It's probably because I was there."

Modified from Beck, A. T. (1979). *Cognitive therapy and the emotional disorders*. International Universities Press.

Treatment focuses on behavioral targets, beginning with identification of and interventions for suicidal behaviors and then progressing to a focus on interrupting destructive behaviors. Finally, DBT addresses quality-of-life behaviors across a hierarchy of care.

Mindfulness-Based Approaches

Mindfulness involves being fully present in the moment and paying attention to the here and now, without judgment. In our culture, it has become the norm to think about and analyze (or worry) about the future. Many of us also dwell on the past. What tends to get missed is the present.

Table 29.2 **Thought Diary Entry**

Event or Situation	Automatic Thought	Feelings and Behaviors	Alternate Thoughts
I went to my favorite restaurant. The waitress, Rebecca, who I know well, barely acknowledged me.	Rebecca doesn't like me anymore. I must have said something stupid. I wonder who else doesn't like me here.	I felt hurt and left the restaurant more quickly than I usually do.	Rebecca doesn't feel well. She may be upset about something going on in her life. The restaurant was crowded; she may have felt overwhelmed.

Mindfulness-Based Stress Reduction

MBSR has roots in the Buddhist and Hindu traditions. Jon Kabat-Zinn is credited with bringing mindfulness to the Western culture in his MBSR program. The original aim of this program was in treating chronic pain but has progressed to other uses such as major depressive disorders, anxiety disorders, and stress relief.

MBSR can be practiced in formal meditation sessions or informally throughout the day. For instance, individuals can pick one activity they are already doing in the day that they might tend to "zone out" while doing (e.g., brushing their teeth, doing the dishes, taking a shower). The practice is in bringing awareness of that activity to the present. Rather than letting the mind wander, the focus is brought on how all five senses experience that activity.

Mindfulness-Based Cognitive Therapy

MBCT is a focused approach that helps patients to disengage from unhealthy cognitive patterns. The patterns that make individuals vulnerable to relapse of depression are those of rumination, where the mind repetitively focuses on specific negative thoughts. The main skill with MBCT is teaching patients how to shift mental gears.

Unlike conventional CBT, MBCT does not focus on changing core beliefs. Instead it trains individuals to be more aware of physical sensations and of thoughts and feelings as mental events. Individuals come to see thoughts and feelings as aspects of experience which move through awareness but are not necessarily reality.

EYE MOVEMENT DESENSITIZATION AND REPROCESSING THERAPY

EMDR therapy is an evidence-based approach to treat traumatized children and adults. EMDR therapy processes traumatic memories through a specific protocol. The clinician asks the patient to think about the traumatic event. At the same time, the patient attends to other stimulation, such as eye movements, audio tones, or tapping. The combination of thinking and other stimuli brings about neurological and physiological changes that help people process and integrate traumatic memories.

EXPOSURE AND RESPONSE PREVENTION

ERP is used for obsessive–compulsive disorder (OCD), eating disorders, phobias, panic disorders, generalized anxiety disorders, and social anxieties. This approach is similar to the behavioral approach of systematic desensitization but does not use relaxation techniques. This cognitively based therapy involves purposely exposing the individual to the uncomfortable thoughts, images, and situations that bring on anxiety and obsessions. The patient then makes a conscious choice not to engage in the compulsive ritual or behavior. Over time with exposure to the obsession and avoidance of the compulsion, the patient experiences less anxiety and obsessions.

A common metaphor used to explain this therapy is to stop "feeding the lion." In this example, the lion begging for food is viewed as the obsessive thought. Feeding the lion is compared to the compulsion or ritual. When a choice is made to stop "feeding the lion" (i.e., stop the compulsion/ritual), the lion might initially get angry (i.e., anxiety may increase), but then the lion eventually goes away (i.e., anxiety decreases).

INTERPERSONAL THERAPY

Interpersonal therapy is a short-term therapy with a number of sessions between 12 and 16. The assumption with this therapy is that psychiatric disorders are influenced by interpersonal interactions and a social context. The goal of interpersonal therapy is to reduce or eliminate psychiatric symptoms by improving interpersonal functioning and satisfaction with social relationships.

Interpersonal therapy has been proven to be successful in the treatment of depression, particularly related to grief and loss, interpersonal conflict, role transitions, and deficits related to interpersonal skills. Treatment is based on the notion that disturbances in important interpersonal relationships (or a deficit in one's capacity to form those relationships) can play a role in initiating or maintaining clinical depression. In interpersonal psychotherapy, the therapist identifies the nature of the problem to be resolved and then selects strategies consistent with that problem area.

BEHAVIORAL THERAPY

Behavioral therapy is based on the assumption that changes in maladaptive behavior can occur without insight into the underlying cause. This approach works best when it is directed at specific problems and the goals are well defined. Behavioral therapy is effective in treating people with phobias, alcohol use disorder, schizophrenia, and many other conditions. Five types of behavior therapy are modeling, operant conditioning, systematic desensitization, aversion therapy, and biofeedback.

Modeling

In modeling, the therapist provides a role model for specific behaviors, and the patient learns through imitation. The therapist may do the modeling, provide another person to model the behaviors, or present a video for the purpose. For example, clinicians can help patients reduce their phobias about nonpoisonous snakes. They do this by having them first view close-up filmed encounters between people and snakes. Afterward they view live encounters between people and snakes.

Similarly, some behavioral therapists demonstrate patterns of behavior that might be more effective than those usually engaged in and then have the patients practice these new behaviors. For example, a student who does not know how to ask a professor for an extension on a term paper may watch the therapist portray a potentially effective way of making the request. The clinician would then help the student practice the new skill in a similar role-playing situation.

Operant Conditioning

Operant conditioning is the basis for behavior modification and uses positive reinforcement to increase desired behaviors. For example, when desired goals are achieved or behaviors are performed, patients might be rewarded with tokens. These tokens can be exchanged for food, small luxuries, or privileges. This reward system is known as a token economy.

Operant conditioning has been useful in improving the verbal behaviors of children with mute, autistic, and developmentally disabled conditions. In patients with severe and persistent mental illness, behavior modification has helped increase levels of self-care, social behavior, group participation, and more.

A familiar example of positive reinforcement is a mother who takes her preschooler to the grocery store, and the child starts acting out, demanding candy, nagging, crying, and yelling. Table 29.3 lists three ways that the child's behavior can be reinforced.

Table 29.3 **Behavioral Reinforcement Approaches**

Action	Result
1. The mother gives the child the candy.	The child continues to use this behavior. This is positive reinforcement of negative behavior.
2. The mother scolds the child.	Acting out may continue, because the child receives attention. This positively rewards negative behavior.
3. The mother ignores the acting out but gives attention to the child when he is acting appropriately.	The child gets a positive reward for appropriate behavior.

Systematic Desensitization

Systematic desensitization is another behavioral modification therapy that involves engaging in tasks customized to address the patient's specific fears. It is similar to ERP, but the behavioral aspect of practicing relaxation techniques is added. Systematic desensitization involves four steps:

1. The patient's fear is broken down into its components by exploring the particular stimulus cues to which the patient reacts. For example, certain situations may precipitate a phobic reaction, whereas others do not. Crowds at parties may be problematic, whereas similar numbers of people in other settings do not cause the same distress.

2. The patient is exposed to the fear little by little. For example, a patient who has a fear of flying is introduced to short periods of visual presentations of flying—first with still pictures, then with videos, and finally in a busy airport. The situations are confronted while the patient is in a relaxed state. Gradually, over a period of time, exposure is increased until anxiety about or fear of the object or situation has ceased.

3. The patient is instructed in how to design a hierarchy of fears. For a fear of flying, a patient might develop a set of statements representing the stages of a flight, order the statements from the most fearful to the least fearful, and use relaxation techniques to reach a state of relaxation while progressing through the list.

4. The patient practices these techniques every day.

Aversion Therapy

Aversion therapy is used to treat disorders such as alcohol use disorder and, paraphilic disorders, and behaviors such as shoplifting, violent and aggressive behavior, and self-mutilation. Aversion therapy pairs a negative stimulus with a specific target behavior, thereby suppressing the behavior. This treatment may be used when other, less drastic, measures have failed to produce the desired effects.

Simple examples of extinguishing undesirable behavior through aversion therapy include painting unpleasant-tasting substances on the fingernails for nail biting or thumbsucking. Other examples of aversive stimuli are chemicals that induce nausea and vomiting, unpleasant odors, unpleasant verbal stimuli (e.g., descriptions of disturbing scenes), costs or fines in a token economy, and denial of positive reinforcement (e.g., isolation).

Before initiating any aversive protocol, the therapist, treatment team, or society must answer the following questions:

- Is this therapy in the best interest of the patient?
- Does its use violate the patient's rights?
- Is it in the best interest of society?

If the therapist believes aversion therapy is the most appropriate treatment, it is important to have ongoing supervision, support, and evaluation of those administering it the therapy.

Biofeedback

Through the use of sensitive instrumentation, biofeedback provides objective information regarding muscle activity, brain waves, skin temperature, heart rate, blood pressure, and other bodily functions. Indicators of the particular internal physiological process are detected and amplified by a sensitive recording device. An individual can achieve greater voluntary control over phenomena once considered to be exclusively involuntary if knowing, through an auditory or visual signal, whether a somatic activity is increasing or decreasing.

The use of biofeedback was once reserved for clinicians with specialized training. Now, with increasingly sophisticated technology, most people can use some form of biofeedback independently. Exercise trackers and smartwatches provide users with the ability to track sleep patterns and heart rates. Clip-on devices tracks respiration changes that indicate tension. A companion application (app) suggests relaxation techniques such as meditation. A hand-held device that measures skin conductance (sweat) that indicates stress also comes with an app that teaches calming techniques.

Heart rate variability (HRV) testing has become popular to monitor stress and recovery. This method uses a chest strap to measure heart rate and a third-party app for data analysis to show the slight variations in time between beats. It is usually quantified out of 100 points to simplify information to the user. When stressed, the HRV is low. When relaxed, the HRV is high. Individuals can obtain a baseline HRV measure and then use stress-relieving techniques such as relaxation, mindfulness, and physical activity to raise the HRV.

ACCEPTANCE AND COMMITMENT THERAPY

Acceptance and commitment therapy (ACT) evolved from behavioral therapy, CBT, and mindfulness concepts. It is beneficial for individuals who struggle with rumination over life's difficulties with a goal of increasing psychological flexibility. During ACT, patients are guided to replace the internal struggle of emotions with acceptance of these feelings and work toward life goals. The six areas of focus in ACT are:

- Acceptance: allowing negative feelings and emotions to exist without trying to avoid or change them
- Cognitive defusion: noticing thoughts and feelings, without judgment, and learning techniques to deal with them in a nonthreatening way
- Being present: bringing full awareness and attention to the present moment
- Self as context (observing self): awareness of the "you" that experiences life and realization that one is more than an individual emotion or experience
- Values: positive qualities that the individual wants to work toward
- Committed action: setting goals and taking actions that align with personal values

MOTIVATIONAL INTERVIEWING

Motivational interviewing is an approach based on the transtheoretical or stages of change theory. It has gained popularity in its use as a brief, long-term, and supplementary intervention, particularly in the treatment of substance use disorders. It uses a person-centered approach to strengthen motivation for change. A key premise to motivational interviewing is that the individual makes the choice to engage in treatment.

Individuals may be at stage one, precontemplation, and need assistance in admitting there is a problem. If they have acknowledged the problem, contemplation, they may still not be ready to address it. The goal of treatment is to assist in the development of awareness and a commitment. Preparation, or getting ready, and action, or changing, take place in early treatment phases. The maintenance stage is the ongoing commitment to a recovery program.

MILIEU THERAPY

Milieu (mil'yōo) is a word of French origin (mi "middle" + lieu "place") and refers to surroundings and physical environment. In a therapeutic context, it refers to the overall environment and interactions within that environment. It is an all-inclusive term that recognizes the people (patients and staff), the setting, the structure, and the emotional climate as important to healing. Regardless of whether the setting involves treatment of children, adult patients in a psychiatric hospital, individuals in a substance use residential treatment center, or patients in a psychiatric day treatment program, a well-managed milieu offers a sense of security and promotes healing. Structured aspects of the milieu include scheduled activities, rules, assigned personnel, and environment.

GROUP THERAPY

Group therapy is an evidence-based practice that allows multiple patients to be treated at the same time. Members benefit from the knowledge, insights, and life experience of both the leader and participants. A therapeutic group is a safe setting to learn new ways of relating to other people and to practice communication skills. Groups can also promote feelings of belonging and a sense of cohesiveness (e.g., "We're in this together.").

Group work is characterized by both content and process. Group content is the actual words that are used in the setting. Group process is the term used to describe everything else that goes on in a group. Group process refers to the way group members interact with one another, such as being supportive, interruptive, or silent.

Registered nurses lead groups for the purpose of education, tasks, and support. Advanced practice registered nurses are educated in the provision of theoretically based group therapy.

Nurse leaders set the foundation for open communication and mutual respect. The degree to which the leader controls the direction of the group depends on the group's needs. Autocratic leaders do not encourage much interaction and exert control over the group. This leadership style works best for time-limited tasks such as community meetings. Democratic leaders promote group interaction while maintaining the role of leader. This style works well in most groups in the psychiatric setting. Laissez-faire leaders allow the group to control its direction. This works well in creative groups such as art or horticulture groups.

Yalom and Leszcz (2005) identify core principles that make a group therapeutic. These curative (healing) factors are powerful aspects of group work success. Table 29.4 summarizes these curative factors.

Table 29.4 **Curative Factors in Group Therapy**

Curative Factor	Description
Interpersonal learning	Members gain insight into themselves based on the feedback from others during later group phases.
Catharsis	Through experiencing and expressing feelings, therapeutic discharge of emotions is shared.
Instillation of hope	The leader shares optimism about successes of group treatment, and members share their improvements.
Universality	Members realize that they are not alone with their problems, feelings, or thoughts.
Imparting of information	Participants receive formal teaching by the leader or advice from peers.
Altruism	Members gain or profit from giving support to others, leading to improved self-value.
Corrective experience of primary family	Members repeat patterns of behavior in the group that they learned in their families; with feedback from the leader and peers, they learn about their own behavior.
Socializing techniques	Members learn new social skills based on others' feedback and modeling.
Imitative behavior	Members may copy behavior from the leader or peers and can adopt healthier habits.
Group cohesiveness	Group member feels connected to the other members, the leader, and the group as a whole; members can accept positive feedback and constructive criticism.
Existential resolution	Members examine aspects of life (e.g., loneliness, mortality, responsibility) that affect everyone in constructing meaning.

From Yalom, I. D., & Leszcz, M. (2005). *The theory and practice of group psychotherapy* (5th ed.). Basic Books.

CHAPTER 30

Brain Stimulation Therapies

Although medication is the foundation of somatic (physical) treatments for psychiatric disorders and psychiatric symptoms, other options are available. Brain stimulation therapy began in 1938 when electroshock therapy was used to treat most every psychiatric condition. Since then brain stimulation therapies have become more sophisticated and are even considered high technology. These therapies all involve activating or inhibiting the brain directly with electricity. The following brain stimulation therapies are discussed in this chapter:

- Electroconvulsive therapy (ECT)
- Repetitive transcranial magnetic stimulation (rTMS)
- Magnetic seizure therapy (MST)
- Vagus nerve stimulation (VNS)
- Deep brain stimulation (DBS)

ELECTROCONVULSIVE THERAPY

Despite being a highly effective somatic treatment for psychiatric disorders, ECT has a bad reputation. This may be related, in part, to the outdated practice of restraining a conscious individual while inducing a full-blown seizure. In fact, before paralytic drugs, more than 30% of ECT patients experienced compression fractures of the spine (Welch, 2016). Given the current sophistication of anesthetic and paralytic agents, ECT is actually not dramatic and is quite effective.

Indications

ECT has US Food and Drug Administration (FDA) approval for depressive symptoms associated with major depressive disorder or bipolar disorder in individuals aged 13 years and older. Using ECT for depressive symptoms accounts for about 65% of the procedures. However, since the FDA does not regulate the practice of medicine, practitioners may use ECT for other conditions such as schizophrenia, schizoaffective disorder, and mania.

Risk Factors

Using ECT requires patients and clinicians to weigh the risk of using this method versus the risk of suicide and diminished quality of life. Several conditions pose risks and require careful workup and management. Because the heart can be stressed at the onset of the seizure and for up to 10 minutes after, careful assessment and management in hypertension, congestive heart failure, cardiac arrhythmias, and other cardiac conditions are warranted (Welch, 2016). ECT also stresses the brain as a result of increased cerebral oxygen, blood flow, and intracranial pressure. Conditions such as brain tumors and subdural hematomas may increase the risk when using ECT.

Procedure

The procedure for ECT is explained to the patient, and informed consent is obtained if the patient is being treated voluntarily. For a patient treated involuntarily, permission may be obtained from the next of kin, although in some states such treatment must be court-ordered. The patient is usually given a general anesthetic to induce sleep and a muscle-paralyzing agent to prevent muscle distress and fractures.

Patients have a pre-ECT workup that includes chest x-ray, an electrocardiogram (ECG), a urinalysis, a complete blood count, blood urea nitrogen, and an electrolyte panel. Benzodiazepines are discontinued before the procedure because they will interfere with the seizure process.

An electroencephalogram (EEG) monitors brain waves, and an ECG monitors cardiac responses. Brief seizures (30–60 seconds) are induced by an electrical current (as brief as 1 second) transmitted through electrodes attached to one or both sides of the head.

The usual course of ECT for an individual with major depressive disorder is two or three treatments per week to a total of 6 to 12 treatments. Continuation of ECT along with medication may help to de-crease relapse rates.

Potential Adverse Reactions

Patients wake about 15 minutes after the procedure and are often confused and disoriented for several hours. The nurse and family may need to orient the patient frequently during the course of treatment. Most people experience what is called retrograde amnesia, which is a loss of memory of events leading up to and including the treatment itself.

REPETITIVE TRANSCRANIAL MAGNETIC STIMULATION

rTMS is a noninvasive modality used in the treatment of major depressive disorder. The rTMS system is an electromagnetic device that painlessly delivers a rapidly pulsed magnetic field to the cerebral cortex. These magnetic pulses activate neurons without inducing a seizure.

Indications

In 2008 the FDA approved the use of rTMS for major depressive disorder. Specifically, this treatment is approved for adult patients who have failed to achieve satisfactory improvement from one prior antidepressant medication at or above the minimal effective dose and duration in the current episode. rTMS may also be a promising treatment for generalized anxiety disorder.

Risk Factors

With the exception of braces and dental fillings, individuals with non-removable metal in their heads should not receive rTMS. This procedure could result in the metal moving, heating up, or malfunctioning. Examples of metals include:
- Aneurysm clips or coils
- Stents in the neck or brain
- Deep brain stimulators
- Electrodes
- Metallic implants in ears and eyes
- Shrapnel or bullet fragments in or near the head
- Facial tattoos with metallic or magnetic-sensitive ink

Procedure

Outpatient treatment with rTMS takes about 30 minutes and is typically administered 5 days a week for 4 to 6 weeks. Patients are awake and alert during the procedure. An electromagnet is placed on the patient's scalp, and short, magnetic pulses pass into the prefrontal cortex of the brain. These pulses are similar to those used for magnetic resonance imaging (MRI) but are more focused. The pulses cause electrical charges to flow and induce neurons to fire or become active. During the procedure, patients feel a slight tapping or knocking in the head, contraction of the scalp, and tightening of the jaws.

Potential Adverse Reactions

After the procedure, patients may feel pain on the scalp at the site of the stimulation due to muscle contraction. Headache, fatigue, and lightheadedness may occur. No neurological deficits or memory problems have been noted. Seizures are a rare complication of rTMS. Most of the common side effects of rTMS are mild and include scalp tingling and discomfort at the administration site.

MAGNETIC SEIZURE THERAPY

MST combines certain elements from both ECT and rTMS. Like rTMS, MST uses magnetic pulses instead of electricity to stimulate a precise area of the brain (National Institute of Mental Health, 2016). Like ECT, MST induces a seizure. The seizure is accomplished by using higher-frequency pulses than the ones given in rTMS.

The goal of MST is to achieve the effectiveness of ECT while reducing its cognitive side effects. ECT leads to a much more widespread seizure induction. This widespread effect is probably responsible for cognitive problems after ECT. MST uses a more focal seizure expression with less involvement of hippocampal and deep brain structures.

Indications

Although MST is in the early stages of testing for psychiatric disorders, results are promising. Recent research indicates that MST has been effective in triggering remission in 30% to 40% of individuals treated for major depressive disorder and bipolar disorder. It is also being investigated as a treatment for schizophrenia and obsessive–compulsive disorder.

Procedure

The patient must be anesthetized and given a muscle relaxant to prevent movement during the procedure. The motor activity of the right foot is assessed visually to track the duration of the motor seizure. An EEG is used to track seizure activity in the brain. Up to 600 pulses are delivered. Generally, two or three MST sessions are delivered each week. Some research reports using a total of 24 sessions or continued use until symptoms abate.

Potential Adverse Reactions

Common side effects after MST are headache, dizziness, nausea, vomiting, muscle aches, and fatigue. These side effects can be explained by anesthesia exposure and the induction of a seizure. Studies in both animals and humans have found that as compared to ECT, MST produces the following:

- Fewer memory side effects
- Shorter seizures
- A shorter recovery time

VAGUS NERVE STIMULATION

The use of VNS originated as a treatment for epilepsy. Clinicians noted that in addition to decreasing seizures, VNS also seemed to improve mood in a population who normally experiences higher rates of depression. The theory behind VNS relates to the action of the vagus nerve, the longest cranial nerve, which extends from the brainstem to organs in the neck, chest, and abdomen. Electrical stimulation of the vagus nerve results in higher levels of neurotransmitters, thereby improving mood and also enhancing the action of antidepressants.

Indications

Nearly a decade after VNS was approved for use in Europe, the FDA granted approval for its use in the United States for treatment-resistant depression. The efficacy of VNS in treating depression is still being established. Other potential applications of VNS include anxiety, obesity, and pain.

Procedure

The surgery to implant VNS is typically an outpatient procedure. A pacemaker-like device is implanted surgically into the left chest wall. The device is connected to a thin flexible wire that is threaded up and wrapped around the vagus nerve on the left side of the neck. After surgery, an infrared magnetic wand is held against the chest, while a personal computer or personal digital assistant is used to program the frequency of pulses. Pulses are usually delivered for 30 seconds, every 5 minutes, 24 hours a day. Antidepressant action usually occurs in several weeks.

Potential Adverse Reactions

The implantation of VNS is a surgical procedure, carrying with it the risks inherent in any surgical procedure (e.g., pain, infection, sensitivity to anesthesia). One side effect of VNS therapy is related to the proximity of the lead to the vagus nerve, which is adjacent to the laryngeal and pharyngeal branches of the left vagus nerve. Voice alteration occurs in nearly 60% of patients. Other side effects include neck pain, cough, paresthesia, and dyspnea. These side effects tend to decrease with time. The device can be temporarily turned off by placing a special magnet over the implant. This may be especially helpful when engaging in public speaking or heavy exercise.

DEEP BRAIN STIMULATION

DBS is a treatment whereby electrodes are surgically implanted into specific areas of the brain to stimulate those regions identified to be underactive in depression. Electrical pulses are delivered continuously and are believed to reset the malfunctioning area of the brain.

Indications

DBS has FDA approval for Parkinson's disease. It has also been approved for humanitarian use in treatment-resistant obsessive–compulsive disorder and is used off-label in major depressive disorder. One of the challenges is identifying the optimal neuroanatomical target in the brain.

Procedure

As in VNS, a device is implanted in the chest wall that is designed to provide electrical stimulation. It differs from VNS in that electrodes are implanted directly into the brain to modify brain activity. Before the procedure, the head is shaved and then attached with screws to a frame to prevent movement. The patient is awake during the procedure to provide the surgeon with feedback.

Two holes are drilled into the head under a local anesthetic. A slender tube is threaded to specific areas, of the brain and electrodes are inserted. In the case of major depressive disorder, several areas of the brain have been targeted by DBS. In the case of obsessive–compulsive disorder, the electrodes are placed in the ventral capsule and ventral striatum, the areas of the brain believed to be associated with obsessive thoughts and compulsive behavior.

After placement, the patient provides feedback and then is placed under general anesthesia. The electrodes are then attached to wires inside the body that run from the head to the chest. A pair of battery-operated generators is implanted in the chest that continuously delivers electrical pulses to stimulate the brain.

Potential Adverse Reactions

DBS is a minimally invasive procedure and carries risks associated with any type of brain surgery. For example, the procedure may lead to the following:
- Bleeding in the brain or stroke
- Infection
- Disorientation or confusion
- Unwanted mood changes
- Movement disorders
- Lightheadedness
- Sleep disturbances

Because of its recent introduction, it is likely that not all side effects have been identified.

References

Alzheimer's Association. (2019). *Stages of Alzheimer's*. Retrieved from https://www.alz.org/alzheimers-dementia/stages

Alzheimer's Association. (2021). 2021 *Alzheimer's Disease Facts and Figures*. Retrieved from, https://www.alz.org/alzheimers-dementia/facts-figures

American Nurses Association, American Psychiatric-Mental Health Nurses Association, & the International Society of Psychiatric-Mental Health Nurses. (2014). *Psychiatric-mental health nursing: Scope and standards of practice* (2nd ed.). American Nurses Association.

American Psychiatric Association. (2013). *Diagnostic and statistical manual of mental disorders* (5th ed.). American Psychiatric Association.

Beck, A. T. (1979). *Cognitive therapy and the emotional disorders*. International Universities Press.

Brown, R. L., & Rounds, L. A. (1995). Conjoint screening questionnaires for alcohol and drug abuse. *Wisconsin Medical Journal*, *94*, 135–140.

Brownell, K. D., & Walsh, B. T. (2017). *Eating disorders and obesity*. Guilford.

Caplan, G. (1964). *Principles of preventive psychiatry*. Basic Books.

Centers for Disease Control and Prevention. (2018). *Data and Statistics Fatal Injury Report for 2017*. Retrieved from https://webappa.cdc.gov/cgi-bin/broker.exe

Centers for Disease Control and Prevention. (2021). Provisional mortality data—United States, 2020. *Weekly*, *70*(14), 519–522. https://www.cdc.gov/mmwr/volumes/70/wr/mm7014e1.htm#:~:text=COVID%2D19%20death%20rates%20were%20highest%20among%20males%2C%20older%20adults,causes%20of%20death%20(6).

Christensen, D. L., Bilder, D. A., Zahorodny, W., Pettygrove, S., Durkin, M. S., Fitzgerald, R. T., … Yeargin-Allsopp, M. (2016). Prevalence and characteristics of autism spectrum disorder among 4-year old children in the Autism and Developmental Disabilities Monitoring Network. *Journal of Developmental Behavioral Pediatrics*, *37*(1), 1–8. https://doi.org/10.1097/DBP.0000000000000235.

Danielson, M. L., Bitsko, R. H., Ghandour, R. M., Holbrook, J. R., Kogan, M. D., & Blumberg, S. J. (2018). Prevalence of parent-reported ADHD diagnosis and associated treatment among US children and adolescents. *Journal of Clinical Child and Adolescent Psychology, 47*(2), 199–212.

Donnelly, B., Touyz, S., Hay, P., Burton, A., Russell, J., & Caterson, I. (2018). Neuroimaging in bulimia nervosa and binge eating disorder: A systematic review. *Journal of Eating Disorders, 6*, 30. https://doi.org/10.1186/s40337-018-0187-1.

Ebert, D. H., Finn, C. T., & Smoller, J. W. (2016). Genetics and psychiatry. In T. A. Stern, M. Fava, & T. E. Wilens (Eds.), *Massachusetts General Hospital comprehensive clinical psychiatry* (2nd ed., pp. 681). Saunders.

Erikson, E. H. (1963). *Childhood and society.* Norton.

Gordon, C., & Bereson, E. V. (2016). The doctor-patient relationship. In T. A. Stern, M. Fava, & T. E. Wilens (Eds.), *Massachusetts General Hospital comprehensive clinical psychiatry* (2nd ed., pp. 1–7). Saunders.

Gummin, D. D., Mowry, J. B., Spyker, D. A., Brooks, D. E., Osterthaler, K. M., & Banner, W. (2018). 2017 Annual report of the American association of poison control centers' National Poison Control Data System (NPDS): 35th Annual report. *Clinical Toxicology, 56*(12), 1213–1415.

Harrington, B. C., Jimerson, M., Haxton, C., & Jimerson, D. C. (2015). Initial evaluation, diagnosis, and treatment of anorexia nervosa and bulimia nervosa. *American Family Physician, 91*(1), 46–52.

Hays, J. S., & Larson, K. (1963). *Interacting with patients.* Macmillan.

Herling, S. F., Greve, I. E., Vasilevskis, E. E., Egerod, I., Bekker Mortensen, C., Møller, A. M., … Thomsen, T. (2018). Interventions for preventing intensive care unit delirium in adults. *Cochrane Database of Systematic Reviews, 11*, CD009783. https://doi.org/10.1002/14651858.CD009783.pub2.

Hudson, J. I., Hiripi, E., Pope, H. G., & Kessler, R. C. (2012). The prevalence and correlates of eating disorders in the National Comorbidity Survey Replication. *Biological Psychiatry, 61*(3), 348–358. https://doi.org/10.1016/j.biopsych.2006.03.040.

International Council of Nurses. (2019). *International Classification for Nursing Practice Catalog.* Retrieved from https://www.icn.ch/sites/default/files/inline-files/ICNP2019-DC.pdf

Kerr, K. L., Moseman, S. E., Avery, J. A., Bodurka, J., Zucker, N. L., & Simmons, W. K. (2016). Altered insula activity during visceral interoception in weight-restored patients with anorexia nervosa. *Neuropsychopharmacology*, *41*(2), 521–528. https://doi.org/10.1038/npp.2015.174.

Kessler, R. C., Berglund, P., Demler, O., Jin, R., Merikangas, K. R., & Walters, E. E. (2006). Lifetime prevalence and age-of-onset distributions of DSV-IV disorders in the National Comorbidity Survey Replication. *Archives of General Psychiatry*, *62*(6), 593–602.

Kübler-Ross, E. (1973). *On death and dying*. Routledge.

Linehan, M. M. (1993). *Cognitive behavioral treatment of borderline personality disorder*. New York, NY: Guilford.

Lock, J. (2015). An update on evidence-based psychosocial treatments for eating disorders in children and adolescents. *Journal of Clinical Child & Adolescent Psychology*, *44*(5), 707–721. https://doi.org/10.1080/15374416.2014.971458.

Mahler, M. S., Pine, F., & Berman, A. (1975). *The psychological birth of the human infant*. Basic Books.

Maslow, A. H. (1972). *The farther reaches of human nature*. Viking.

Mehler, P. S., & Andersen, A. E. (2017). *Eating disorders* (3rd ed.). Johns Hopkins.

Memon, A., Rogers, I., Fitzsimmons, S. M. D. D., Carter, B., Strawbridge, R., Hidalgo-Mazzei, D., & Young, A. H. (2020). Association between naturally occurring lithium in drinking water and suicide rates: Systematic review and meta-analysis of ecological studies. *British Journal of Psychiatry*, *217*(6), 667–678. https://doi.org/10.1192/bjp.2020.128.

Merikangas, K. R., He, J. P., Burstein, M., Swanson, S. A., Avenevoli, S., Cui, L., … Swendsen, J. (2010). Lifetime prevalence of mental disorders in U.S. adolescents: Results from the National Comorbidity Survey Replication–Adolescent Supplement (NCS-A). *Journal of the American Academy of Child Adolescent Psychiatry*, *49*(10), 980–989.

Mitchell, J. E., King, W. C., Courcoulas, A., Dakin, G., Elder, K., Engel, S., … Wolfe, B. (2015). Eating behavior and eating disorders in adults before bariatric surgery. *International Journal of Eating Disorder*, *48*(2), 215–222. https://doi.org/10.1002/EAT.22275.

Modi, S., Dharaiya, D., Schultz, L., & Varelas, P. (2016). Neuroleptic malignant syndrome: Complications, outcomes, and mortality. *Neurocritical Care, 24*(1), 97–103. https://doi.org/10.1007/s12028-015-0162-5.

Myrick, D., & Erney, T. (1984). *Caring and sharing: Becoming a peer evaluator*. Educational Media.

National Center for Complementary and Integrative Health. (2020). *Chamomile*. Retrieved from https://www.nccih.nih.gov/health/chamomile

National Council of State Boards of Nursing. (2018a). *A Nurse's Guide to Professional Behaviors*. Retrieved from https://www.ncsbn.or/ProfessionalBoundaries_Complete.pdf.

National Council of State Boards of Nursing. (2018b). *NCLEX-RN® examination: Test plan for the National Council Licensure Examination for Registered Nurses*. Chicago, IL: National Council of State Boards of Nursing.

National Council of State Boards of Nursing. (2021). *NCSBN Clinical Judgment Measurement Model*. Retrieved from https://www.ncsbn.org/14798.htm

National Eating Disorder Association. (2018). *Glossary*. Retrieved August 9, 2018, from https://www.nationaleatingdisorders.org/learn/glossary

National Institute of Mental Health. (2012). *Older Adults: Depression and Suicide Facts*. Retrieved from http://www.nimh.nih.gov/health/publications/older-adults-and-depression/older-adults-and-depression_141998.pdf.

National Institute of Mental Health. (2016). *Brain Stimulation Therapies*. Retrieved from https://www.nimh.nih.gov/health/topics/brain-stimulation-therapies/brain-stimulation-therapies.shtml

National Institute on Alcohol Abuse and Alcoholism. (n.d.). *What is a standard drink?* https://www.niaaa.nih.gov/alcohols-effects-health/overview-alcohol-consumption/what-standard-drink#:~:text=In%20the%20United%20States%2C%20one,which%20is%20about%2040%25%20alcohol

National League for Nursing. (2015). *Debriefing Across the Curriculum*. Retrieved from https://www.nln.org/docs/default-source/about/nln-vision-series-(position statements)/nln-vision-debriefing-across-the-curriculum.pdf?sfvrsn=).

Peplau, H. E. (1952). *Interpersonal relations in nursing: Offering a conceptual frame of reference for psychodynamic nursing*. New York: Putnam.

Peplau, H. E. (1968). A working definition of anxiety. In S. F. Burd & M. A. Marshall (Eds.), *Some clinical approaches to psychiatric nursing* (pp. 323–327). Macmillan.

Peplau, H. E. (1999). *Interpersonal relations in nursing: A conceptual frame of reference for psychodynamic nursing.* New York, NY: Springer.

Posner, K., Brent, D., Lucas, C., Gould, M., Stanley, B., Brown, G., … Mann, J. (2009). *Columbia-Suicide Severity Rating Scale.* Retrieved from http://www.integration.samhsa.gov/clinical-practice/Columbia_Suicide_Severity_Rating_Scale.pdf.

Prins, A., Bovin, M.J., Kimerling, R., Kaloupek, D.G., Marx, B.P., Pless Kaiser, A., & Schnurr, P.P. (2015). *The Primary Care PTSD Screen for DSM-5 (PC-PTSD-5).* Retrieved from http://www.ptsd.va.gov/professional/assessment/screens/pc-ptsd.asp

Quality and Safety Education for Nurses (QSEN) Institute. (2012). *QSEN Competencies.* Retrieved from http://qsen.org/competencies/pre-licensure-ksas

Rosenvinge, J., & Petterson, G. (2015). Epidemiology of eating disorders part II: An update with special reference to the DSM-5. *Advances in eating disorders, 3*(2), 198–220.

Sadock, B. J., Sadock, V. A., & Ruiz, P. (2015). *Kaplan & Sadock's synopsis of psychiatry* (11th ed.). Philadelphia, PA: Wolters Kluwer.

Shear, K., Jin, R., Ruscio, A. M., Walters, E. E., & Kessler, R. C. (2006). Prevalence and correlates of estimated DSM-IV child and adult separation anxiety disorder in the national comorbidity survey replication. *American Journal of Psychiatry, 163*(6), 1074–1083. https://doi.org/10.1176/appi.ajp.163.6.1074.

Siddiqi, N., Harrison, J. K., Clegg, A., Teale, E. A., Young, J., Taylor, J., & Simpkins, S. A. (2016). Interventions for preventing delirium in hospitalised non-ICU patients. *Cochrane Database of Systematic Reviews, 3,* CD005563. https://doi.org/10.1002/14651858.

Skodol, A. E., Bender, D. S., & Oldham, J. M. (2019). Personality pathology and personality disorders. In L. W. Roberts (Ed.), *Textbook of psychiatry* (6th ed., pp. 711–747). Washington, DC: American Psychiatric.

Spielman, A., & Glovinsky, P. (2004). A conceptual framework of insomnia for primary care providers: Predisposing, precipitating, and perpetuating factors. *Sleep Medicine Alert, 9*(1), 1–6.

Stein, D. J., Lim, C. C. W., Roest, A. M., de Jonge, P., Aguilar-Gaxiola, S., Al-Hamzawi, A., … Xavier, M. (2017). The cross-national epidemiology of social anxiety disorder: Data from the World Mental Health Survey Initiative. *BMC Medicine*, *15*(143), 1–21. https://doi.org/10.1186/s12916-017-0889-2.

Stone, D. M., Simon, T. R., Fowler, K. A., Kegler, S. C., Yuan, K., Holland, K. M., & Crosby, A. E. (2018). Vital signs: Trends in state suicide rates—United States, 1999–2016 and circumstances contributing to suicide—27 states, 2015. *Morbidity and Mortality Weekly Report*, *67*, 617–624. https://dx.doi.org/10.15585/mmwr.mm6722a1external icon.

Stroebe, M., & Schut, H. (1999). The dual process model of coping with bereavement: Rationale and description. *Death Studies*, *23*(3), 197–224. https://doi.org/10.1080/074811899201046.

Substance Abuse and Mental Health Service Administration. (2018). *National Survey on Drug Use and Health*. Retrieved from https://www.samhsa.gov/data/release/2018-national-survey-drug-use-and-health-nsduh-releases.

Substance Abuse and Mental Health Services Administration. (2020). *National Survey on Drug Use and Health*. Retrieved from https://www.samhsa.gov/data/release/2019-national-survey-drug-use-and-health-nsduh-releases.

Substance Abuse and Mental Health Service Administration. (2021). *Screening, Brief Intervention, and Referral to Treatment (SBIRT)*. Retrieved from https://www.samhsa.gov/sbirt.

US Census Bureau. (2019). *Selected Social Characteristics in the United States*. Retrieved from https://data.census.gov/cedsci/table?tid=ACSDP5Y2019.DP02&hidePreview=true

US Department of Health and Human Services. (2012). *Use of Psychiatric Medications in Pregnancy and Lactation*. Retrieved from https://www.guideline.gov/summaries/summary/12490.

US Department of Justice. (2013). *Crime in the United States 2013: Rape*. Retrieved from https://ucr.fbi.gov/crime-in-the-u.s/2013/crime-in-the-u.s.-2013/violent-crime/rape

US Department of Veteran Affairs. (2017). *Management of Posttraumatic Stress Disorder and Acute Stress Reaction*.

Retrieved from https://www.healthquality.va.gov/guidelines/MH/ptsd/VADoDPTSDCPGFinal012418.pdf

US Department of Veteran Affairs. (2018). *PTSD: How Common is PTSD in Adults?* Retrieved from https://www.ptsd.va.gov/understand/common/common_adults.asp.

US Food and Drug Administration. (2021). *Online Label Repository.* Retrieved from https://labels.fda.gov/.

Wardenaar, K. J., Lim, C. C. W., Al-Hamzawi, A. O., Alonso, J., Andrade, L. H., Benjet, C., … de Jonge, P. (2017). The cross-national epidemiology of specific phobia in the World Mental Health Surveys. *Psychological Medicine, 47*(10), 1744–1760. https://doi.org/10.1017/S0033291717000174.

Welch, C. A. (2016). Electroconvulsive therapy. In T. A. Stern, M. Fava, T. E. Wilens, & J. F. Rosenbaum (Eds.), *Comprehensive clinical psychiatry* (2nd ed.). St. Louis, MO: Elsevier.

Whitney, D. G., & Peterson, M. D. (2019). U.S. and state prevalence of mental health disorders and disparities of mental health care use in children. *JAMA Pediatrics, 173*(4), 389–391. https://doi.org/10.1001/jamapediatrics.2018.5399.

World Health Organization. (2019). *Depression.* Retrieved from https://www.who.int/news-room/fact-sheets/detail/depression

Yalom, I. D., & Leszcz, M. (2005). *The theory and practice of group psychotherapy* (5th ed.). New York, NY: Basic Books.

Zipfel, S., Giel, K. E., Bulik, C. M., Hay, P., & Schmidt, U. (2015). Anorexia nervosa: Aetiology, assessment, and treatment. *The Lancet Psychiatry, 2*(12), 1099–1111.

Patient-Centered Assessment

A patient-centered assessment such as this can be used to structure admission data. Key findings from an initial assessment provide direction for developing a nursing care plan. It is important to supplement most of the checkboxes included in this assessment tool with additional descriptions of abnormal findings. The assessment begins with general information, then covers essential information (e.g., substance use and sleep), and progresses to the more detailed mood and cognitive domains.

GENERAL INFORMATION

Name (or initials):

Age:

Gender identity: Sex assigned at birth:

Preferred pronoun: Sexual orientation:

Race:

☐ White ☐ Black or African American ☐ American Indian or Alaska Native

☐ Asian ☐ Native Hawaiian or Other Pacific Islander

Ethnicity:

☐ Non-Hispanic, Latino, or Spanish origin ☐ Hispanic, Latino, or Spanish origin

Language:

☐ English ☐ English as second language ☐ Need for interpreter/translator ☐ Other:

Height: Weight: Recent weight gain/loss (amount):

Marital status: ☐ Single ☐ Married ☐ Cohabitating ☐ Divorced ☐ Other:

Education: ☐ <High school ☐ High school

☐ Some associates/technical/trade ☐ Associates/-technical/trade

☐ Some undergraduate ☐ Undergraduate

☐ Some graduate ☐ Graduate
Employment: ☐ Currently employed ☐ Full-time
    ☐ Part-time ☐ Unemployed
Occupation:
Residence: ☐ Rents ☐ Owns home ☐ Other:
Lives with:

PRESENTING PROBLEM

The presenting problem is the patient's own words as to the reason for being admitted or entering into treatment. Use a question such as, "What is the reason you are being admitted (or treated) here?" Once a problem is identified you can use the patient's terms and phrases during the assessment.

RELEVANT HISTORY

1. Do you have any health problems?
2. Do you have allergies?
3. Do any family members have psychiatric problems?
4. Do you have a history of emotional, physical, or sexual abuse and/or neglect?
5. Have you ever experienced a traumatic event or traumatic events?

PSYCHIATRIC HISTORY

Treatment Dates	Therapist/Facility	Outcome

History of suicidality (ideation, attempt, method):
Current suicidality (ideation, plan, means):
History of violence/homicidality:
Current thoughts of violence/homicidality:

History of self-injury (e.g., cutting, head banging):
Current self-injury:

MEDICATION (INCLUDING OVER-THE-COUNTER)

Medication	Dose	Frequency	Dates of Use

ALCOHOL/SUBSTANCE USE

History of alcohol and/or substance use (when it started, how
   often, how much, legal problems associated with it):
Treatment for alcohol and/or substance use:
Current alcohol and/or substance use (how often, how
   much, last use):

RELIGIOUS, SPIRITUAL, SOCIAL, AND CULTURAL ASSESSMENT

1. What do you think are the causes of [insert chief
   complaint]?
2. Do you have a spiritual or religious affiliation?
3. What aspects of your spirituality or religious practices
   do you find most helpful?
4. Who are your main personal or social supports?
5. Are there practices within your culture that address
   [insert chief complaint]?
6. Are there restrictions on medical interventions or diet
   based on your spiritual, religious, or cultural beliefs
   and customs?

STRENGTHS, GOALS, AND COPING

Ask the patient to identify three strengths.

   1. _____
   2. _____
   3. _____

Ask the patient to identify three goals for hospitalization/ treatment.

1. _____
2. _____
3. _____

Ask the patient to identify coping methods for stress, anxiety, and anger.

SLEEP PATTERN

Quantity: ☐ 0 to 2 hours ☐ 2 to 4 hours ☐ 4 to 6 hours ☐ 6 to 8 hours ☐ 9+ hours

Initiation: ☐ No problem falling asleep ☐ Difficulty falling asleep

Maintenance: ☐ Continuous sleep ☐ Wakes repeatedly ☐ Wakes and has difficulty returning to sleep

Quality: ☐ Refreshing ☐ Not refreshing

APPEARANCE

Eye contact: ☐ Direct ☐ Poor ☐ Intermittent ☐ Staring ☐ Intense

Pupils: ☐ Normal ☐ Constricted ☐ Dilated

Age: ☐ Appears stated age ☐ Appears older than stated age

Posture: ☐ Neutral ☐ Slouched ☐ Straight ☐ Tense

Gait: ☐ Normal ☐ Shuffling ☐ Staggering ☐ Spastic

Attire: ☐ Neat ☐ Unkempt ☐ Appropriate ☐ Inappropriate attire

Hygiene: ☐ Good ☐ Neglected

Skin: ☐ Healthy ☐ Impaired integrity

ATTITUDE

☐ Cooperative ☐ Engaged ☐ Disengaged ☐ Defensive ☐ Guarded ☐ Elusive ☐ Poor historian

BEHAVIOR

Psychomotor: ☐ Normal ☐ Hyperactive ☐ Restless ☐ Agitated ☐ Retarded

Movement: ☐ Akathisia ☐ Catatonia ☐ Echopraxia ☐ Waxy flexibility

☐ Verbal tics ☐ Motor tics ☐ Fine hand tremor ☐ Course hand tremor ☐ Dystonia

☐ Tardive dyskinesia (attach Abnormal Involuntary Movement Scale [AIMS] from Chapter 22)

MOOD

Mood is assessed by asking the patient, "How do you feel?" and then summarized by the nurse.

☐ Euthymic (normal) ☐ Depressed ☐ Sad ☐ Euphoric (elated) ☐ Angry

☐ Irritable ☐ Anxious ☐ Fearful ☐ Apathetic ☐ Anhedonic ☐ Alexithymic (unable to describe mood)

AFFECT

Affect is determined by observations of the nurse.

☐ Appropriate to situation ☐ Inappropriate to situation

☐ Congruent with mood ☐ Incongruent with mood

☐ Even ☐ Intense ☐ Blunt ☐ Flat ☐ Heightened ☐ Dramatic

☐ Constricted ☐ Fixed ☐ Immobile ☐ Labile

SPEECH

Presence: ☐ Present ☐ Absent/mute ☐ Aphasic

Rate: ☐ Slow ☐ Hesitant ☐ Normal ☐ Rapid ☐ Pressured

Volume: ☐ Soft ☐ Normal ☐ Loud

Articulation: ☐ Clear ☐ Mumbled ☐ Garbled ☐ Overemphasis ☐ Stuttered

Speech patterns: ☐ Echolalia (repeating others' words) ☐ Palilalia (repeating own words) ☐ Neologisms (creating new words)

THOUGHT PROCESSES

☐ Poverty of thought ☐ Normal quantity of thought ☐ Overabundance of thought

☐ Retarded ☐ Perseveration ☐ Circumstantiality ☐ Tangentiality ☐ Loose associations

☐ Flight of ideas ☐ Logical ☐ Disorganized ☐ Blocking ☐ Concrete thinking

THOUGHT CONTENT

Delusions: ☐ Paranoid ☐ Ideas of reference
     ☐ Persecutory ☐ Grandiose ☐ Erotomanic
☐ Somatic ☐ Jealousy ☐ Control ☐ Guilt ☐ Poverty
     ☐ Nihilistic ☐ Religious
Outside control: ☐ Thought broadcasting ☐ Thought
     withdrawal ☐ Thought insertion
Intrusive thoughts: ☐ Obsessions ☐ Phobias
Preoccupation: ☐ Suicidality ☐ Aggression ☐ Homicidality
     ☐ Suspicions ☐ Fears

PERCEPTIONS

Hallucinations: ☐ Auditory ☐ Visual ☐ Tactile
     ☐ Olfactory ☐ Gustatory
Auditory hallucinations: ☐ Inside own head
     ☐ Outside own head ☐ Pleasant/positive ☐ Negative
     ☐ Insulting ☐ Command ☐ Distractible
Frequency:
Other: ☐ Illusions ☐ Depersonalization ☐ Derealization
     ☐ Déjà vu

COGNITION

Alertness: ☐ Alert ☐ Clouded ☐ Drowsy ☐ Stuporous
Orientation: ☐ Person ☐ Time ☐ Date ☐ Place ☐ Situation
Attention and concentration:
Serial sevens (counting backward from 100 by 7s)
☐ Able ☐ Makes mistakes ☐ Unable
Spelling a five-letter word (such as world) backward
☐ Able ☐ Makes mistakes ☐ Unable
Memory:
Immediate memory (repeating a set of words)
☐ Able ☐ Makes mistakes ☐ Unable
Short-term memory (repeating a set of words after an interval)
☐ Able ☐ Makes mistakes ☐ Unable
Long-term memory (recalling a historical or geographical fact)
☐ Able ☐ Makes mistakes ☐ Unable
Cognitive/visual functioning:
Complex task (draw the face of a clock)
☐ Able ☐ Makes mistakes ☐ Makes many mistakes
     ☐ Unable

INSIGHT

Recognition of psychiatric disorder
☐ Insight intact ☐ Some insight ☐ Insight absent
Participation in care decisions
☐ Actively participates ☐ Some participation
    ☐ No participation ☐ Resists participation
Understands that symptoms are part of a psychiatric disorder
☐ Insight intact ☐ Some insight ☐ Insight absent

JUDGMENT

☐ Judgment intact ☐ Judgment fair ☐ Judgment
    impaired ☐ Judgment critically impaired

APPENDIX B

Integrative Care

Disorder	Therapy	Description
Anxiety	Natural products/ herbs	Supplements, vitamins, minerals, and herbs/ botanicals are used to reduce anxiety. Examples: • Kava: rare cases of hepatotoxicity • L-theanine: increases GABA and alpha activity • 5-HTTP: may be used for panic attacks
	Aromatherapy	Essential oils are used to enhance physical and mental well-being and for healing. Guidelines for safe use include dilution rates, caution with ingestion and use around eyes, and obtaining training for use in pregnancy, lactation, and with children. Examples: • Roman chamomile • Clary sage • Lavender • Mandarin • Neroli • Vetiver

Disorder	Therapy	Description
	Exercise	Exercise releases endorphins, provides distraction, and reduces tension. Exercise alters dopamine, serotonin, and norepinephrine; increases brain-derived neurotrophic factor; and reduces oxidative stress levels.
	Mind–body therapies: yoga, mindfulness-based stress reduction	Techniques such as yoga and mindfulness are used to enhance the mind's positive impact on the body. A specific yoga breathing technique may reduce obsessive–compulsive disorder symptoms.
	Expressive therapies	Music promotes relaxation and decreases autonomic arousal.
	Virtual reality–graded exposure therapy	Virtual images stimulate anxiety, which is paired with relaxation exercises.
	Electroencephalogram (EEG) or electromyography (EMG) biofeedback	Scalp sensors measure brain activity and patients learn how to regulate the body's responses to stress.
	Heart rate variability biofeedback	Heart rate changes are measured, and feedback promotes increased variability, lowers stress levels, and improves overall well-being.

(Continued)

Disorder	Therapy	Description
Attention-Deficit/ Hyperactivity Disorder (ADHD)	Diet/nutrition	Food colorings, additives, sugar, and certain food allergens are avoided to decrease symptoms of ADHD.
	Natural products/ herbs	Supplements, vitamins, minerals, and herbs/ botanicals are used to decrease symptoms of ADHD. Examples: • Omega-3 fatty acids: high doses may decrease symptom severity • Zinc: may decrease hyperactivity • Acetyl-L-carnitine: may decrease symptoms of inattention
	EEG biofeedback	Scalp sensors measure brain activity, and patients learn how to regulate body responses. Symptoms of inattention, impulsivity, and hyperactivity are decreased.
	Mind–body therapies	Techniques such as yoga, mindfulness, and massage enhance the mind's positive impact on the body and decrease symptoms of ADHD.
	Exercise	Physical activity is used to reduce the symptoms of ADHD.
Bipolar	Natural products/ herbs	Supplements, vitamins, minerals, and herbs/ botanicals are used to help stabilize mood.

Disorder	Therapy	Description
		Example: • Omega-3 fatty acids: decrease mood swings when taken with a mood stabilizer
	Exercise	Physical activity is used to decrease symptoms of mania.
Depression	Natural products/ herbs	Supplements, vitamins, minerals, and herbs/ botanicals are used to improve mood. Examples: • St. John's wort: mild to moderate depression • Omega-3 fatty acids: in conjunction with antidepressants • SAMe: moderate to severe depression with or without antidepressants; risk of serotonin syndrome
	Exercise	Physical activity improves depressive symptoms.
	Bright light therapy	Light boxes decrease melatonin, reducing the symptoms of depression.
	Mind–body therapies: yoga	Yoga is an effective treatment for major depressive disorder.
	Diet/nutrition	Regular meals consisting of fish, fruit, raw or cooked vegetables, and omega-3 fatty acids reduces depression. Vitamin D supplementation may reduce depressive symptoms.

(Continued)

Disorder	Therapy	Description
	Massage therapy	A broad group of medically valid therapies involving rubbing or moving the skin are used to reduce depressive symptoms.
	Repetitive transcranial magnetic stimulation (rTMS)	Stimulation of the brain using a magnet on the scalp is used to help improve refractory depression.
	Intermittent theta-burst stimulation (iTBS)	A more intense form of rTMS reduces refractory depression.
Posttraumatic Stress Disorder (PTSD)	Virtual reality–graded exposure therapy	Virtual environments are used for progressive exposure therapy. Virtual environments may be even more effective than medication in PTSD and decrease symptoms by 30%.
	Acupuncture	May reduce symptoms of PTSD. Needles are inserted in the skin at key points (meridians) to modulate the flow of qi.
	Eye movement desensitization and reprocessing (EMDR)	Patients explore disturbing memories while simultaneously focusing on external stimuli such as eye movements or hand tapping.
Schizophrenia	Natural products/herbs	Supplements, vitamins, minerals, and herbs/botanicals are used to alleviate symptoms of schizophrenia.

Disorder	Therapy	Description
		Examples: • Omega-3 fatty acids • Folic acid: reduces positive and negative symptoms • Thiamine: used in conjunction with an antipsychotic • Glycine: improves functioning and decreases negative symptoms • Ginkgo biloba: used in conjunction with an antipsychotic.
	Mind–body therapies: yoga	Yoga enhances the positive interaction between the mind and body, which helps to decrease agitation and anxiety.
	Avatar therapy	Patients converse with an avatar that represents the hallucination. Avatar becomes less derogatory and more submissive over time, reducing the severity of the auditory hallucinations (Craig et al., 2018).
Substance Use	Diet/nutrition	Relapse is reduced with diets low in sugar and caffeine and high in omega-3 fatty acids.
	Natural products	Supplements, vitamins, minerals, and herbs/botanicals are used to help reduce cravings, withdrawal, and the effect of substances on the body.

(Continued)

Disorder	Therapy	Description
		Examples: • Amino acids such as taurine and L-tryptophan decrease cravings and help with withdrawal. • SAMe may decrease the risk of liver damage. • Kudzu decreases cravings and can help prevent relapse.
	EMG, thermal EMG, and EEG biofeedback	Patients are able to view the activity in the muscles and brain and learn how to self-regulate the body's response to stress. Biofeedback may decrease the relapse rate of alcohol use disorder.
	Exercise	Physical activity may decrease the relapse rate of alcohol use disorder.
	Mind–body therapies: yoga	Yoga enhances the positive interaction between mind and body, which helps to decrease agitation and anxiety and reduces relapse.
	Cranioelectrotherapy stimulation (CES)	A weak electrical current in the head and neck reduces the severity of withdrawal for alcohol and opiates.

DSM-5 Classification With ICD-10-CM Codes

Psychiatric disorders in the *Diagnostic and Statistical Manual of Mental Disorders*, 5th edition (*DSM-5*) are listed in this appendix. Before each disorder name, the International Classification of Disease, 10th edition with Clinical Modification (ICD-10-CM) codes are provided. Blank lines indicate that the ICD-10-CM code is not applicable. For some disorders, the code can be indicated only according to the subtype or specifier. After chapter titles and disorder names, page numbers for the corresponding text or criteria in the *DSM-5* are included in parentheses.

Note that for all mental disorders related to another medical condition, clinicians identify the name of the other medical condition. The diagnosis becomes the name of the psychiatric disorder with "due to [the medical condition]."

NEURODEVELOPMENTAL DISORDERS (31)

Intellectual Disabilities (33)

—.—	Intellectual Disability (Intellectual Developmental Disorder) (33)
	Specify current severity:
F70	Mild
F71	Moderate
F72	Severe
F73	Profound
F88	Global Developmental Delay (41)
F79	Unspecified Intellectual Disability (Intellectual Developmental Disorder) (41)

Communication Disorders (41)

F80.9	Language Disorder (42)
F80.0	Speech Sound Disorder (44)
F80.81	Childhood-Onset Fluency Disorder (Stuttering) (45)
	Note: Later-onset cases are diagnosed as 307.0 (F98.5) Adult-Onset Fluency Disorder.
F80.82	Social (Pragmatic) Communication Disorder (47)
F80.9	Unspecified Communication Disorder (49)

Autism Spectrum Disorder (50)

F84.0	Autism Spectrum Disorder (50)
	Specify if: Associated with a known medical or genetic condition or environmental factor; Associated with another neurodevelopmental, mental or behavioral disorder
	Specify current severity for Criterion A and Criterion B: Requiring very substantial support, Requiring substantial support, Requiring support
	Specify if: With or without accompanying intellectual impairment, With or without accompanying language impairment, With catatonia (use additional code 293.89 [F06.1])

Attention-Deficit/Hyperactivity Disorder (59)

—.—	Attention-Deficit/Hyperactivity Disorder (59)
	Specify whether:
F90.2	Combined presentation
F90.0	Predominantly inattentive presentation
F90.1	Predominantly hyperactive/impulsive presentation
	Specify if: In partial remission
	Specify current severity: Mild, Moderate, Severe
F90.8	Other Specified Attention-Deficit/Hyperactivity Disorder (65)
F90.9	Unspecified Attention-Deficit/Hyperactivity Disorder (66)

Specific Learning Disorder (66)

—.—	Specific Learning Disorder (66)
	Specify if:

F81.0	With impairment in reading (specify if with word reading accuracy, reading rate or fluency, reading comprehension)
F81.81	With impairment in written expression (specify if with spelling accuracy, grammar and punctuation accuracy, clarity or organization of written expression)
F81.2	With impairment in mathematics (specify if with number sense, memorization or arithmetic facts, accurate or fluent calculation, accurate math reasoning)
	Specify current severity: Mild, Moderate, Severe

Motor Disorders (74)

F82	Developmental Coordination Disorder (74)
F98.4	Stereotypic Movement Disorder (77)
	Specify if: With self-injurious behavior, Without self-injurious behavior
	Specify if: Associated with a known medical or genetic condition, neurodevelopmental disorder, or environmental factor
	Specify current severity: Mild, Moderate, Severe

Tic Disorders

F95.2	Tourette's Disorder (81)
F95.1	Persistent (Chronic) Motor or Vocal Tic Disorder (81)
	Specify if: With motor tics only, With vocal tics only
F95.0	Provisional Tic Disorder (81)
F95.8	Other Specified Tic Disorder (85)
F95.9	Unspecified Tic Disorder (85)

Other Neurodevelopment Disorders (86)

| F88 | Other Specified Neurodevelopmental Disorder (86) |
| F89 | Unspecified Neurodevelopmental Disorder (86) |

SCHIZOPHRENIA SPECTRUM AND OTHER PSYCHOTIC DISORDERS (87)

The following specifiers apply to Schizophrenia Spectrum and Other Psychotic Disorders where indicated:

F21	Schizotypal (Personality) Disorder (90)
F22	Delusional Disorder (90)
	Specify whether: Erotomanic type, Grandiose type, Jealous type, Persecutory type, Somatic type, Mixed type, Unspecified type
	Specify if: With bizarre content
F23	Brief Psychotic Disorder (94)
	Specify if: With marked stressor(s), Without marked stressor(s), With postpartum onset
F20.81	Schizophreniform Disorder (96)
	Specify if: With good prognostic features, Without good prognostic features
F20.9	Schizophrenia (99)
——.——	Schizoaffective Disorder (105)
	Specify whether:
F25.0	Bipolar type
F25.1	Depressive type
——.——	Substance/Medication-Induced Psychotic Disorder (110)
	Note: See the criteria set and corresponding recording procedures for substance-specific codes and ICD-10-CM coding.
	Specify if: With onset during intoxication, With onset during withdrawal
——.——	Psychotic Disorder Due to Another Medical Condition^c (115)
	Specify whether:
F06.2	With delusions
F06.0	With hallucinations
F06.1	Catatonia Associated With Another Mental Disorder (Catatonia Specifier) (119)
F06.1	Catatonic Disorder Due to Another Medical Condition (120)
F06.1	Unspecified Catatonia (121)
	Note: Code first 781.99 (R29.818) other symptoms involving nervous and musculoskeletal systems.
F28	Other Specified Schizophrenia Spectrum and Other Psychotic Disorder (122)
F29	Unspecified Schizophrenia Spectrum and Other Psychotic Disorder (122)

BIPOLAR AND RELATED DISORDERS (123)

The following specifiers apply to Bipolar and Related Disorders where indicated:

—.—	Bipolar I Disorder (123)
—.—	Current or most recent episode manic
F31.11	Mild
F31.12	Moderate
F31.13	Severe
F31.2	With psychotic features
F31.73	In partial remission
F31.74	In full remission
F31.9	Unspecified
F31.0	Current or most recent episode hypomanic
F31.73	In partial remission
F31.74	In full remission
F31.9	Unspecified
—.—	Current or most recent episode depressed
F31.31	Mild
F31.32	Moderate
F31.4	Severe
F31.5	With psychotic features
F31.75	In partial remission
F31.76	In full remission
F31.9	Unspecified
F31.9	Current or most recent episode unspecified
F31.81	Bipolar II Disorder[a] (132)
	Specify current or most recent episode: Hypomanic, Depressed
	Specify course if full criteria for a mood episode are not currently met: In partial remission, In full remission
	Specify severity if full criteria for a mood episode are not currently met: Mild, Moderate, Severe
F34.0	Cyclothymic Disorder (139)
	Specify if: With anxious distress
—.—	Substance/Medication-Induced Bipolar and Related Disorder (142)
	Note: See the criteria set and corresponding recording procedures for substance-specific coded and ICD-10-CM coding.
	Specify if: With onset during intoxication, With onset during withdrawal

Continued

——.——	Bipolar and Related Disorder Due to Another Medical Condition (145)
	Specify if:
F06.33	With manic features
F06.33	With manic- or hypomanic-like episode
F06.33	With mixed features
F31.89	Other specified Bipolar and Related Disorder (148)
F31.9	Unspecified Bipolar and Related Disorder (149)

DEPRESSIVE DISORDERS (155)

The following specifiers apply to Depressive Disorders where indicated:

F34.81	Disruptive Mood Dysregulation Disorder (156)
——.——	Major Depressive Disorder (160)
——.——	Single episode
F32.0	Mild
F32.1	Moderate
F32.2	Severe
F32.3	With psychotic features
F32.4	In partial remission
F32.5	In full remission
F32.9	Unspecified
——.——	Recurrent episode
F33.0	Mild
F33.1	Moderate
F33.2	Severe
F33.3	With psychotic features
F33.41	In partial remission
F33.42	In full remission
F33.9	Unspecified
F34.1	Persistent Depressive Disorder (Dysthymia) (168)
	Specify if: In partial remission, In full remission
	Specify if: Early onset, Late onset
	Specify if: With pure dysthymic syndrome; With persistent major depressive episode; With intermittent major depressive episodes, with current episode; With intermittent major depressive episodes, without current episode
	Specify current severity: Mild, Moderate, Severe

F32.81	Premenstrual Dysphoric Disorder (171)
—.—	Substance/Medication-Induced Depressive Disorder (175)
	Note: See the criteria set and corresponding recording procedures for substance-specific codes and ICD-10-CM coding.
	Specify if: With onset during intoxication, With onset during withdrawal
—.—	Depressive Disorder Due to Another Medical Condition (180)
	Specify if:
F06.31	With depressive features
F06.32	With major depressive-like episode
F06.34	With mixed features
F32.89	Other Specified Depressive Disorder (183)
F32.9	Unspecified Depressive Disorder (184)

ANXIETY DISORDERS (189)

F93.0	Separation Anxiety Disorder (190)
F94.0	Selective Mutism (195)
—.—	Specific Phobia (197)
	Specify if:
F40.218	Animal
F40.228	Natural environmental
—.—	Blood-injection-injury
F40.230	Fear of blood
F40.231	Fear of injections and transfusions
F40.232	Fear of other medical care
F40.233	Fear of injury
F40.248	Situational
F40.298	Other
F40.10	Social Anxiety Disorder (Social Phobia) (202)
	Specify if: Performance only
F41.0	Panic Disorder (208)
—.—	Panic Attack Specifier (214)
F40.00	Agoraphobia (217)
F41.1	Generalized Anxiety Disorder (222)
—.—	Substance/Medication-Induced Anxiety Disorder (226)
	Note: See the criteria set and corresponding recording procedures for substance-specific codes and ICD-10-CM coding.

Continued

	Specify if: With onset during intoxication, With onset during withdrawal, With onset after medication use
F06.4	Anxiety Disorder Due to Another Medical Condition (230)
F41.8	Other Specified Anxiety Disorder (233)
F41.9	Unspecified Anxiety Disorder (233)

OBSESSIVE–COMPULSIVE AND RELATED DISORDERS (235)

The following specifiers apply to Obsessive–Compulsive and Related Disorders where indicated:

F42.2	Obsessive–Compulsive Disorder[a] (237)
	Specify if: Tic-related
F45.22	Body Dysmorphic Disorder[a] (242)
	Specify if: With muscle dysmorphia
F42.3	Hoarding Disorder[a] (247)
	Specify if: With excessive acquisition
F63.2	Trichotillomania (Hair-Pulling Disorder) (251)
F42.4	Excoriation (Skin-Picking) Disorder (254)
—.—	Substance/Medication-Induced Obsessive–Compulsive and Related Disorder (257)
	Note: See the criteria set and corresponding recording procedures for substance-specific codes and ICD-10-CM coding.
	Specify if: With onset during intoxication, With onset during withdrawal, With onset after medication use
F06.8	Obsessive–Compulsive and Related Disorder Due to Another Medical Condition (260)
	Specify if: With obsessive–compulsive disorder–like symptoms, With appearance preoccupations, With hoarding symptoms, With hair-pulling symptoms, With skin-picking symptoms
F42.8	Other Specified Obsessive–Compulsive and Related Disorder (263)
F42.9	Unspecified Obsessive–Compulsive and Related Disorder (264)

[a]Specify if: With good or fair insight, With poor insight, With absent insight/delusional beliefs

TRAUMA-AND STRESSOR-RELATED DISORDERS (265)

F94.1	Reactive Attachment Disorder (265)
	Specify if: Persistent
	Specify current severity: Severe
F94.2	Disinhibited Social Engagement Disorder (268)
	Specify if: Persistent
	Specify current severity: Severe
F43.10	Posttraumatic Stress Disorder (includes Posttraumatic Stress Disorder for Children 6 Years and Younger) (271)
	Specify whether: With dissociative symptoms
	Specify if: With delayed expression
F43.0	Acute Stress Disorder (280)
—.—	Adjustment Disorder (286)
	Specify whether:
F43.21	With depressed mood
F43.22	With anxiety
F43.23	With mixed anxiety and depressed mood
F43.24	With disturbance of conduct
F43.25	With mixed disturbance of emotions and conduct
F43.20	Unspecified
F43.8	Other Specified Trauma- and Stressor-Related Disorder (289)
F43.9	Unspecified Trauma- and Stressor-Related Disorder (290)

DISSOCIATIVE DISORDERS (291)

F44.81	Dissociative Identity Disorder (292)
F44.0	Dissociative Amnesia (298)
	Specify if:
F44.1	With dissociative fugue
F48.1	Depersonalization/Derealization Disorder (302)
F44.89	Other Specified Dissociative Disorder (306)
F44.9	Unspecified Dissociative Disorder (307)

SOMATIC SYMPTOM AND RELATED DISORDERS (309)

F45.1	Somatic Symptom Disorder (311)
	Specify if: With predominant pain
	Specify if: Persistent
	Specify current severity: Mild, Moderate, Severe

Continued

F45.21	Illness Anxiety Disorder (315)
	Specify whether: Care-seeking type, Care-avoidant type
—.—	Conversion Disorder (Functional Neurological Symptom Disorder) (318)
	Specify symptom type:
F44.4	With weakness or paralysis
F44.4	With abnormal movement
F44.4	With swallowing symptoms
F44.4	With speech symptom
F44.5	With attacks or seizures
F44.6	With anesthesia or sensory loss
F44.6	With special sensory symptom
F44.7	With mixed symptoms
	Specify if: Acute episode, Persistent
	Specify if: With psychological stressor (specify stressor), Without psychological stressor
F54	Psychological Factors Affecting Other Medical Conditions (322)
	Specify current severity: Mild, Moderate, Severe, Extreme
F68.10	Factitious Disorder (324)
F68.A	Factitious Disorder Imposed on Another
	Specify: Single episode, Recurrent episodes
F45.8	Other Specified Somatic Symptom and Related Disorder (327)
F45.9	Unspecified Somatic Symptom and Related Disorder (327)

FEEDING AND EATING DISORDERS (329)

The following specifiers apply to Feeding and Eating Disorders where indicated:

—.—	Pica[a] (329)
F98.3	In children
F50.89	In adults
F98.21	Rumination Disorder (332)
F50.82	Avoidant/Restrictive Food Intake Disorder (334)
—.—	Anorexia Nervos (338)
	Specify whether:
F50.01	Restricting type
F50.02	Binge-eating/purging type
F50.2	Bulimia Nervos (345)

F50.81	Binge-Eating Disorder (350)
F50.89	Other Specified Feeding or Eating Disorder (353)
F50.9	Unspecified Feeding or Eating Disorder (354)

ELIMINATION DISORDERS (355)

F98.0	Enuresis (355)
	Specify whether: Nocturnal only, Diurnal only, Nocturnal and diurnal
F98.1	Encopresis (357)
	Specify whether: With constipation and overflow incontinence, Without constipation and overflow incontinence
——.——	Other Specified Elimination Disorder (359)
N39.498	With urinary symptoms
R15.9	With fecal symptoms
——.——	Unspecified Elimination Disorder (360)
R32	With urinary symptoms
R15.9	With fecal symptoms

SLEEP–WAKE DISORDERS (361)

The following specifiers apply to Sleep–Wake Disorders where indicated:

G47.00	Insomnia Disorder (362)
	Specify if: With nonsleep disorder mental comorbidity, With other medical comorbidity, With other sleep disorder
G47.10	Hypersomnolence Disorder (368)
	Specify if: With mental disorder, With medical condition, With another sleep disorder
——.——	Narcolepsy (372)
	Specify whether:
G47.419	Narcolepsy without cataplexy but with hypocretin deficiency
G47.411	Narcolepsy with cataplexy but without hypocretin deficiency
G47.419	Autosomal dominant cerebellar ataxia, deafness, and narcolepsy
G47.419	Autosomal dominant narcolepsy, obesity, and type 2 diabetes
G47.429	Narcolepsy secondary to another medical condition

Breathing-Related Sleep Disorders (378)

G47.33	Obstructive Sleep Apnea Hypopnea (378)
—.—	Central Sleep Apnea (383)
	Specify whether:
G47.31	Idiopathic central sleep apnea
R06.3	Cheyne–Stokes breathing
G47.37	Central sleep apnea comorbid with opioid use
	Note: First code opioid use disorder, if present.
	Specify current severity
—.—	Sleep-Related Hypoventilation (387)
	Specify whether:
G473.34	Idiopathic hypoventilation
G47.35	Congenital central alveolar hypoventilation
G47.36	Comorbid sleep-related hypoventilation
	Specify current severity
—.—	Circadian Rhythm Sleep–Wake Disorders (390)
	Specify whether:
G47.21	Delayed sleep phase type (391)
	Specify if: Familial, Overlapping with non-24-hour sleep–wake type
G47.22	Advanced sleep phase type (393)
	Specify if: Familial
G47.23	Irregular sleep–wake type (394)
G47.24	Non-24-hour sleep–wake type (396)
G47.26	Shift work type (397)
G47.20	Unspecified type

Parasomnias (399)

—.—	Nonrapid Eye Movement Sleep Arousal Disorders (399)
	Specify whether:
F51.3	Sleepwalking type
	Specify if: With sleep-related eating, With sleep-related sexual behavior (sexsomnia)
F51.4	Sleep terror type
F51.5	Nightmare Disorder (404)
	Specify if: During sleep onset
	Specify if: With associated nonsleep disorder, With associated other medical condition, With associated other sleep disorder
G473.52	Rapid Eye Movement Sleep Behavior Disorder (407)
G25.81	Restless Legs Syndrome (410)
—.—	Substance/Medication-Induced Sleep Disorder (413)

	Note: See the criteria set and corresponding recording procedures for substance-specific codes and ICD-10-CM coding.
	Specify whether: Insomnia type, Daytime sleepiness type, Parasomnia type, Mixed type
	Specify if: With onset during intoxication, With onset during discontinuation/withdrawal
G47.09	Other Specified Insomnia Disorder (420)
G47.00	Unspecified Insomnia Disorder (420)
G47.19	Other Specified Hypersomnolence Disorder (421)
G47.10	Unspecified Hypersomnolence Disorder (421)
G47.8	Other Specified Sleep–Wake Disorder (421)
G47.9	Unspecified Sleep–Wake Disorder (422)

SEXUAL DYSFUNCTIONS (423)

The following specifiers apply to Sexual Dysfunctions where indicated:

F52.32	Delayed Ejaculation (424)
F52.21	Erectile Disorder (426)
F52.31	Female Orgasmic Disorder (429)
	Specify if: Never experienced an orgasm under any situation
F52.22	Female Sexual Interest/Arousal Disorder (433)
F52.6	Genito-Pelvic Pain/Penetration Disorder (437)
F52.0	Male Hypoactive Sexual Desire Disorder (440)
F52.4	Premature (Early) Ejaculation (443)
——.——	Substance/Medication-Induced Sexual Dysfunction (446)
	Note: See the criteria and corresponding recording procedures for substance-specific codes ICD-10-CM coding.
	Specify if: With onset during intoxication, With onset during withdrawal, With onset after medication use
F52.8	Other Specified Sexual Dysfunction (450)
F52.9	Unspecified Sexual Dysfunction (450)

GENDER DYSPHORIA (451)

——.——	Gender Dysphoria (452)
F64.2	Gender Dysphoria in Children
	Specify if: With a disorder of sex development
F64.0	Gender Dysphoria in Adolescents and Adults
	Specify if: With a disorder of sex development
	Specify if: Posttransition

Continued

	Note: Code the disorder of sex development if present, in addition to gender dysphoria.
F64.8	Other Specified Gender Dysphoria (459)
F64.9	Unspecified Gender Dysphoria (459)

DISRUPTIVE, IMPULSE-CONTROL, AND CONDUCT DISORDERS (461)

F91.3	Oppositional Defiant Disorder (462)
	Specify current severity: Mild, Moderate, Severe
F63.81	Intermittent Explosive Disorder (466)
—.—	Conduct Disorder (469)
	Specify whether:
F91.1	Childhood-onset type
F91.2	Adolescent-onset type
F91.9	Unspecified onset
	Specify if: With limited prosocial emotions
	Specify current severity: Mild, Moderate, Severe
F60.2	Antisocial Personality Disorder (476)
F63.1	Pyromania (476)
F63.3	Kleptomania (478)
F91.8	Other Specified Disruptive, Impulse-Control, and Conduct Disorder (479)
F91.9	Unspecified Disruptive, Impulse-Control, and Conduct Disorder (480)

SUBSTANCE-RELATED AND ADDICTIVE DISORDERS (481)

The following specifiers and note apply to Substance-Related and Addictive Disorders where indicated:

Substance-Related Disorders (483)

Alcohol-Related Disorders (490)

—.—	Alcohol Use Disorder (490)
	Specify current severity:
F10.10	Mild
F10.11	Mild, in early or sustained remission
F10.20	Moderate
F10.21	Moderate, in early or sustained remission
F10.20	Severe
F10.21	Severe, in early to sustained remission

—.—	Alcohol Intoxication (497)
F10.129	With use disorder, mild
F10.229	With use disorder, moderate or severe
F10.929	Without use disorder
—.—	Alcohol Withdrawal (499)
F10.239	Without perceptual disturbances
F10.232	With perceptual disturbances
—.—	Other Alcohol-Induced Disorder (502)
F10.99	Unspecified Alcohol-Related Disorder (503)

Caffeine-Related Disorders (503)

F15.929	Caffeine Intoxication (503)
F15.93	Caffeine Withdrawal (506)
—.—	Other Caffeine-Induced Disorder (508)
F15.99	Unspecified Caffeine-Related Disorder (509)

Cannabis-Related Disorders (509)

—.—	Cannabis Use Disorder (509)
	Specify current severity:
F12.10	Mild
F12.11	Mild, in early or sustained remission
F12.20	Moderate
F12.21	Moderate, in early or sustained remission
F12.20	Severe
F12.21	Severe, in early or sustained remission
—.—	Cannabis Intoxication (516)
	Without perceptual disturbances
F12.129	With use disorder, mild
F12.229	With use disorder, moderate or severe
F12.929	Without use disorder
	With perceptual disturbances
F12.122	With use disorder, mild
F12.222	With use disorder, moderate or severe
F12.922	Without use disorder
F12.288	Cannabis Withdrawal, with moderate or severe use disorder (517)
F12.93	Without use disorder
—.—	Other Cannabis-Induced Disorders (519)
F12.99	Unspecified Cannabis-Related Disorder (519)

Hallucinogen-Related Disorders (520)

—.—	Phencyclidine Use Disorder (520)
	Specify current severity:
F16.10	Mild
F16.11	Mild, in early or sustained remission
F16.20	Moderate
F16.21	Moderate, in early or sustained remission
F16.20	Severe
F16.21	Severe, in early or sustained remission
—.—	Other Hallucinogen Use Disorder (523)
	Specify the particular hallucinogen
	Specify current severity:
F16.10	Mild
F16.11	Mild, in early or sustained remission
F16.20	Moderate
F16.21	Moderate, in early or sustained remission
F16.20	Severe
F16.21	Severe, in early or sustained remission
—.—	Phencyclidine Intoxication (527)
F16.129	With use disorder, mild
F16.229	With use disorder, moderate or severe
F16.292	Without use disorder
—.—	Other Hallucinogen Intoxication (529)
F16.129	With use disorder, mild
F16.229	With use disorder, moderate or severe
F16.929	Without use disorder
F16.983	Hallucinogen Persisting Perception Disorder (531)
—.—	Other Phencyclidine-Induced Disorder (532)
—.—	Other Hallucinogen-Induced Disorder (532)
F16.99	Unspecified Phencyclidine-Related Disorder (533)
F16.99	Unspecified Hallucinogen-Related Disorder (533)

Inhalant-Related Disorder (533)

—.—	Inhalant Use Disorder (533)
	Specify the particular inhalant
	Specify current severity:
F18.10	Mild
F18.11	Mild, in early or sustained remission
F18.20	Moderate
F18.21	Moderate, in early or sustained remission
F18.20	Severe
F18.21	Severe, in early or sustained remission
—.—	Inhalant Intoxication (538)
F18.129	With use disorder, mild

F18.229	With use disorder, moderate or severe
F18.929	Without use disorder
—.—	Other Inhalant-Induced Disorder (540)
F18.99	Unspecified Inhalant-Related Disorder (540)

Opioid-Related Disorders (540)

—.—	Opioid Use Disorder (541)
	Specify if: On maintenance therapy, In a controlled environment
	Specify current severity:
F11.10	Mild
F11.11	Mild, in early or sustained remission
F11.20	Moderate
F11.21	Moderate, in early or sustained remission
F11.20	Severe
F11.21	Severe, in early or sustained remission
—.—	Opioid Intoxication (546)
	Without perceptual disturbances
F11.129	With use disorder, mild
F11.229	With use disorder, moderate or severe
F11.929	Without use disorder
	With perceptual disturbances
F11.122	With use disorder, mild
F11.222	With use disorder, moderate or severe
F11.922	Without use disorder
F11.23	Opioid Withdrawal (547)
F11.93	Without use disorder
—.—	Other Opioid-Induced Disorder (549)
F11.99	Unspecified Opioid-Related Disorder (550)

Sedative-, Hypnotic-, or Anxiolytic-Related Disorders (550)

—.—	Sedative, Hypnotic, or Anxiolytic Use Disorder (550)
	Specify current severity:
F13.10	Mild
F13.11	Mild, in early or sustained remission
F13.20	Moderate
F13.21	Moderate, in early or sustained remission
F13.20	Severe
F13.21	Severe, in early or sustained remission
—.—	Sedative, Hypnotic, or Anxiolytic Intoxication (556)
F13.129	With use disorder, mild

Continued

F13.229	With use disorder, moderate or severe
F13.929	Without use disorder
——.——	Sedative, Hypnotic, or Anxiolytic Withdrawal (557)
F13.229	Without perceptual disturbances
F13.232	With perceptual disturbances
F13.931	With delirium, without moderate or severe use disorder
F13.932	With perceptual disturbances, without use disorder
F13.939	With perceptual disturbances, without use disorder
——.——	Other Sedative-, Hypnotic-, or Anxiolytic-Induced Disorder (560)
F13.99	Unspecified Sedative-, Hypnotic-, or Anxiolytic-Related Disorder (560)

Stimulant-Related Disorders (561)

——.——	Stimulant Use Disorder (561)
	Specify current severity:
	Mild
F15.10	Amphetamine-type substance
F15.11	Amphetamine-type substance, in early or sustained remission
F14.10	Cocaine
F14.11	Cocaine, in early or sustained remission
F15.10	Other or unspecified stimulant
F15.11	Other or unspecified stimulant, in early or sustained remission
——.——	Moderate
F15.20	Amphetamine-type substance
F15.21	Amphetamine-type substance, in early or sustained remission
F14.20	Cocaine
F14.21	Cocaine, in early or sustained remission
F15.20	Other or unspecified stimulant
F15.21	Other or unspecified stimulant, in early or ustained remission
——.——	Severe
F15.20	Amphetamine-type substance
F15.21	Amphetamine-type substance, in early or sustained remission
F14.20	Cocaine
F14.21	Cocaine, in early to sustained remission
F15.20	Other or unspecified stimulant
F15.21	Other or unspecified stimulant, in early or sustained remission

—.—	Stimulant Intoxication (567)
	Specify the specific intoxicant
—.—	Amphetamine or other stimulant, Without perceptual disturbances
F15.129	With use disorder, mild
F15.229	With use disorder, moderate or severe
F15.929	Without use disorder
—.—	Cocaine, Without perceptual disturbances
F14.129	With use disorder, mild
F14.229	With use disorder, moderate or severe
F14.929	Without use disorder
—.—	Amphetamine or other stimulant, With perceptual disturbances
F15.122	With use disorder, mild
F15.222	With use disorder, moderate or severe
F15.922	Without use disorder
—.—	Cocaine, With perceptual disturbances
F14.122	With use disorder, mild
F14.222	Without use disorder, moderate or severe
F14.922	Without use disorder
—.—	Stimulant Withdrawal (569)
	Specify the specific substance causing the withdrawal syndrome
F15.23	Amphetamine or other stimulant
F15.93	Without use disorder
F14.23	Cocaine
—.—	Other Stimulant-Induced Disorder (570)
—.—	Unspecified Stimulant-Related Disorder (570)
F15.99	Amphetamine or other stimulant
F14.99	Cocaine

Tobacco-Related Disorders (571)

—.—	Tobacco Use Disorder (571)
	Specify if: On maintenance therapy, In a controlled environment
	Specify current severity:
Z72.0	Mild
F17.200	Moderate
F17.200	Moderate, in early or sustained remission
F17.200	Severe
F17.200	Severe, in early or sustained remission
F17.203	Tobacco Withdrawal (575)
—.—	Other Tobacco-Induced Disorder (576)
F17.209	Unspecified Tobacco-Related Disorder (577)

Other (or Unknown) Substance-Related Disorders (577)

—.—	Other (or Unknown) Substance Use Disorder (577)
	Specify current severity:
F19.10	Mild
F19.10	Mild, in early or sustained remission
F19.20	Moderate
F19.20	Moderate, in early or sustained remission
F19.20	Severe
F19.20	Severe, in early or sustained remission
—.—	Other (or Unknown) Substance Intoxication (581)
F19.129	With use disorder, mild
F19.229	With use disorder, moderate or severe
F19.229	Without use disorder
F19.23	Other (or Unknown) Substance Withdrawal (583)
F19.939	Without use disorder
—.—	Other (or Unknown) Substance-Induced Disorders (584)
F19.99	Unspecified Other (or Unknown) Substance-Related Disorder (585)

Non–Substance-Related Disorders (585)

F63.0	Gambling Disorder (585)
	Specify if: Episodic, Persistent
	Specify current severity: Mild, Moderate, Severe

NEUROCOGNITIVE DISORDERS (591)

—.—	Delirium (596)
	Specify whether:
—.—	Substance intoxication delirium
—.—	Substance withdrawal delirium
—.—	Medication-induced delirium
F05	Delirium due to another medical condition
F05	Delirium due to multiple etiologies
	Specify if: Acute, Persistent
	Specify if: Hyperactive, Hypoactive, Mixed level of activity
R41.0	Other Specified Delirium (602)
R41.0	Unspecified Delirium (602)

Major and Mild Neurocognitive Disorders (602)

Specify whether due to: Alzheimer's disease, Frontotemporal lobar degeneration, Lewy body disease, Vascular disease, Traumatic brain injury, Substance/medication use, human immunodeficiency virus (HIV) infection, Prion disease, Parkinson's disease, Huntington's disease, Another medical condition, Multiple etiologies, Unspecified

Major or Mild Neurocognitive Disorder Due to Alzheimer's Disease (611)

—.—	Probable Major Neurocognitive Disorder Due to Alzheimer's Disease
	Note: Code first 331.0 (G30.9) Alzheimer's disease
F02.81	With behavioral disturbance
F02.80	Without behavioral disturbance
G31.9	Possible Major Neurocognitive Disorder Due to Alzheimer's Disease
G31.84	Mild Neurocognitive Disorder Due to Alzheimer's Disease

Major or Mild Frontotemporal Neurocognitive Disorder (614)

—.—	Probable Major Neurocognitive Disorder Due to Frontotemporal Labor Degeneration
	Note: Code first 331.19 (G31.09) Frontotemporal disease.
F02.81	With behavioral disturbance
F02.80	Without behavioral disturbance
G31.9	Possible Major Neurocognitive Disorder Due to Frontotemporal Labor Degeneration
G31.84	Mild Neurocognitive Disorder Due to Frontotemporal Labor Degeneration

Major or Mild Neurocognitive Disorder With Lewy Bodies (618)

—.—	Probable Major Neurocognitive Disorder With Lewy Bodies
	Note: Code first 331.82 (G31.83) Lewy body disease.
F02.81	With behavioral disturbance
F02.80	Without behavioral disturbance

Continued

G31.9	Possible Major Neurocognitive Disorder With Lewy Bodies
G31.84	Mild Neurocognitive Disorder With Lewy Bodies

Major or Mild Vascular Neurocognitive Disorder (621)

—.—	Probable Major Vascular Neurocognitive Disorder
	Note: No additional medical code for vascular disease.
F01.51	With behavioral disturbance
F01.50	Without behavioral disturbance
G31.9	Possible Major Vascular Neurocognitive Disorder
G31.84	Mild Vascular Neurocognitive Disorder

Major or Mild Neurocognitive Disorder Due to Traumatic Brain Injury (624)

—.—	Major Neurocognitive Disorder Due to Traumatic Brain Injury
	Note: For ICD-10-CM, code first S06.2X9S diffuse traumatic brain injury with loss of consciousness of unspecified duration, sequela.
F02.81	With behavioral disturbance
F02.80	Without behavioral disturbance
G31.84	Mild Neurocognitive Disorder Due to Traumatic Brain Injury

Substance-/Medication-Induced Major or Mild Neurocognitive Disorder[a] (627)

Note: No additional medical code. See the criteria set and corresponding recording procedures for substance-specific codes and ICD-10-CM coding.

Specify if: Persistent

Major or Mild Neurocognitive Disorder Due to HIV Infection (632)

—.—	Major Neurocognitive Disorder Due to HIV Infection
	Note: Code first 042 (B20) HIV infection.
F02.81	With behavioral disturbance
F02.80	Without behavioral disturbance
G31.84	Mild Neurocognitive Disorder Due to HIV Infection

Major or Mild Neurocognitive Disorder Due to Prion Disease (634)

—.—	Major Neurocognitive Disorder Due to Prion Disease
	Note: Code first 046.79 (A81.9) Prion disease.
F02.81	With behavioral disturbance
F02.80	Without behavioral disturbance
G31.84	Mild Neurocognitive Disorder Due to Prion Disease

Major or Mild Neurocognitive Disorder Due to Parkinson's Disease (636)

—.—	Major Neurocognitive Disorder Probably Due to Parkinson's Disease
	Note: Code first 332.0 (G20) Parkinson's disease.
F02.81	With behavioral disturbance
F02.80	Without behavioral disturbance
G31.9	Major Neurocognitive Disorder Possibly Due to Parkinson's Disease
G31.84	Mild Neurocognitive Disorder Due to Parkinson's Disease

Major or Mild Neurocognitive Disorder Due to Huntington's Disease (638)

—.—	Major Neurocognitive Disorder Due to Huntington's Disease
	Note: Code first 333.4 (G10) Huntington's disease.
F02.81	With behavioral disturbance
F02.80	Without behavioral disturbance
G31.84	Mild Neurocognitive Disorder Due to Huntington's Disease

Major or Mild Neurocognitive Disorder Due to Another Medical Condition (641)

—.—	Major Neurocognitive Disorder Due to Another Medical Condition
	Note: Code first the other medical condition.
F02.81	With behavioral disturbance
F02.80	Without behavioral disturbance
G31.84	Mild Neurocognitive Disorder Due to Another Medical Condition

Major or Mild Neurocognitive Disorder Due to Multiple Etiologies (642)

—.—	Major Neurocognitive Disorder Due to Multiple Etiologies
	Note: Code first all the etiological medical conditions (with the exception of vascular disease).
F02.81	With behavioral disturbance
F02.80	Without behavioral disturbance
G31.84	Mild Neurocognitive Disorder Due to Multiple Etiologies

Unspecified Neurocognitive Disorder (643)

R41.9	Unspecified Neurocognitive Disorder

PERSONALITY DISORDERS (645)

Cluster A Personality Disorders

F60.0	Paranoid Personality Disorder (649)
F60.1	Schizoid Personality Disorder (652)
F21	Schizotypal Personality Disorder (655)

Cluster B Personality Disorders

F60.2	Antisocial Personality Disorder (659)
F60.3	Borderline Personality Disorder (663)
F60.4	Histrionic Personality Disorder (667)
F60.81	Narcissistic Personality Disorder (669)

Cluster C Personality Disorders

F60.6	Avoidant Personality Disorder (672)
F60.7	Dependent Personality Disorder (675)
F60.5	Obsessive–Compulsive Personality Disorder (678)

Other Personality Disorders

F07.0	Personality Change Due to Another Medical Condition (682)
	Specify whether: Labile type, Disinhibited type, Aggressive type, Apathetic type, Paranoid type, Other type, Combined type, Unspecified type

| F60.89 | Other Specified Personality Disorder (684) |
| F60.9 | Unspecified Personality Disorder (684) |

PARAPHILIC DISORDERS (685)

The following specifier applies to Paraphilic Disorders where indicated:

F65.3	Voyeuristic Disorder[a] (686)
F65.2	Exhibitionistic Disorder[a] (689)
	Specify whether: Sexually aroused by exposing genitals to prepubertal children, Sexually aroused by exposing genitals to physically mature individuals, Sexually aroused by exposing genitals to prepubertal children and to physically mature individuals
F65.81	Frotteuristic Disorder[a] (691)
F65.51	Sexual Masochism Disorder[a] (694)
	Specify if: With asphyxiophilia
F65.52	Sexual Sadism Disorder[a] (695)
F65.4	Pedophilic Disorder (697)
	Specify whether: Exclusive type, Nonexclusive type
	Specify if: Sexually attracted to males, Sexually attracted to females, Sexually attracted to both
	Specify if: Limited to incest
F65.0	Fetishistic Disorder[a] (700)
	Specify: Body part(s), Nonliving object(s), Other
F65.1	Transvestic Disorder[a] (702)
	Specify if: With fetishism, With autogynephilia
F65.89	Other Specified Paraphilic Disorder (705)
F65.9	Unspecified Paraphilic Disorder (705)

[a]Specify if: In a controlled environment, In full remission

OTHER MENTAL DISORDERS (707)

F06.8	Other Specified Mental Disorder Due to Another Medical Condition (707)
F09	Unspecified Mental Disorder Due to Another Medical Condition (708)
F99	Other Specified Mental Disorder (708)
F99	Unspecified Mental Disorder (708)

MEDICATION-INDUCED MOVEMENT DISORDERS AND OTHER ADVERSE EFFECTS OF MEDICATION (709)

G21.11	Neuroleptic-Induced Parkinsonism (709)
G21.19	Other Medication-Induced Parkinsonism (709)
G21.0	Neuroleptic Malignant Syndrome (709)
G24.02	Medication-Induced Acute Dystonia (711)
G25.71	Medication-Induced Acute Akathisia (711)
G24.01	Tardive Dyskinesia (712)
G24.09	Tardive Dystonia (712)
G25.71	Tardive Akathisia (712)
G25.1	Medication-Induced Postural Tremor (712)
G25.79	Other Medication-Induced Movement Disorder (712)
—.—	Antidepressant Discontinuation Syndrome (712)
T43.205A	Initial encounter
T43.205D	Subsequent encounter
T43.205S	Sequelae
—.—	Other Adverse Effect of Medication (714)
T50.905A	Initial encounter
T50.905D	Subsequent encounter
T50.905S	Sequelae

OTHER CONDITIONS THAT MAY BE A FOCUS OF CLINICAL ATTENTION (715)

Relational Problems (715)

Problems Related to Family Upbringing (715)

Z62.820	Parent–Child Relational Problem (715)
Z62.891	Sibling Relational Problem (716)
Z62.29	Upbringing Away From Parents (716)
Z62.898	Child Affected by Parental Relationship Distress (716)

Other Problems Related to Primary Support Group (716)

Z63.0	Relationship Distress With Spouse or Intimate Partner (716)
Z63.5	Disruption of Family by Separation or Divorce (716)
Z63.8	High Expressed Emotion Level Within Family (716)
Z63.4	Uncomplicated Bereavement (716)

Abuse and Neglect (717)

Child Maltreatment and Neglect Problems (717)

Child Physical Abuse (717)
Child Physical Abuse, Confirmed (717)
| T743.12XA | Initial encounter |
| T74.12XD | Subsequent encounter |

Child Physical Abuse, Suspected (717)
| T76.12XA | Initial encounter |
| T76.12XD | Subsequent encounter |

Other Circumstances Related to Child Physical Abuse (718)
Z69.010	Encounter for mental health services for victim of child abuse by parent
Z69.020	Encounter for mental health services for victim of nonparental child abuse
Z62.810	Personal history (past history) of physical abuse in childhood
Z69.011	Encounter for mental health services for perpetrator of parental child abuse
Z69.021	Encounter for mental health services for perpetrator of nonparental child abuse

Child Sexual Abuse (718)
Child Sexual Abuse, Confirmed (718)
| T74.22XA | Initial encounter |
| T74.22XD | Subsequent encounter |
Child Sexual Abuse, Suspected (718)
| T76.22XA | Initial encounter |
| T76.22XD | Subsequent encounter |

Other Circumstances Related to Child Sexual Abuse (718)
Z69.010	Encounter for mental health services for victim of child sexual abuse by parent
Z69.020	Encounter for mental health services for victim of nonparental child sexual abuse
Z62.810	Personal history (past history) of sexual abuse in childhood
Z69.011	Encounter for mental health services for perpetrator of parental child sexual abuse
Z69.021	Encounter for mental health services for perpetrator of nonparental child sexual abuse

Child Neglect (718)
Child Neglect, Confirmed (718)
| T74.02ZA | Initial encounter |
| T74.02XD | Subsequent encounter |

Child Neglect, Suspected (719)
| T76.02XA | Initial encounter |

Continued

T76.02XD	Subsequent encounter

Other Circumstances Related to Child Neglect (719)

Z69.010	Encounter for mental health services for victim of child neglect by parent
Z69.020	Encounter for mental health services for victim of nonparental child neglect
Z62.812	Personal history (past history) of neglect in childhood
Z69.011	Encounter for mental health services for perpetrator of parental child neglect
Z69.021	Encounter for mental health services for perpetrator of nonparental child neglect

Child Psychological Abuse (719)
Child Psychological Abuse, Confirmed (719)

T74.32XA	Initial encounter
T74.32XD	Subsequent encounter

Child Psychological Abuse, Suspected (719)

T76.32XA	Initial encounter
T76.32XD	Subsequent encounter

Other Circumstances Related to Child Psychological Abuse (719)

Z69.010	Encounter for mental health services for victim of child psychological abuse by parent
Z69.020	Encounter for mental health services for victim of nonparental child psychological abuse
Z62.811	Personal history (past history) of psychological abuse in childhood
Z69.011	Encounter for mental health services for perpetrator of parental child psychological abuse
Z69.021	Encounter for mental health services for perpetrator of nonparental child psychological abuse

Adult Maltreatment and Neglect Problems (720)

Spouse or Partner Violence, Physical (720)
Spouse or Partner Violence, Physical, Confirmed (720)

T74.11XA	Initial encounter
T74.11XD	Subsequent encounter

Spouse or Partner Violence, Physical, Suspected (720)

T76.11XA	Initial encounter
T76.11XD	Subsequent encounter

Other Circumstances Related to Spouse or Partner Violence, Physical (720)

Z96.11	Encounter for mental health services for victim of spouse or partner violence, physical

| Z91.410 | Personal history (past history) of spouse or partner violence, physical |
| Z69.12 | Encounter for mental health services for perpetrator of spouse or partner violence, physical |

Spouse or Partner Violence, Sexual (720)

Spouse or Partner Violence, Sexual, Confirmed (720)

| T74.21XA | Initial encounter |
| T74.21XD | Subsequent encounter |

Spouse or Partner Violence, Sexual, Suspected (720)

| T76.21XA | Initial encounter |
| T76.21XD | Subsequent encounter |

Other Circumstances Related to Spouse or Partner Violence, Sexual (720)

Z69.81	Encounter for mental health services for victim of spouse or partner violence, sexual
Z91.410	Personal history (past history) of spouse or partner violence, sexual
Z69.12	Encounter for mental health services for perpetrator of spouse or partner violence, sexual

Spouse or Partner Neglect (721)

Spouse or Partner Neglect, Confirmed (721)

| T47.01XA | Initial encounter |
| T74.01XD | Subsequent encounter |

Spouse or Partner Neglect, Suspected (721)

| T76.01XA | Initial encounter |
| T76.01XD | Subsequent encounter |

Other Circumstances Related to Spouse or Partner Neglect (721)

Z69.11	Encounter for mental health services for victim of spouse or partner neglect
Z91.412	Personal history (past history) of spouse or partner neglect
Z69.12	Encounter for mental health services for perpetrator of spouse or partner neglect

Spouse or Partner Abuse, Psychological (721)

Spouse or Partner Abuse, Psychological, Confirmed (721)

| T74.31XA | Initial encounter |
| T74.31XD | Subsequent encounter |

Spouse or Partner Abuse, Psychological, Suspected (721)

| T76.31XA | Initial encounter |
| T76.31XD | Subsequent encounter |

Other Circumstances Related to Spouse or Partner Abuse, Psychological (721)

| Z69.11 | Encounter for mental health services for victim of spouse or partner psychological abuse |

Continued

Z91.411	Personal history (past history) of spouse or partner psychological abuse
Z69.12	Encounter for mental health services for perpetrator of spouse or partner psychological abuse

Adult Abuse by Nonspouse or Nonpartner (722)

Adult Physical Abuse by Nonspouse or Nonpartner, Confirmed (722)

T74.11XA	Initial encounter
T74.11XD	Subsequent encounter

Adult Physical Abuse by Nonspouse or Nonpartner, Suspected (722)

T76.11XA	Initial encounter
T76.11XD	Subsequent encounter

Adult Sexual Abuse by Nonspouse or Nonpartner, Confirmed (722)

T74.21XA	Initial encounter
T74.21XD	Subsequent encounter

Adult Sexual Abuse by Nonspouse or Nonpartner, Suspected (722)

T76.21XA	Initial encounter
T76.21XD	Subsequent encounter

Adult Psychological Abuse by Nonspouse or Nonpartner, Confirmed (722)

T74.31XA	Initial encounter
T74.31XD	Subsequent encounter

Adult Psychological Abuse by Nonspouse or Nonpartner, Suspected (722)

T76.31XA	Initial encounter
T76.31XD	Subsequent encounter

Other Circumstances Related to Adult Abuse by Nonspouse or Nonpartner (722)

Z69.81	Encounter for mental health services for victim of nonspousal adult abuse
Z69.82	Encounter for mental health services for perpetrator of nonspousal adult abuse

Educational and Occupational Problems (723)

Educational Problems (723)

Z55.9	Academic or Educational Problem (723)

Occupational Problems (723)

Z56.82	Problem Related to Current Military Deployment Status (723)
Z56.9	Other Problem Related to Employment (723)

Housing and Economic Problems (723)

Housing Problems (723)

Z59.0	Homelessness (723)
Z59.1	Inadequate Housing (723)
Z59.2	Discord With Neighbor, Lodger, or Landlord (723)
Z59.3	Problem Related to Living in a Residential Institution (724)

Economic Problems (724)

Z59.4	Lack of Adequate Food or Safe Drinking Water (724)
Z59.5	Extreme Poverty (724)
Z59.6	Low Income (724)
Z59.7	Insufficient Social Insurance or Welfare Support (724)
Z59.9	Unspecified Housing or Economic Problem (724)

Other Problems Related to the Social Environment (724)

Z60.0	Phase of Life Problem (724)
Z60.2	Problem Related to Living Alone (724)
Z60.3	Acculturation Difficulty (724)
Z60.4	Social Exclusion or Rejection (724)
Z60.5	Target of (Perceived) Adverse Discrimination or Persecution (724)
Z60.9	Unspecified Problem Related to Social Environment (725)

Problems Related to Crime or Interaction With the Legal System (725)

Z65.4	Victim of Crime (725)
Z65.0	Conviction in Civil or Criminal Proceedings Without Imprisonment (725)
Z65.1	Imprisonment or Other Incarceration (725)
Z65.2	Problems Related to Release From Prison (725)
Z65.3	Problems Related to Other Legal Circumstances (725)

Other Health Service Encounters for Counseling and Medical Advice (725)

Z70.9	Sex Counseling (725)
Z71.9	Other Counseling or Consultation (725)

Problems Related to Other Psychosocial, Personal, and Environmental Circumstances (725)

Z65.8	Religious or Spiritual Problem (725)
Z64.0	Problems Related to Unwanted Pregnancy (725)
Z64.1	Problems Related to Multiparity (725)
Z64.4	Discord With Social Service Provider, Including Probation Officer, Case Manager, or Social Service Worker (725)
Z65.4	Victim of Terrorism or Torture (725)
Z65.5	Exposure to Disaster, War, or Other Hostilities (725)
Z65.8	Other Problem Related to Psychosocial Circumstances (725)
Z65.9	Unspecified Problem Related to Unspecified Psychosocial Circumstances (725)

Other Circumstances of Personal History (726)

Z91.49	Other Personal History of Psychological Trauma (726)
Z91.5	Personal History of Self-Harm (726)
Z91.82	Personal History of Military Deployment (726)
Z91.89	Other Personal Risk Factors (726)
Z72.9	Problem Related to Lifestyle (726)
Z72.811	Adult Antisocial Behavior (726)
Z72.810	Child or Adolescent Antisocial Behavior (726)

Problems Related to Access to Medical and Other Health Care (726)

Z75.3	Unavailability or Inaccessibility of Health Care Facilities (726)
Z75.4	Unavailability or Inaccessibility of Other Helping Agencies (726)

Nonadherence to Medical Treatment (726)

Z91.19	Nonadherence to Medical Treatment (726)
E66.9	Overweight or Obesity (726)
Z76.5	Malingering (726)
Z91.83	Wandering Associated With a Mental Disorder (727)
R41.83	Borderline Intellectual Functioning (727)

Index

Page numbers followed by "*f*" indicate figures, "*t*" indicate tables, and "*b*" indicate boxes.

NURSING DIAGNOSES BY CHAPTER

International Council of Nurses. (2019). *International Classification of Nursing Practice*. Retrieved from https://www.icn.ch/what-we-do/projects/ehealth-icnptm/icnp-browser